doctor ken

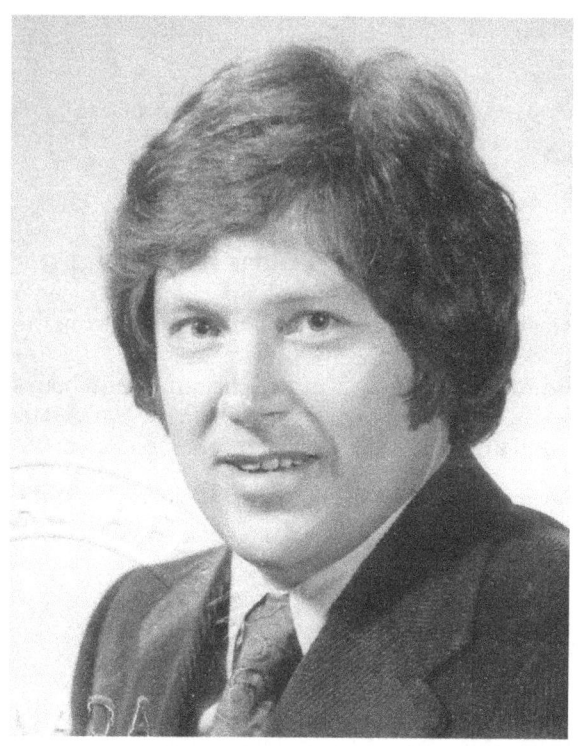

Kehnroth Schramm, M.D. 1932 – 2004

doctor ken

a true story about a man and the Hippocratic Oath

Story told by H.T.A. Heisler with *Writings by doctor ken*

doctor ken

Author and Editor of Doctor Kehnroth Schramm's notebooks:
H.T.A. Heisler

Cover design and artwork: H.T.A. Heisler

Permissions granted for publishing in this book:

Carl Leggo - poem
Bob and Carol Bean - photo of Ken
Maria Hay - cover photo of The Rose
Richard Schramm
William A. McLachlan
Henry C. Wood
College of Physicians and Surgeons of British Columbia - articles
University of Toronto Press - book excerpts
Canwest - newspaper articles
Dartmouth College - song

TABLE OF CONTENTS

Introduction

part one

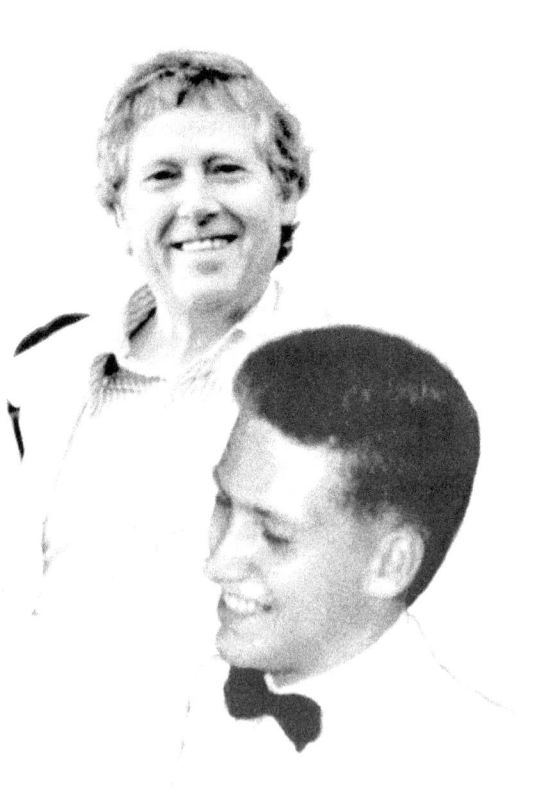

Introduction

It is written in the Hippocratic Oath, that a physician shall do no harm and keep his patients' secrets to himself. The Hippocratic Oath demands physicians to be truthful in their promise; otherwise they should not be admitted to do the work of a physician.

Why tell the truth? It is written in the Bible, John 8:32 "And ye shall know the truth, and truth shall make you free." The man who said those words was persecuted and crucified.

To tell the truth is why this book is written and is meant to give truth freedom. Sometime it takes enormous strength to be truthful and to stand alone rather than be a follower. This story is about the physician who stood strong in truth, stood alone, and was persecuted. It examines medical ethics, legal ethics and social issues.

This story is completely based on real events, actual conversations, and written papers. The story is about the determination of Kehnroth Schramm, M.D. to protect his Hippocratic Oath and his patients, and of the woman who tried to protect him. This is a story about enduring love– in many hues.

Ken was a generous, humble man. He preferred to teach and work as a healer without expecting monetary or personal benefit. Ruthless people obsessed with greed, power and lack of respect for the Hippocratic Oath made Doctor Schramm their target, causing a never-ending struggle; they caused damage to his reputation by their distortions of truth in their struggle to gain control of Ken and extort money from him. Doctor Schramm refused to compromise his ethics.

The promise to do no harm and keep patients' secrets has traditionally been a right of passage into practicing medicine. Some present day medical schools and medical students are balking at the idea of taking the Hippocratic Oath. They say it does not fit present day society and perhaps society should think about the implications of no oath.

The story, creative non-fiction written in third person, was a literary decision.

H.T.A. Heisler

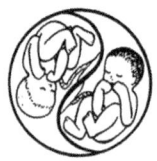

part one

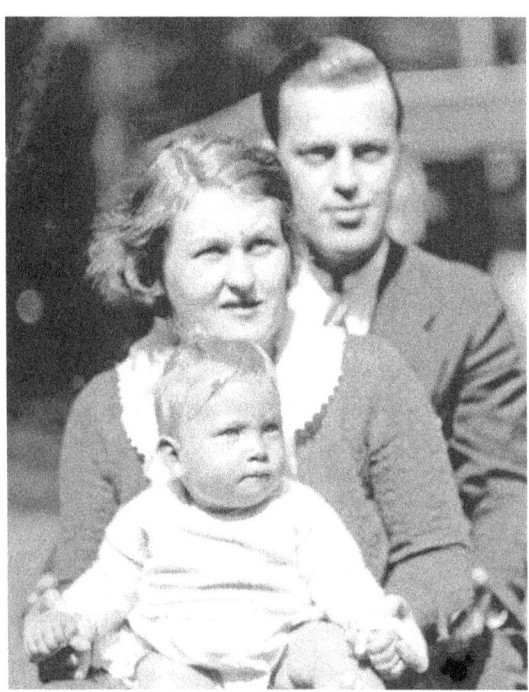

Kehnroth Schramm with his parents

1

In the Beginning

1958

TIME – DESTINY – ENERGY – PROMISE – SOUND will amalgamate this auspicious day in the making of a new physician. Born with a calling, Kehnroth Schramm has lived his life in pursuit of his destiny – of this morning. Wearing a blue robe that swayed around his soft-soled shoes, and carrying in his hand a square blue cap with the long tassel swinging to his rhythm, he walked quickly through the inner hallway of the potent, grey stone Vermont University Medical School. He paused a moment at a doorway to position the symbol of graduation on his head, then took a deep breath as he entered the next chapter of his life.

In a room filled with light and fresh Spring air through open windows, he took his place in the assembly to pledge to live by the morals of the Hippocratic Oath in work and in private life for his whole life.

Facing the graduates, an elder read out the preamble:

"In our profession it is a custom, established more than two thousand years ago, that no man may be admitted to its honors, who has not first expressly taken upon himself its obligations. Now, therefore, in behalf of your elders, I call upon you to take, as we have taken before you, the oath which bears the name of Hippocrates. The language in which our predecessor first pronounced it is no longer spoken but still we find no nobler words than the most ancient in which to hand down the traditions of our calling."

The elder lifted his hand to invite voices of the thirty-nine graduates to unite as one and to vibrate within the room and out the open window across the campus.

"I do solemnly swear, each to whatever we hold most sacred:

"That I will be loyal to the Profession of Medicine and just and generous to it members;

"That I will lead my life and practice my art in uprightness and honor;

"That into whatsoever house I shall enter, it shall be for good of the sick to the utmost of my power, I hold myself far aloof from wrong, from corruption, from the tempting of others to vice;

"That I will exercise my art solely for the cure of my patients, and will give no drug, perform no operation for a criminal purpose, even if solicited; far less suggest it;

"That whatsoever I shall see or hear of the lives of men which is not fitting to be spoken, I will keep inviolably sacred."

The elder physician said, "Let each candidate raise his right hand in acquiescence."

With profound reverence, Kehn raised his right hand to this defining moment and voiced, *"These things I do swear."*

The symbolism of a birth had just happened. Though he had lived the life of a physician honoring the Hippocratic Oath for the past four years, now the Hippocratic Oath was indelibly sealed on his body and soul.

It has been known that monks and priests the world over achieve higher consciousness through the vibration of sound and the sound of Aum is the sound of Creation. The sound of the Hippocratic Oath is mightier than the walls of the school; though invisible, the vibration has a life of its own, carrying Kehn's promise out through the shimmering green sentry of old trees that witnessed each new physician declaring the oath, and out across the earth into eternity.

OUT ON THE LAWN with the brick and stone of the medical school as a backdrop, the graduating class gathered for their official class photo. Kehn sat third from the right in the front row. The colour of his eyes matched the blue of his robe and his blond hair that curled except when cut short, as it was this day, glistened under the blue cap in the warm June sun. Twenty-five year old, Kehn was a man who spoke softly but earnestly about his devotion to making a better world for all.

From his seat, he saw his parents waiting patiently across the lawn as the photographer prepared his camera. Kehn smiled at them as the large black camera poised on a tripod made snapping noises. The sound brought back comical thoughts of his mother's father... a grandfather seriously opinionated about the world he lives in and a hobbyist photographer who took photos with a camera just like this one while making promises to eat chocolate ice cream in heaven.

The images of this day would be a printed reminder of the completion of one phase of life and the start of another. Kehn was headed for Specialty studies in Paediatrics. Babies, children, and their parents were his first love in medicine.

Kehn's mother, with blond curls bouncing and Baby Brownie camera in hand, made a dash to greet him as the group disbanded.

Kehn smiled. "Hi, Mom."

"Doctor Kehn," she proudly greeted him, "I need my own snapshot of you on this special day."

Another memory was created with a click.

THAT DAY – THAT PROMISE and the man who made it are the reasons for telling this story.

Years later, on the west coast of Canada, the photo taken by Kehn's mother stood on Daisy's desk. Concentrating on the photo, Daisy was trying to put all that happened in perspective to be able to tell the story.

Kehn and Daisy met in the summer of 1969. Their lives circled around each other for the next twelve years until they came together as though drawn into a predestined union to become life-companions.

Kehn then told her, "You will write my story."

It was a startling statement. Looking into serious blue eyes, she was mystified at his prophetic tone but it provoked an overpowering question.

"How... what would I write?"

He simply answered, "You will write about my life and my work."

Her mind had swirled the known facts. Her roots were in the Canadian Prairies. She knew nothing about Vermont or New York and had never been to medical school.

THE 1958 GRADUATION PHOTO of thirty-nine new physicians was one of several photos and neat piles of notebooks and papers written by Kehn that Daisy had been sorting through. Among the papers, she found the poem she wrote for him in 1981 after their lives came together for the third time. She had wondered if he ever read it and was surprised that he actually kept it for another quarter of a century. Raising her gaze again to the framed picture, her hand followed to rest on his hands. She remembered the feel of his hands and how gently they would touch people and animals, and how they most often held a book... and held a pen to write in black ink, as he loved to do...

Picking up another small photo, Daisy paused in surprise to see that as a young boy sitting with his brothers on a lush lawn, Kehn wore shoes that buckled. The look in Kehn's eyes told a tale of unhappiness or distrust when the photo was taken; something had gone wrong. But the shoes solved a long-standing puzzle that Daisy had since her own childhood.

On a corner of her desk was another framed picture copied from a larger poster of two unknown children walking hand in hand through the forest into the light. The poster had become a symbol of Kehn and Daisy's relationship.

After years of crossing paths, the day came when there was *Knowing* from some far-reaching memory where past, present and future all became one. They knew each other as though they had been together before and this was a continuation of oneness, a unity in an unexplained universe. There was a coming home.

Life is like a giant puzzle; the meaning of pieces and events become clearer over time when looking at the big picture. How much is destiny? Where and how is the plan of life made? In other words, where were we before we were born? These are age-old questions.

But what happened? What brought them to this point? How could the promise Kehn made by taking the Hippocratic Oath that day in 1958 be the reason Kehn would also lose his life?

Reaching to stroke his blond hair, Daisy imagined reaching through the cold glass barrier to him... the warm, real, remembered *him*. Over many years of knowing Kehn, a man determined to honour his Hippocratic Oath, the story to tell had become clear.

She began the long days and nights of writing...

2

Early Memories

NOVEMBER 20TH, 1932. A car moved slowly through the streets of White Plains, New York to the sound of slushy snow under its tires and slapping of windshield wipers trying to keep the windshield clear. The car stopped under a street lamp at the hospital entrance. August Schramm, a young, handsomely tall blond man stepped out of the car and dashed to open the passenger door.

His wife Jean leaned on him as she stepped out, pausing with a contraction. They were apprehensive and excited about the birth of their first baby. She looked up into the wet, white snowflakes that clumped together in big puffs falling toward her through the light. The cool wetness felt good on her face; in anticipation of giving birth she imagined it to be a refreshing spray of eternal blessings that under the overhead streetlight fanned out over her, protecting her with a blanket of sparkling light. As the contraction passed, August held her protectively, not allowing her footing to slip as they walked slowly toward and through the large, heavy doors into the hospital lobby.

Jean was swiftly whisked away in a wheelchair through another set of big doors by white-coated staff. Left behind, August, looked anxiously and confused at the blank closed doors. His wife was gone too fast. He was alone, no longer able to protect his wife. The void was large. He looked down at his black boots, noting that he stood in puddles of water from melted snow over top of a shiny stone floor.

IN THE EARLY HOURS of the morning a son was born. The doctor immediately became distressed as he laid the baby down on a flat, hard surface. Under his breath, he muttered, "Oh, God! Spina Bifida."

"It's a good thing the mother is out for a while," the nurse stated crisply. "Anesthesia is such a blessing."

The anesthetist was quietly stunned but kept his mind on his own job.

"This boy may not make it," the doctor muttered while suctioning the baby boy and examining him closer with the nurse looking on.

"And if he does?" she asked.

"We would not expect him to have much of a life. He has a large opening in his cervical spine, leaking spinal fluid... a cone shaped head... retained fluid in his head... possible brain damage..."

And so it was in the early hours of November 21st, 1932, a boy was born with a destiny of becoming a physician.

[ks notebook] "I wish my parents had known what they were doing when they made me on Valentine's Day, 1932 -- a child of love. I don't remember when I first asked where did I come from but I'm still asking and I still want to know not so much where babies come from as where did I come from, why am I here, and where am I going? The Tibetans believe we choose our parents as we make our own way from one lifetime to another until one at a time, each of us becomes a fully human person able to stop time and break the cycle of pain and desire, desire and pain. What did my mother and my father desire when they made me? What did they suffer because of their desires for themselves and for me in the midst of the Great Depression; the year Franklin Roosevelt became President of the United States. I was born with congenital cervical spina bifida and meningococcal that could have killed me by infection, paralyzed, dumbed and immobilized me with hydrocephalus, water on the brain... relates me through my medical embryological text books to others born with similar conditions at least since the Egyptians... their hieroglyphic text.

"...At birth I met Death and Love. My Dad had just received a cut in pay, which meant the family would have even less money for medical, food, housing, and other necessary expenses. My scars were invisible to me when my mother told me the story of their fears before my surgery that I would die, or be crippled or retarded. For good luck, I was named after Dr. Charles Kehnroth, (my father's grandfather)."

EXTRACT FROM BLAIRSTOWN PRESS of **June 14, 1905**, announcing Kehn's grandfather's marriage.

KEHNROTH-SCHRAMM

On June 7th a wedding... took place at Holy Trinity, one of New York's stately and beautiful churches. Franziska Katharina Kehnroth, younger daughter of Dr. C.H. Kehnroth, was married to Mr. August Schramm, Jr. of New York. The golden haired girl who was once a student at Blair Academy made a beautiful and queenly bride. It was one of those occasions when everything seemed to be in unison and harmony...

[ks notebook] "Great grandfather, Dr. Charles Kehnroth was a practicing physician in England, teacher and Master at several schools in the Americas and West Indies, and in the Crimean War was a Lieutenant in the English Army and received Victorian Cross for bravery. I believe he was also a homeopathic physician who later became professor at Blair Academy, a Congregational school, where my parents met each other at summer church camp as teenagers.

"His surgeon friend used his skill and Gray's Anatomy [book] to repair my spine under local anaesthesia when I was ten days old.

"Growing up I had no difficulty in walking or running or any other visible handicap from the birth defect and surgery. My name Schramm and my circumcision also relate me to Judaism and the Holocaust.

"My [mother's] family story of Pilgrim Puritans coming to Cape Cod in November 1620 and being helped by an Abernaki, named Squanto, to learn to live on Turtle Island relates us to the genocide of North America, to Henry Wadsworth Longfellow, who wrote Song of Hiawatha which, justifying that genocide as progress, the Courtship of Miles Standish which tells of our relatives John and Priscilla Alden (passengers of the Mayflower), also ancestor of Samuel Morrison, U.S. historian of Christopher Columbus and U.S. history teacher of Page Smith, who at Dartmouth College, 'the Indian School' my brothers and I attended..."

"Wounded loon
will fly soon
will soon fly

"I remember the sun warming me with golden light through bars of my crib when I was three years old and my brother was six months old, playing in baby talk, birds and dogs singing music in my heart, waking to hear strange noises. I do not know as once I knew life's secret languages. My earliest memory, real to me as anything I have ever dreamt or seen or thought or said, I relive now in my desire to know and speak the languages of life. I experience everyone and thing I see, hear, think, remember, and imagine as alive. I did not know that others do not have "naturally" the same sense of life that I see in children's eyes and play.

"Sunbeams warm
Light golden bathing
Singing birds
Calling dogs
Baby babbling brooks
Speaking loves
Lost meanings
Ask Me born
Breathing life
Wonder"

"Every morning is a rebirth of this dream (memory work) which calling called me to be a doctor, teacher, healer with words. Later I found this calling to be a shaman's dream, speaking with life in animals and light healing poetry.

"My grandfather wanted a boy, so when my mother (Mom) was born, he taught her to be a boy. My mother taught me to do all the household chores and was afraid to let me be afraid. She pushed me to do things I was afraid to do, like speak to strangers. I learned to face my fears. I crawled around the attic alone in the dark until I was no longer afraid of the dark. I climbed trees, rocks and ropes until I wasn't afraid of heights. I think my mother and I together, as eldest children and as companions in the kitchen, pushed fear deeper inside us where we could no longer feel it. I was afraid to cry, to get angry, to fight or to run away for fear of other peoples' opinions and hurts and angers...

"...Health as happiness in everyday life has been the focus of my thought since birth. The embryological defect in the fusion of the cervical vertebral bonding was explained to me as a birth defect due to unknown causes. I was the oldest of five children, two brothers followed by two sisters, none of who had any similar defects. My brothers and I inherited bad teeth from our maternal grandfather because our adult teeth came in with soft transparent enamel so that the orange colored dentine was visible and we were teased at school"

A NEW BABY BROTHER intruded on Kehn's early relationship with his mother. Though he enjoyed his brother's company, he experienced loss when sent to school at age four while his brother stayed home.

Meanwhile, he studied fervently, was an avid reader, kept up on world events even as a small child, but was too shy to speak in school. He did not go to the toilet while at school; instead he rushed home to the safety of his own bathroom and family, holding his full bladder all the way. Tap dancing school was thought to build Ken's self esteem.

His mother's constant pushing into difficult situations so that Kehn could be ready for the real world as the physician he would surely become, accomplished what years later would be Kehn's ability to tackle the scariest situations head on. Regardless of the pain he would cause himself, Kehn became a warrior for causes he believed in, especially when he saw people being hurt by a society that curtailed freethinking and did not take care of the needy and sick.

LIVING ON THE edge of a forest in 1941 provided a favorite play area for Kehn and his brothers. Six-year-old Dick was on the bicycle seat behind Kehn, legs flailing wide as Kehn stood on the pedals to steer down a small hill. At the bottom of the hill a small rock launched the front wheel into the air. Suddenly, they were planted in the ground. Pausing to contemplate the situation and realizing there was no blood spilling anywhere, Kehn reached a hand to Dick, who avoided help by scrambling to his feet.

"Whew, I'm still alive! Did you dump me on purpose?"

"Of course not! Are you hurt?"

"Nah," Dick replied.

"Well, I didn't dump us on purpose." But the question had Kehn wondering briefly if in some unconscious way he did do it on purpose to make up for being displaced by his brother. He decided it was a dumb idea. He would not deliberately hurt his brother or anyone for that matter, but the incident would remain vivid in Kehn's mind about how an accident could provoke such emotional questions.

The boys laughed. They wandered through the forest on foot, wheeling the bike alongside. Their young voices resonated with the forest as they loudly expressed their pride of resilience to the mishap.

Kehn stopped to lay a hand on a tree for a moment. "Listen, I feel this tree is talking. It is trying to tell the world, "Save me! Don't let me become toilet paper!"

The boys laughed again as they knelt down, leaning ears against the tree to listen.

Seeing a friend through the trees, Dick jumped up and took off running, as so often happened After watching the boys disappear from the forest, Kehn laid on the ground, pondering aloneness while viewing the sky through the lace of green leaves. The gently swaying canopy above looked like Grandmother's lace that she made with her own hands out of a ball of string by making tiny quick movements with a small silver hook. Her lace would grow like magic. He wondered if women looked at nature and came up with the idea of making lace. Grandmother... thinking of her was comfort. The forest provided the quiet time to meditate and question what life is all about... a time to feel personal spirituality.

His mother's voice in the distance penetrated the silence, calling him to come home.

BATHED AND DRESSED in new sailor suits, Kehn and Dick along with their parents were about to get into the family car.

"You boys look so nice. Just a minute while I take a picture of you." Mother smiled proudly as she snapped the picture with her Baby Brownie camera.

Moments later, the boys were reluctant passengers in the back seat of a moving vehicle. To Kehn, even the motor had a determined sound. He blurted out, "I don't want to have my tonsils out!"

"Neither do I!" Dick was glad Kehn took the lead.

"Oh, it will be alright." Mother's voice had a bright lilt that was supposed to make the boys feel okay. "Afterward, you will get to eat all the ice-cream and jelly you want for a couple of days."

"Dick needs to have his tonsils out." Father's head bobbed as he talked, trying to turn his head to see the boys behind him but keeping his eyes on the road at the same time. "And the doctor thought you may as well have them out together."

"I don't need my tonsils out," Kehn answered. "They don't bother me." Frustrated, seeing only the back of his parents' heads, Kehn tugged at his suit. "And I don't like this monkey suit. And I don't care about ice-cream."

Mother turned to look at the boys. "You want to look nice and smart for the nurses and doctor, don't you?"

"No!" Kehn despondently looked out the window, feeling jailed as the car traveled down the dirt road heading for the hospital while leaving a dusty plume in the air behind. Contemplating running on getting out of the car, he wondered where to? Could he run to the forest? Could he run to the Indians? He was trapped.

INSIDE THE HOSPITAL LOBBY, they approached a large desk. Then a nurse in a crisp blue and white striped dress, white apron and cap came toward the family. The rustle of her heavily starched clothing was heard before her words.

"Welcome, boys. You are here to have your tonsils out, right? Then you can eat jelly and ice-cream." Her voice was annoyingly over-cheery.

"I don't want my tonsils out!" Kehn was adamant, "I don't want ice-cream or jelly!"

"Oh, come now. It is no big deal. You will be out of here in no time." The nurse turned to Jean and August. "You can leave now. We will take care of the boys."

"Don't leave!" Dick shouted.

The nurse took his small hand in hers. "But they have to go home."

Kehn asked, "Why?"

"That's the way we do things. Your parents will pick you up in a few days. We don't need them now." That information was supposed to be reassuring to the boys but had the opposite effect as they were led away from their parents.

THE FOLLOWING MORNING Kehn woke up in a hospital bed, realizing that not only his throat hurt but also his penis was in terrible pain. He tried to lift the sheet to see why. Groggy, hardly able to speak, he asked the nurse who was tending to Dick in another bed, "Why do I hurt there?"

The nurse walked quickly toward him and grabbed at Kehn's arms to keep his hands from going under the sheet.

"Now, dear, you are all right. Just don't touch."

"What happened?" Kehn asked, "Why does it hurt?"

"You had an operation."

"What... kind... of an operation?"

"Well, you had your tonsils out and..." she hesitated, "well... you had a circumcision."

"Circumcision?"

Turning her head away from Kehn to look at Dick, the nurse said, "Dick is waking, I'll be back later. Just don't touch!" With that order the nurse walked away, leaving Kehn by himself to deal with his shock and pain.

Tears flowed down Kehn's face as he lay in the bed feeling horribly trapped, deceived, his body engulfed in pain. He wondered what right anyone had to do anything with private parts of his body. He felt raped. He felt violated to the depth of his soul and he was alone with his feelings. Even though he felt on display with nurses and doctors coming and going, no one talked with him.

AT HOME AGAIN, in the privacy of the bathroom, nine-year-old Kehn cleaned and bandaged his penis by himself. Streams of tears ran down his face. He was afraid friction of his pants would cause even more pain. Bandages were strewn around the sink as he tried to make a wearable bandage for his wounded penis.

MORNING SUNSHINE poured in through the kitchen window, splattering brilliant patches on the floor between Kehn and his mother as they faced each other.

"You told me I was going to have my tonsils out! You made me wear a sailor suit and then you let them circumcise me. You deceived me!"

"I was doing what I was told to do."

"By who?"

"The doctor. I did not want to hurt you."

"But you did! Why was I circumcised?"

"So that you would look like other boys."

"I was okay the way I was."

"Other boys were circumcised at birth. You had to have a hole at the back of your neck fixed, so you never got circumcised. It was overlooked at the time."

"Why did they get circumcised?"

"Because that's what they do with baby boys."

"Why? Are we Jewish?"

"No. They say it is cleaner."

"I was clean."

"Yes, but the doctor thought so long as you were under the anesthetic, they might as well do it all together."

"Why did I need my tonsils out?"

"Because Dick was having his out."

"That's a dumb reason."

"That's just what they do to kids. They say you don't need tonsils."

"So I had my tonsils taken out because Dick needed to have his out. I had a circumcision because other boys had a circumcision. I did not need even one of those operations. You deceived me! How can I ever trust you again?"

"I was only following medical advice."

"Oh, fine. One doctor saves my life; the other mangles me for life. I'll be scarred forever!" Kehn was unable to control the tears, his voice raised a pitch, "When I'm a doctor, I won't hurt people! I will heal them, not hurt them... and you watch, I'll fight those doctors who hurt people! And I'll never lie to people! Never!" Walking away, he threw one last *"Never!"* over his shoulder.

OFTEN ON A SUNDAY afternoon the family piled into the car for the hour's drive to visit maternal grandparents in their large white house surrounded by an expansive green lawn and tall old trees. Kehn was close with his gentle maternal grandmother. He looked forward to the visits to feel her much needed non-judgmental nurturing.

Grandfather provided the spice of life by expressing his strong opinions and not so generous nature. He was a hard-nosed, self-made, wealthy businessman and proud of it.

[ks notebook] "I was not as close to him as to my grandmother but I identified myself more with him than with my own father because he was a 19th century individual, a Social Darwinist and Teddy Roosevelt admirer."

A THIRD BROTHER was now drawing on his mother's attention. One-year-old Donny had joined his older brothers to sit wide-eyed on the grass, waiting for the click of the camera.

Grandfather's head was under a black drape that hid both him and his camera. Then there was the familiar loud clicking sound and his head reappeared.

Grandfather was pleased. "Good! Well done! You boys will appreciate these pictures some day."

Grandfather took the film plate out of the large black Hassleblad camera, placing it in a black case and folded up his equipment as the boys watched. The long process always intrigued the boys. "Now we can have chocolate ice cream." Grandfather's eyes twinkled.

Dick jumped up in excitement. "Yeah, and we can all go to heaven and eat chocolate ice cream like you always tell us."

"Yes, Dick, I intend to go to heaven and eat as much chocolate ice cream as I like... and your Grandmother won't be able to tell me how much. I will look down on you guys and laugh because I will be eating all that chocolate ice cream, and I know you guys will one day join me... to eat ice cream. Right Kehn?"

"I have to fix the world first," Kehn answered.

"Kehn, I suppose that's a good thing. But that's a giant chore for one man. The best one man can hope for is that he makes a little dent in this world."

"I want to do more than make a dent. People lie."

Grandfather laughed, "And I'll watch you from heaven while you change the world. I'll be eating my ice cream without any worries." Then his laughter abruptly stopped. His voice lowered as he leaned toward Kehn, "You're still upset about your circumcision, aren't you, son."

It was nice to have someone identify the problem and not just cover it up. With that realization some pent up stress was released from Kehn's chest. He looked down at his feet in buckled shoes among the blades of green grass. "Yeah."

"I could see it in your eyes through my camera. Son, I don't blame you. I would be upset, too. Damned upset!"

Kehn was surprised by the sudden recognition of his painful turmoil. He silently savored the moment, and then took up his responsibility to his brother again and turned to Donny, "Come on."

They all crossed the lawn together like a parade. Grandfather and his gear led the way. Kehn brought up the rear to make sure his small brother followed safely.

Dick asked, "Grandfather, where is heaven?"

"Right now, it is going to be in the kitchen if Grandmother will let me have a big bowl of chocolate ice cream."

Inside the kitchen, Grandfather and Dick sat at the big, heavy-legged table topped with Grandmother's handiwork – a cloth embroidered with many colourful flowers. Kehn carefully rubbed a finger over the silk threads of a pink flower that he had watched his Grandmother embroider when he was younger. Now it was another way to feel his Grandmother. He laid the small book he had been carrying on the tablecloth and helped Donny onto a chair before seating himself. The smell of chocolate ice cream filled the air as Grandmother served it in bowls painted with red roses and gold rims.

Grandfather motioned with his hand, "Another scoop for me, please, Grandmother."

"Now you know it is not good for your waistline." Grandmother scooped more ice cream into a bowl.

Grandfather winked at the boys. "Thank you, Grandmother."

Dick reached for his bowl. "Grandfather is going to heaven and eat all the ice-cream he wants."

Grandmother smiled, "Yes, Dick. He always says that."

Grandfather nodded his head toward Kehn. "And Kehn is going to fix the world. No more lies in *this* world!"

Kehn felt Grandmother's gentle hand on his head. "Kehn is going to be a doctor just like his great grandfather. Dr. Kehnroth saved your life, Kehn. You were named after him and you will be like him... a good, honest man."

"Yes, I know..." Kehn's voice drifted off as his eyes looked past the open window into the outdoors. Deep in thought as he ate his ice cream, he whispered on an outgoing breath, "I kno-o-o-w..."

"What are you reading these days, Kehn?" Grandmother's question brought him out of reverie. She had been looking at the title on the table.

"I found John Dewey. This book is called Human Nature and Conduct."

"Isn't that a little hard for you to read?" Grandmother expressed her surprise. "You're ten years old and usually that book is read at college."

Dick answered, "Kehn always reads that kind of stuff."

"I'm able to read it. I want to know who we are... why we are... what are we doing here. I'm trying to understand what makes human beings the way we are. Men go to war instead of working things out without hurting anyone. And you know what makes me upset is that leaders send men into war instead of fighting it out between themselves. Innocent people get killed. Families are broken up. And the leaders sit back in their offices and feel none of it."

Grandmother became animated, waving a hand in the air, "Greed. That's what makes people go to war. Take Hitler, he got greedy and now we are at war."

"I want to understand our history. Why is a man like that in power?"

Grandmother asked, "Do they talk about this in school?"

"They talk about the war but not about philosophy. My mother is the only person who I can really talk to about these things."

Dick had been listening intently and responded again, "Yeah, Mom and Kehn talk a lot about his books. Kehn keeps pictures from magazines about the war in his pirate box under his bed."

Grandfather looked surprised. "Is that so? And what do you intend to do with them, Kehn?"

"I'm trying to figure out how to change the world. I need to understand what is going on. I want to help poor people and sick people."

"That's big ideas for a boy your age. Your mother has a good head. One day she'll make a million."

"Money?" Kehn asked, "What good is money? People are important, not money."

With an exaggerated motion of his whole body, Grandfather took a small, folded bundle of paper money out of his pocket and smacked it on the table so hard it bounced. "You need money in your pocket to be someone in this society. Everything costs money. You will need a house for your family and if you work hard, you too can have a nice house like this one. You will need money to go to medical school."

Kehn's eyebrows went up. He was digesting his Grandfather's overt reaction as Grandmother stepped close to Kehn's side, coming between Kehn and Grandfather. She said, "You certainly are an unusual boy... a strong willed boy... a smart boy." Kehn felt his Grandmother protective arm wrap around his shoulders.

The boys' parents, walking arm in arm along the country road, could be seen through the window.

Grandmother saw them. "Your parents are so lucky to have all three of you. They'll be back from their walk any minute. Let's start dinner. Kehn, will you help?"

Grandfather noticed the couple through the window and shook his head. "Your parents are still lovebirds even after all these years and three children. I have to give your headstrong mother credit. She certainly knows what she wants. I guess you take after her, my boy."

Those words were unspoken reminders that Grandfather had objected to his daughter marrying a poor, motherless boy from the farm, regardless that the boy had come from a lineage of nobility. Kehn had heard all about it by overhearing family conversations. August Schramm had no family money to rely on when he married fair-haired Jean Richards. Grandfather Richards was not sympathetic, challenging his daughter to make her own money as he had raised her to do.

IT WAS WRITTEN in information gathered by sisters of Kehn's father, aunts Marie Frances and Augusta (Dolly) Schramm and brother of Kehn's father, uncle Arthur E. Schramm:

Dr. Charles Henry Kehnroth, [Kehn's paternal great grandfather, the man he was named after] father of Franziska Katharina Kehnroth Schramm, [Kehn's grandmother] died of Brights Disease at French Hospital in New York, July 2, 1906. He had finished only a few days ago his twelfth year as a Master at Berkeley School and for the ten preceding years, he had been Professor of Modern Languages and Drawing at Blair Academy, Blairstown, N.J. In the Crimean War, he was a Lieutenant in the English Army and received the Victoria Cross for Bravery. In 1860, he was graduated from Erlanger University in Germany. He practiced medicine in London and, in 1870, received the Honorary Degree of LLD. From London University. He taught in the Colonies about 20 years, partly in Nova Scotia, as Professor of Modern Languages, and partly in the West Indies where he was Head Master successively at St. John's Academy, Bel Retiro Academy and Potsdam Grammar School. My mother, [Kehn's paternal grandmother] Franziska Katharina Schramm was traced back to: Sir William and Jane Keith, Lieutenant Governor of the colonial Pennsylvania and Delaware, 1669-1749.

FAMILY TREE

Sir William Keith and Lady Ann Keith (married 1704)
Jane (Yules) born in London 1708 [married James Jules]
Elizabeth [married John Merrick Williams of Westmoorland]
Raby Williams
Joseph Williams
Frances Williams [Kehn's great grandmother -- married Dr. Charles Kehnroth]
Katherine (Franziska Katherina Kehnroth) [Kehn's grandmother -- married August A. Schramm]
August Schramm [Kehn's father -- married Jean Richards]
Kehnroth Schramm [and two brothers and two sisters]

[Excerpt from old letter] ...and Lady Keith are now their heirs and possessors of their Title and Honors. Sir Robert Keith was the brother of Mrs. Jane Yules who was my Grandmother. My dear Mother was her fifth daughter, named Elizabeth, and was afterwards married to John Merrick Williams of Westmoorland, proprietor of one of the largest sugar estates there, known as the Retreat. He was of a Welsh family, and the older brand of which likewise possessed large estates in Westmoorland by the names of [?] and Anglesia.

[Excerpt from a letter written January 4, 1764]

Sir William Keith was 12 years Governor of Pennsylvania in America while under the English Government.

He was likewise Surveyor General of the Colonies and patented a great deal of land for Government. The Keiths are said to have founded the College of Aberdeen and were near relations of Earl Marischall and Field Marischall Keith. Sir William Keith's paternal seat was in the shire of Aberdeen in Scotland, Ludguthown. Lord Marshall's and Lord Wigton's families were settled near them...

* * *

[Another excerpt from the early 1800s] ...Lady Keith was a Miss Newberry of Kent. She appears to have had a fortune, for there were conveyances of Lands and Tenements to Sir William Keith on their marriage; and she had likewise houses in London that rented for 300 (pounds?) a year. They had likewise possessions in Pennsylvania. They had six sons and one daughter, Jane, born in London, 1708, who married a Mr. Yules from Jamaica, after her father was appointed Governor of Pennsylvania; and to their grief brought her to Jamaica, where she had a large family...

THE KEITH LINEAGE traced back through the mother and grandmothers of Kehn's father to old, powerful and colourful families in Scotland. Kehn's father's father, a man who loved to sing and did perform in musicals on stage, became a widower when his wife Franziska Katharina Kehnroth Schramm died in 1919 of the influenza epidemic. He struggled financially to raise his six children aged 2 to 13 to adulthood on his own. He worked as an accountant and needed to be mother and father to his children. He was greatly admired by extended family for his triumph of keeping the family together. But that history had been lost on Kehn's maternal Grandfather.

GROWING UP WITH STORIES of an illustrious family history on both sides of his family – stories of people who participated in the building of America and especially the physician/educator he was name after, and to top that off – his own mother's example of self-determination, Kehn grew up with knowledge that determination and work could accomplish change when necessary.

[ks notebook] "My neck was repaired surgically when I was ten days old delaying the inevitable circumcision till I was nine years old and my tonsils were removed. I could not tell which hurt the most, my throat or my penis. I felt betrayed by my mother who had as usual made light of my planned pain, (~John Dewey's religious mother?) buying us sailor suits and taking our picture (my brother and mine) before admitting us to the hospital. Prior to that I felt betrayed by my mother for giving birth to my brother when I was two and a half years old and packing me off to school when I was four and a half years old. School was a frightening place devoid of family and room to play or run. I was so 'shy' I didn't speak in school until I was eleven and my grade six teacher encouraged me to present my historical research on famous people of the Second World War to the class. From then on I became class president at the various public schools I attended. School was compulsory background for my education as a physician."

3

A World at War

[ks notebook] "I was just coming into my teens, getting erect on my way to the pencil sharpener. Roosevelt died, and The War ended in Europe May '45 before school was out. We went to Victory Parades in New York City. News reels showed starving Jews dying in Nazi concentration camps. In early August the U.S. dropped The Bomb on Hiroshima. I remember The News: 100,000 KILLED. To prove they weren't sorry and it wasn't a mistake, Our Great Leaders dropped a more powerful Bomb on Nagasaki. World War II was over. World War III was starting unless we stopped it. That's what I thought..."

WHILE PLAYING in the forest near their house, the sound of a car approaching interrupted the boys' laughter.

"Hey, listen. Someone's coming." Dick pointed, "I see a car."

Kehn recognized the car, "Oh, good, it's uncle Bob." The boys ran toward home.

Uncle Bob stepped out of the car as the boys approached.

"Hi, Uncle Bob!" Kehn and Dick called out in unison.

Head down and deep in thought, Uncle Bob had not heard the boys. He walked slowly toward the house.

"I wonder what's wrong!" Kehn whispered.

The boys ran fast to follow Uncle Bob through the door into the kitchen where mother was cooking dinner. Uncle Bob continued to stand close to the door. On seeing family, tears rolled down his cheeks.

Barely audible, he asked, "Have you heard?"

"Heard what?" Jean asked.

Uncle Bob's words exploded from his mouth, "We bombed Japan!"

"Yes, we have heard," Jean's voice was soft.

"I did it!" Uncle Bob sobbed.

Jean's eyes got big, "You? You did not!"

"I did it. I helped make the bomb."

"You? How? I don't understand. You're a scientist, not a bomb maker."

The boys were transfixed.

"The Atom Bomb! I didn't know I was working on an Atom Bomb. I was only working on a part of it. I never saw the whole thing. I didn't know what I was doing would kill thousands of innocent people... women and... children! ...babies! ...melt them to nothing!"

Kehn was aware of the bombs and had been in his own private hell over what the United States had done to innocent Japanese people. He asked, "They tricked you?"

Uncle Bob looked long at Kehn, then took a seat at the kitchen table and laid his head in his hands. "They didn't tell me! I am to blame even if I didn't know. How can I live with that? It is on my soul forever."

Mother asked, "So you came home?

Uncle Bob muttered from inside his hands, "I couldn't stay there. I quit! I can't go back! No job is worth that! This damn war!"

"It's not your fault," Kehn tried to console his uncle.

"Oh, yes it is," Bob answered. "I can't live with this guilt."

Kehn said again, "It's not your fault. You were lied to. You have to forgive yourself."

"You seem older than your twelve years," Uncle Bob shook his head.

Kehn's mother answered, "He does make sense. Kehn is right and he is older than his age in his understanding."

THE MOON REFLECTED light into the quiet bedroom located over the garage where the boys were sleeping, seemingly quite separate from the rest of the house even though it was attached. The silence was disturbed as Kehn became restless, making tortured sounds.

Kehn's nightmare took place in Japan's daylight that suddenly disappeared as a dense, dark grey cloud overtook people who melted to the ground. Babies melted in their mother's arms and became splotches of grey matter on the ground.

The sound woke Dick. "Kehn, what's wrong?"

"Huh? ...Ahh! ...I see all those people melting. There were babies and mothers melting. AhhH! It's awful!"

Dick said, "Our uncle helped make the bomb."

"I know, but he didn't know what he was doing."

"Yes, but he helped."

"Uncle Bob would never kill anything if he knew what he was doing. We all live in the United States. If he is guilty, we all are. How can we live with that? My life will never be the same again."

Kehn lay wide-eyed, staring out the window at the moon in a deep blue-black sky with innocent looking stars twinkling in all their brilliance as though nothing had changed under a country sky.

[ks notebook] "Franklin Roosevelt was the only President I had known until 1945 when Harry Truman became president and decided to drop the first and second atomic bombs on Hiroshima and Nagasaki. One bomb could have been a mistake, two bombs meant: he did it on purpose!

"And so it was that my happy childhood days came to an abrupt end. A circumcision followed by the bombing of Japan. Life would never be the same again for me. My education in community development began in adolescence when I learned that my great uncle, a chemical engineer, had worked on the Manhattan Project, putting his head in the centrifuges to find out what was happening to his chemical mixtures, not knowing the material was radioactive, and without knowing he was building a bomb.

"I was ultimately concerned with the meaning of life in a world divided against itself and hostile to growing life.

"When my Great Uncle Bob discovered he had been used to help make atom bombs, he quit chemical engineering — A Better Living Through Chemistry for the Old Family Religion of his in-law's furniture business. He was not taking any more chances. We stopped worrying about the effects of radioactivity on Uncle Bob's family when his son was born normal. We knew about babies born with birth defects before we knew about radioactivity because I was born with one.

"His oldest brother, my grandfather, Lee Richards, admired Winston Churchill and Teddy Roosevelt, but hated Franklin Roosevelt, my President and even joked he would take out the fireplace unless FDR stopped his fireside chats on the radio.

"At twelve I needed to know about atomic energy, communism and world government. My first research project, interviewing my uncle taught me that decisions affecting the future life on earth were made without even consulting government employed scientists! The only other secret about the bomb was how to mass-produce it.

"Following my conversations with Uncle Bob, I continued to study atomic energy and at thirteen I broke my eight-year silence in school. Since Grade One I hadn't spoken in Class but I began to bring pictures from Life Magazine and my writing into our Current Events Class. Nobody could stop me telling what I somehow knew about the horrors of war and Our Leaders making war on us. Except for secrets the U.S. government kept from its employees, there were no scientific secrets, and the whole world soon learned to mass-produce atomic bombs.

"Later I read of the murder of Jews in concentration camps by Germans and the Genocide of American Indians by Spanish, English and French. I read government publications on Communism where I found the Marxist ethic: 'From each according to his ability, to each according to his need.' I adopted this ethic as my own version of The Golden Rule when I spoke my belief in god to become a member of the Congregational Church of my Pilgrim ancestors. My parents and I disagreed with my grandfather Lee Richards over the need for the church to be a political body, as we believed it had been in 1620 and when Jesus was alive.

"As the eldest of four children in 1946, I joined the United World Federalists with my parents to build a community of families who take responsibility for learning to live together in a world without war, and to help make the United Nations into a world government able to prevent our Mad Leaders from killing all Life on Earth. The idea emerged from my first research project of interviewing my Great Uncle Bob...

"I cried when Roosevelt died – Our President, the only one I knew. I blamed Harry Truman for Hiroshima when I learned from my Uncle who worked on The Manhattan Project that he didn't even know he was working with radioactive chemicals, helping to build an Atom Bomb! Talking with him and reading Public Documents, I learned there were No Secrets for building Atom Bombs only those The Government kept from its Employees and People. I was angry at the so-called Grown-Ups and scared I would not grow up to have a Family of my own and learn to live before all Life died.

"It was thought that I asked too much, thought too much, and I was too much so they sent me away to Work and School.

"Poor Little Boy. Little Boy is what they named the Uranium Bomb that killed the families in Hiroshima. I was Poor. I don't remember ever having any money, but I didn't need it, and I still don't. Growing up I felt rich, some times I thought I would explode I was so full of myself, longing for a Woman to share my life, have Babies, and show those Old Guys they can't take The Future away from Our Grandchildren. I only felt poor because I did not yet have Children. Nor did I have the experience of a Woman yet in order to have Children, though I dreamed of it, yearned for her.

"Stubbornness and determination were mine, inherited from my Mother. Work ethics were strong. I was on a path with much work to be done. In time I would become rich with children in marriage when I could afford to care for a family."

AT THE AGE OF FOURTEEN, Kehn was inside a toilet stall, scrubbing a toilet with a brush and breathing the harsh fumes of the cleaning powder. He paused, listening to the sounds of children laughing and playing outside. With brush in hand, he walked past more toilet stalls yet to be cleaned, to the open doorway to look outside. The day was sunny and hot. He watched children playing in the lake. His brothers were among the children having fun. The boys waved at Kehn. He waved and then went back to work cleaning toilets with the continuous sound of children playing in the background.

[ks notebook] "At age fourteen... I started work at summer camp so that my brothers could be there as guests... general maintenance at first... then as camp counselor for the next three years. My family thought it was good training for me as a future doctor who should know how to take care of people and understand the working poor..."

KEHN WAS SENT AWAY from home to attend Canaan High School and to live with a foster family. To make the best of his situation, Kehn created new activities by playing football instead of running free in the beloved forest.

[ks notebook] "...In Senior High School, my vocation in medicine broadened and deepened to include learning how to prevent the insanity of war and live with all the peoples of the World in peace. Readers Digest, Life, and the books of John Dewey and Lewis Mumford encouraged us to work toward these goals in our New England schooling and 1950's college experience. My high school yearbook motto 'Nihil humani a me alienum puta' is the Latin for 'I consider nothing human is alien to me'."

4

Dartmouth College

A SHY YOUNG MAN of seventeen, going on eighteen, arrived at Dartmouth College campus to begin his journey into higher learning in the autumn of 1950.

Dartmouth College is a colonial and third oldest college in the United States, a member of the Ivy League, located in Hanover, New Hampshire. A Congregational minister established the college in 1769 before the American Revolution. Its charter created a college 'for the education and instruction of Youth of the Indian Tribes in this Land... and also of English Youth and any others.'

[ks notebook] "At Dartmouth College I studied premedical sciences and philosophy... I found my origins in my lived curriculum as a student of studies in philosophy, and anthropology. Dartmouth was a small college where I was able to study the works of the people who cared about society and to test my ideas for the next four years...

I was in the library every chance I had..."

MAGNIFICENT, LARGE MURALS graced the walls of the Dartmouth Baker Library, painted by Jose Clemente Orozco, a guest lecturer in the Art Department in 1932. Initially, he taught the technique of fresco painting by painting a small fresco, entitled 'Man Released from the Mechanistic to the Creative Life', and then went on to paint the series of twenty-four murals called 'The Epic of American Civilization'.

Kehn could usually be found reading beside a mural in the basement reserved book section that had become his comfort zone. He stacked his books on the classic dark wood table and spent hours there.

IT HAD BEEN a learning process to join the social life of the college, different than the comparatively quiet life experience so far. During the first months, Kehn's parents became concerned, making a visit to see first-hand how their shy son was fairing. Their advice was to smoke cigarettes and drink along with the crowds until Kehn established himself in his own right.

Kehn wrote, "...Dartmouth was a place that offered outdoor activity with indoor discussions."

Physically active all his life, it was natural for Kehn to join the Dartmouth Outing Club. Having its start in 1909, it was the oldest collegiate outing club in the United States.

Wearing the green and white colours of the college, usually a green shirt or jacket with the white letters of Dartmouth College, but sometimes white with green letters, Kehn became active in the year-round winter and summer sports. He enjoyed the serenity and peace of gliding through the waters of Connecticut River by canoe, raft or inner tube. He hiked the Appalachian Trail that ran through the town and up into the White Mountains that surround the town, part of the Appalachian Mountains of New Hampshire. With friends he explored the mountains named after past Presidents of the United States and above the tree line where the alpine meadows provided an unobstructed view for miles all around on a clear day. There were hiking trips to visit Franconia Notch canyon, in the White Mountains, formed during the last ice age.

With best friend and dorm roommate, Bob Bean, Kehn sang college songs as they hiked. A favourite song was:

Dartmouth's in town again,
Team, Team, Team,
Echo the old refrain,
Team, Team, Team.
Dartmouth for you we sing,
Dartmouth the echoes ring,
Dartmouth we cheer you.
Wah Who Wah Who Wah!...

Jazzing up the lyrics, they sang:
Dartmouth's in Town Again,
Run, Girls, Run!...

Dartmouth College had a history of tradition and exuberant school spirit. As a men's college, the official song of Dartmouth in the 1950's was 'Men of Dartmouth', and the list of Dartmouth songs was mainly male oriented. Celebrations abounded on weekends. There was the Winter Carnival in February that had been started in 1911 by the Dartmouth Outing Club; it was a few days of winter sports and competitions, and celebrations that attracted women from around the country.

Discovering a physical weakness of any kind came as a surprise in college. While skiing in the Appalachian Mountains, Kehn became aware that his left leg had been affected by Spina Bifida, just enough for it to be weak in controlling the long, heavy wooden downhill skis, causing him to give up on skiing.

For four years a building of brick Dutch colonial architecture, Middle Massachusetts Hall on the Dartmouth College campus was where Kehn lived in dorm residency on the fourth floor with fellow students. The fire escape was fashioned out of heavy hemp ropes coiled by the window, providing fifty feet of rope for *boys* to swing on, especially when beer flowed.

College life was comfortable enough to enable playfulness. Friendships were strong enough to withstand jokes. One evening Kehn and a friend stuffed the small bathroom from floor to ceiling with crumpled newspaper. And then they waited for Bob to arrive home from his date.

Bob arrived and rushed, as usual, to the bathroom only to encounter it filled with crumpled paper. As he pulled paper out of the room, throwing it over his shoulders, he called out, "What have you goofy guys done to me? I just traveled a long way from another college and I need to get in here!"

When Bob emerged refreshed from the bathroom, he laughed, "Some joke, you guys!"

DAYTIME CLASSES, especially philosophy with Eugen Rosenstock-Huessy, lead to many late night discussions in the dorm about the existence of God and the questions around 'what we are doing here and where are we going'. These classes and dorm discussions would be indelible in Kehn's mind; he would want to recreate these times in future wherever he goes.

Bob and Kehn had built a trusting relationship, a friendship that was sustained through Dartmouth years of serious study, exploration of ideas, agreeing and disagreeing, explorations of the surrounding countryside, and goofiness. Ultimately Bob chose Kehn to be his Best Man at his wedding when marrying Carol in 1953, the same girl he dated the night the bathroom was stuffed with paper.

Bob moved out of the dorm into married life that would last him a lifetime. [In future, Bob would serve in the U.S. Army Counterintelligence Corp from 1955 to 1957.]

Two close friends, going in different directions, carry the memory of their friendship for the rest of their lives.

Kehn continued his deep involvement with the Dartmouth Christian Mission, going on 'help trips' to nearby farms to help people in need by performing chores like chopping wood or any other needed chore.

One year to graduation, the work and his studies leading to medical school kept him busy.

[ks notebook] "Already committed to becoming a physician like my great grandfather whose name I was given, I decided that doctor meant science teacher. I would study, learn, and teach whatever was necessary to make the newly formed United Nations work to prevent war and promote health. At Dartmouth College in the 1950's, I studied philosophy with Rosenstock-Huessy who taught us that World War 1 had been a Revolution, a civil war within the body of humankind and we needed to find a moral equivalent to war in services to our families and the family of humankind. In 1939 with Dartmouth students like Page Smith, he founded Camp William James in Vermont, which later became a model for the Peace Corps. As a volunteer and a lay preacher to a small Vermont church, I studied his teachings through personal experience. Page Smith, who co-founded the William James Association a generation after his experience in Camp William James, tells us that great cities of the past were made on a human scale which can be rebuilt in the country by volunteer labor. The Association continues today as an adult educational and land reform movement to share the work of farm families with city and student volunteers to meet the increasing needs of rural areas depleted by urban economic growth and waste. Lewis Mumford's Fourth Migration from the suburbs to make regional cities was planned in the 1920's to accomplish these goals."

REMEMBERING THE DARTMOUTH YEARS in 1990, Kehn wrote:

On writing one's life

How does questioning The Truth change a speaker or writer of a life? In the movie Semi-Tough, Jill asks Burt: 'What do you want to write about? I want to tell The Truth!' 'Oh', she says, 'a work of fiction!' No truth is without fiction because we tell The Truth by telling stories that make our lies and our lives truthful. I write my life as a speech thinker who hears a common sense in stories that name us. We meet Death and Love in stories of our grandparents by learning who is dying, reborn, or alive in our lives. Time stops and generations are crossed when we respond to stories calling us by name and naming things as they are.

I remember with my life not my brain. I began writing my life when I learned that The President of the United States and Commander-in-Chief of Armed Forces, Harry Truman gave the orders in 1945 to drop The Atomic Bomb on Hiroshima, killing a city of 100,000 people. Despite the outcry against this murder of men, women, and children, he ordered another atomic bombing and, in Nagasaki, killed another city full of Japanese people! My childhood died with them. Afraid I would not even get a chance to live before our leaders destroyed all life on earth, I died of anxiety and found I could be alive when I die! I needed time and friends to prevent the madness of total genocide. Life as a question of Death and Love and Rebirth became my first conversion, my passionate ultimate concern in the conversions of my life.

In the colonial tradition of my New England family, I am telling The Truth as best I can in writing my life, a story of my changes, my conversions, the conversations that give meaning to the common sense of everyday life. During High School in New England whenever I asked any questions about the meanings of Life, I was told that I would learn that in college. I received the same answer in College when I was told I would learn about Life in Medical School! In the Joe McCarthy Era, it seemed that anyone who asked questions was named "a communist." Then I met Eugene Rosenstock-Huessy, a speech thinker at Dartmouth College, who told his students: "Remember you are more alive than your most living thought!"

He spoke his book, Out of Revolution: Autobiography of Western Man... Rosenstock taught us a new meaning of responsibility when he told us not to take notes but to listen. His Latin motto "Respondeo etsi mutabor" means "I respond although I will be changed." After my university writings were lost, I wrote to remember Eugen Rosenstock-Huessy, my spiritual grandfather, and my life in poetry I had never forgotten...

KEHN'S MOTHER, with her Baby Brownie camera in hand, caught up with him as the Graduate class of 1954 at Dartmouth College dispersed. "Doctor Kehn, I need my own snapshot of you."

Kehn smiled. "Hi, Mom, I'm not a doctor yet."

"Yes, you are. Pre-med is done. Medical School is next. You're now becoming the doctor you were born to be."

In front of a white clapboard campus building, in his black ceremonial gown and square cap with the tassel floating on the left side of his face, Kehn stood still for his mother. With hands relaxed together in front of his robe he looked into the distance, emanating strength and determination for his future. The click of the camera savored this moment – this milestone and proclaimed it to be in the archives for generations to come.

[ks notebook] "I came to medicine through philosophy at Dartmouth College. As a pre-medical student, I took every course required by *any* medical school in the U.S. or Canada, because I was applying to Dartmouth Medical College, a two-year school that placed students in third year at Harvard and other medical schools. I was determined to balance my science and arts studies so that I could gain historical understanding of the world in which I live. Majoring in philosophy allowed me to get the broadest education I could under the circumstances. When I was accepted by Dartmouth Medical School to begin medical studies in my fourth year, common practice then, I declined the offer so that I could complete my full major in philosophy during my senior year. This enabled me to attend University of Vermont College of Medicine where family physicians taught us by tutorial to become family doctors. I saw medicine as applied philosophy and I still do, with a strong emphasis on history and cross-cultural study. Despite my best efforts, there are important gaps in my knowledge of my own traditions as well as in my knowledge of other cultures, which are my incentives to further formal study in philosophy, history, and anthropology.

"N.B. My grades in philosophy and other Arts courses were consistently a full grade higher than my science classes (which I considered to be memory role classes rather than thinking classes).

"With a BA in Philosophy I left the wonderful years at Dartmouth and my spiritual grandfather, Eugen Rosenstock-Heussy, whose teachings I would carry with me as I went on to another four years at the University of Vermont Medical School... and for the rest of my life."

5

Medical School

*"I experienced my life as a gift from God calling
me to share what I have with others by being a
doctor, a teacher and a physician for families who
want to care for their own in a world that seems
not to care about their lives except as slaves."*
Kehnroth Schramm

UVM INITIALS stand for the Latin term Univeritas Viridis
Montis. Translation: University of the Green Mountains, named
for its location in Burlington, Vermont, on the shores of Lake
Champlain in a valley between the Adirondack and the Green
Mountains. The University of Vermont was established in 1791, the
same year Vermont became the 14th state in the union. It is the
fifth oldest university in New England. Then followed the
establishment of the University of Vermont Medical School in
1822 as the seventh medical college of the United States.

It became the first university with a charter to declare that it
would not give preference to any religion, and the first university
to admit women and African-Americans into Phi Beta Kappa, the
country's oldest collegiate honor society. UVM has been referred
to as an Ivy League school providing an Ivy League experience to
its students.

John Dewey, the American psychologist, philosopher, educator, social critic and political activist that Kehn had been looking up to and whose writings he had studied since childhood had graduated from UVM in 1879. Following Dewey's death in 1952, he was buried beside the chapel on the grounds of UVM just two years earlier than Kehn's arrival on campus.

Kehn was now in Dewey territory and in Dewey's aura of working for the Humanistic movement and world peace.

[ks notebook] "I studied science based medicine at Vermont University. The classes were small enough that we had personal training.

"My first day of classes in Medical School at University of Vermont, I was named Family Health Advisor to a pregnant family with whom I worked all four years of medical study. We made home visits to care for low-income families who attended our clinics in Burlington. I believed the common sense of stories these people told me more than I believed in lab results because of the many mistakes I saw or made in Lab Tests. Our clinical teachers were physicians who taught that A Complete History And Physical Examination is the only way to understand and interpret what a physician smells, hears, sees, and feels in an hour-long interview and examination before doing the lab studies of The Patient...

"...When I was in medical school in Vermont in the fifties, I was called 'the writer' by my teacher of surgery. I wrote as I read to understand the lives of the people, the patients who were teaching me medicine. ...

"I was greatly troubled by the atomic bomb... I determined to teach science. Physicians were called doctor, I learned in my studies of Latin, because doctor meant teacher. I became a teacher and philosopher, reading medieval philosophy in Latin while studying medicine. I was ultimately concerned with the meaning of life in a world divided against itself and hostile to growing life.

"...I think in words, feelings, impassioned conversations, prayers and conversions, with occasional soft images in contrast to the colours of my night dreams. Perhaps that is why I am called to be a healer with words and a maker of history, of true stories to repay my debt to my teachers and discover another world to live in with children and grandchildren. ...

"In 1956, while I was a medical student, my younger brother, also a philosophy major at Dartmouth, gave me The Transformation of Man by Lewis Mumford. While I was learning to diagnose individuals through their personal histories, Mumford was diagnosing culture problems through person history. He challenged me to become a generalist and the challenge is still with me."

IN THE SPRING of 1958, the taking of the Hippocratic Oath at Graduation from the Vermont University Medical School was accompanied by a ceremonial lecture reminding the newly graduated physicians of their commitment to be healers and of their promise to uphold the high ethical standards that must be adhered to in practicing medicine. For Kehn, the taking of the Oath was a confirmed promise written in the energy of creation – beyond himself – to a way of practicing medicine – and, in living life.

INTERNING AS A PEDIATRICIAN in Syracuse, N.Y., Kehn spent as much time as a family needed to discuss their child's medical care. He sat with sick children throughout the night, trying to make up for a system that caused parents to leave their children by themselves in a hospital. He took the time to play with the children while listening to their stories and fears. He spoke at length with parents, giving them time needed.

In the hospital cafeteria while in a line-up, a nurse who had become a friend told Kehn that a child who had suffered scalding burn injuries in a home accident, had just died in the hospital. Seeing Kehn's distressed face, the nurse said, "Oh well, look at it this way, he is in a better place now."

"We need to take better care of children in this present life – the here and now."

"Maybe it was his Karma," she replied. "Maybe it's all okay."

"It's not okay!" The tray with a partial lunch on it slipped out of Kehn's hands. He paused to look at the food spilled on the floor around his shoes. Turning on his heels, he walked out of the cafeteria.

[ks notebook] "My longstanding interest in health as happiness led me naturally into the problems of growth and development in pediatrics, and continuing study of anthropology. My postgraduate training in the following years in New York State was interning in Pediatrics, becoming Assistant Resident Instructor, and receiving Diplomas in Pediatrics. I would have stayed forever in Vermont to study health and eventually to have a baby farm…"

CHILDREN FILLED SEVERAL BEDS in the room. They were happy about a visit by Doctor Kehn.

"How do you spell your name?" a child colouring with crayons asked.

"K-e-h-n, that spells Kehn."

"Doctor Kehn," the child asked, "How do you spell doctor? I'm making you a new colorful name sign to wear."

"d-o-c-t-o-r."

Just then, a doctor in a white coat opened the door wide enough to poke his head into the room. "Doctor, see me in my office."

Kehn nodded toward the man and the door closed again as the head disappeared.

A child lying in bed holding his teddy bear close to his face asked wistfully, "Doctor Kehn, do you have to go?"

Another child laughed, "Was that jack-in-the-box?"

Kehn laughed with the children and answered the child with a teddy bear, "I will stay with you. We can tell each other stories or sing a song."

The child relaxed, "Okay, Doctor Kehn."

The child with the crayons exclaimed, "I'm finishing your name sign. See?" He held up a small piece of paper that read: **doctor ken**

Kehn responded, "It's very nice. I like all the colours. I have a letter *h* in my first name because my longer name is really *Kehnroth* but I think it looks just right without the *h* and it says *Ken* all the same. I've even got a pin in my pocket so we can pin it on my jacket."

Leaning over as the child pinned the tag on his white lapel, he said quietly, "I shall wear it proudly. Thank you."

AS A DOCTOR OF MEDICINE, Kehn had taken the Hippocratic Oath, believing that he would and could live by his Oath for the rest of his life. He was not aware then of how many times and ways his promise would be tested and re-tested for the rest of his life.

The popping head was seated behind his desk. After a superficial greeting he said, "I've been waiting. Taking your time as usual. Oh, I see you have a new nametag. *doctor ken*. Changed the spelling of your name?"

Kehn took a chair in front of the desk. "A child made it for me. This nametag has a lot of meaning to it... for the child and for me."

"I see. Making me wait brings me right to the reason for this meeting. Doctor Schramm, you are the slowest doctor on the ward. We don't have time to waste around here."

Kehn responded, "There is a lot of fear associated with being here. These children and their parents need more doctors to slow down and spend time with them to explain things carefully and alleviate their fears. What we need to do here is open up the hospital for parents to be here with their children around the clock so that children are not left alone with their fears and pain. Sending parents home, away from their children, makes no sense. Children would heal faster with family present. I do spend time with families around their issues and much of the time spent with the children is my own off duty time, making up for the missing families."

The doctor replied with a wry smile, "I like that you are always thinking, pushing the boundaries about how to improve and change things. That is in your favor. It can work against you, too. In other words, you challenge the hierarchy and their security. Many will want to cover their asses by freezing you out."

Ken asked, "What are they afraid of – being human? Taking time to talk instead of just poking and running away? Children need more from us than needles and our backs when they are suffering. Families need understanding and kindness; they need doctors to be real people, not robots looking for how quickly we can find our escape route. I don't intend to change my ways. If I see a need to take my time, I will respond to the people."

"I'm one of your superiors... the so-called hierarchy. I want to help you to get established... get to where you want to be."

Kehn did not answer. A strange feeling washed over Kehn that somehow things did not smell right.

The doctor handed Kehn a piece of notepaper. "Come to my apartment tonight. We'll sort some things out. Here's my address."

THE AIR SMELLED OF WATER. The evening sky had gathered clouds that threatened rain as Kehn, paper in hand, hesitated in front of an apartment building. He opened the heavy unlocked street door and made his way up two flights of stairs and then partway through the hallway. In front of the door he was looking for, he hesitated to acknowledge a feeling of foreboding. Reasoning with himself about good intentions and thinking positively, he knocked.

The door opened. A smiling head topped wine coloured satin lounging pajamas out of which poked large hands waving Kehn in.

Kehn hesitated as even the smile seemed alarming.

"Please, come in. Have a seat, Kehn."

Looking around cautiously, Kehn took a seat on the nearest sofa. The room was unexpectedly luxurious.

"Like a drink? A brandy?" The doctor headed for a cabinet off to the side.

"Thanks. I don't drink on the job."

"Oh, think of this as a social visit," the doctor said as he poured himself a brandy. "You can change your mind and have a drink with me."

"No thanks. I prefer not to drink just now."

The doctor turned to face Kehn. "I keep this little apartment for when I am working late in town." He sipped his drink while talking and sidestepping across the room toward Kehn. "Kehn, you are a good doctor. Where do you want to be as a Pediatrician?"

"I plan to work in Vermont, preferably with poor families, helping with their health and their housing; to help them keep their children healthy."

Towering over Kehn, the doctor asked, "Housing? How the hell do you think you can do that?"

"Health and a healthy home go together."

The doctor sat on the sofa too close for Kehn's comfort. Liquor breath seemed to have stolen all the oxygen from the air.

"Kehn, you are an idealist. Always the idealist! Let's get real here. You're a doctor, what the hell do you know about their housing? What the hell does being a Pediatrician have to do with housing the patients?"

"If you take a person out of a sick situation and treat him or her, then put that person back into a sick home, that person is most likely to get sick again."

The doctor laid his hand on Kehn's knee. Kehn pulled his knee away as panic set in.

The doctor continued moving closer until his face was only inches away from Kehn's face, breathing liquor directly into Kehn's face. He again laid his hand on Kehn, this time high on his thigh. "Oh, come on now. I can help your career. You think by spending extra time with the kids and their parents, you can solve that? Look at it this way, you can go places and I can help you."

Kehn glanced quickly around the room. Seeing an open window with what looked like a metal fire escape on the other side, Kehn took a leap of faith and dashed across the room and out the window only hoping there would be a bottom. He raced down the fire escape feeling lucky that it almost reached the ground. He leaped the last few feet to the cement below and luckily landed on his feet.

The doctor had followed to the window, calling out to Kehn's back, "You're making a big mistake, Kehn! Your career is finished!"

A light rain had started to fall. In shock, Kehn caught his breath as he walked the streets. Digesting the meaning of the encounter, he realized that the threat just hurtled at him would have consequences.

As he wandered the darkened wet street, he wondered how to overcome this situation. What next? The man was clearly in violation of all ethics of his profession as a doctor and teacher, and of his position. He had violated Kehn's human rights and dignity. The reality was that this particular man was in a position to be able to block registration as a Pediatrician.

Kehn realized it would be a losing battle for him. After years of work and having earned Diplomas in Pediatrics, Kehn made the decision to leave Pediatrics rather than fight this war.

HAVING MET ANTHROPOLOGIST Margaret Mead had a long and deep effect on Kehn. She had taken his hand and told him that his gentleness would be well liked by Samoan people and suggested he could work with them. In the depths of his being, the idea of being a medical anthropologist was growing larger and taking hold. While continuing work on his Doctorate in Anthropology at Cornell University, Ken worked part time for the next six months as Resident Doctor at Sage Hospital, Cornell University.

[ks notebook] "While working as a physician at the Student Health Service of Cornell University in 1960, I discovered Joseph Needham's Science and Civilization in China which deepened my interest in history and philosophy of science and medicine. My subsequent studies in psychiatry at Syracuse with Tom Szasz, Ernest Becker, Stanley Diamond and Marvin Harris further encouraged that interest cross-culturally, I found parallels among Mumford, Needham and Radin... I want to explore in depth..."

6

Choosing a Wife

[ks notebook] "...Because I came to medicine and pediatrics from philosophy and religion, I practiced medicine as philosophy, healing and learning with words, in the Feast of Life as freedom to know the truth by our own efforts and divine grace. I have never doubted that man's duty and destiny is to become divinely human, a loving father, capable of sharing and giving his life if needed for a loved one."

HAVING SPENT YEARS working while studying, and studying while working, it was time for Kehn to fulfill his dream. He searched in earnest for the woman who might share his life and work, and to make a safe home for their children.

People from the university gathered in the evenings at the nearby cafe, eating and dancing to a jukebox. It became a familiar place to Kehn as he dated several women.

He seemed to gravitate toward blonds in his search. Kehn was with a pretty, blond woman as they sipped sodas and joined others on the small dance floor. Later, while walking her home along a quiet street, they stopped to sit on a low stone wall to talk in the quiet of the evening.

"I want to marry you," she announced.

Kehn looked at his shoes for a moment, then responded, "Marriage to me means children, family, a lifetime commitment, responsibility."

"Lifetime? Children? I want children. Commitment is so long as things work out, isn't it?"

"Commitment is working things out! You would be asking me to change who I am for anything less than that." After a moment of silence he said, "You're not ready to marry someone like me."

Proposals were plentiful – eight in all, but finding the right mate for his goals in life proved difficult; each girlfriend eventually bit the dust.

THE HOSPITAL CAFETERIA was crowded with white-coated doctors and nurses in starched caps and aprons over dresses and that made soft rustling sounds. Kehn, in his white jacket, was quietly eating lunch at a table. He was relaxing, casually watching the nurses walk by and listening to the rhythmic music of their whispering starched skirts and softness of their steps. Carolyn, a fair-haired student-nurse with bright blue eyes walked by. Her skirt swayed with the movement of her hips. He watched and found himself imagining her hips having ample room to bear children nicely. There was energy about her that he liked.

THE NIGHT WAS WARM. Large old trees, with leaves shimmering silver in the moonlight, lined the quiet street where Kehn lived in a rented room in a large, brown house across the road from the medical school campus. He was sleeping with the window open after a long workday.

An unusual sound woke him. Drowsily, he opened his eyes to see through the darkness of the room, a figure of a woman climbing into the room through his window, just faintly highlighted from behind by the moonlight. Coming out of the shadow as she approached, he recognized the woman he had dreamed of. He asked, "Why me?"

IN THE YEAR OF 1961, vivacious, bright, beautiful, bold, and smart Carolyn Wernz won Kehn's heart. Carolyn... whose hips had him imagining his children borne of them... became his wife. Hopes and dreams of a family were becoming a reality for Kehn.

The wedding ceremony over, wedding photos were being taken. Kehn, Carolyn and the young male Minister who performed the ceremony stood together in front of a photographer who was slipping black plates in and out of his large, black camera. Carolyn leaned toward the Minister while Kehn was slightly off to one side. Already Kehn felt the gap between himself and his new wife. At the end of the photo session, Carolyn leaned back toward Kehn, whispering, "Don't worry, if it doesn't work out, we can always get a divorce."

Jolted by the statement, Kehn was concerned his divorce was pending on the same day he got married. The irony was that this noncommittal of a lifelong marriage was exactly what he had been avoiding in other women.

From that day forward, the wedding photo was a continual reminder of drenched hopes and dreams, and of the work Kehn would have to do to retrieve them.

There was much Kehn enjoyed about his wife – her talent as an artist, her shining light that he hoped would carry her through the life of being married to a busy doctor and having babies. In the early days of marriage, he wanted to encourage her artistic talents. He posed nude for her to draw and paint.

A son was born. All his life, Kehn had been worried about passing on a congenital defect because of Spina Bifida, but the baby was perfectly healthy and beautifully formed. Kehn was relieved and extremely happy.

[ks notebook] "Actions speak louder than words. Silence is pregnant with meaning. Birds, trees, plants, insects and mammals, even stones and some machines, like cars, are part of nature's dialogue with humanity.

"Reading and writing the signs of my life by trial and error, I find books inviting me to remember my past and imagine my future; whose authors teach living as children, students, warriors, teachers, parents, farmers, workers, doctors, scientists, historians, artists, or writers. Some are "bibles" teaching great-grandparents,

grandparents, parents, peers, and children how to do it: how to be human, somehow making sense of the mysteries of life and death. Writing is dying and reading is a rebirth of writer and reader. Exercising our powers of imagining in self-making knowledge, we bring childhood and ancestors to life in time for our children to become teachers of health as human happiness and freedom in the family of life."

MEANWHILE, IN THE middle of the flat Canadian prairies, a girl had been born in the summer of 1937. As a child, she loved to kick off her shoes and run barefoot, but she would sometimes look down and experience a surreal phenomenon – always the same. She could clearly see her feet standing in the black prairie gumbo covered in wheat, weeds or golden dandelions, but in her mind she was keenly aware of feet in buckled shoes standing in green grass. Somehow she always knew that the grass was in New York State. She would raise her eyes to the sky and wonder. It was as though a magnet from that direction continually pulled on her. As much as she loved the sunny, golden prairie that turned white in winter and became her glistening playground, she always felt a profound loneliness, as though someone who should be part of her life was missing and could be found in those buckled shoes.

All through childhood and into womanhood, she would lie on her back in her parents' garden or in the weeds of grandparents' farmyard, or in the pure white snow looking past the colour of the sky, deep into space for answers – wondering about the make-up of the universe, trying to figure out where we come from and where we are going; wondering what will happen to earthlings when all the toilet paper or the fossil fuels run out, and always, always wondering about the fair-haired boy of her daydreams. At night, while in bed, she imagined the whistle and chugging sound of the nearby trains would take her to the boy so far away.

At the age of eighteen in February of 1956, she married the boyfriend she knew since aged fourteen. He was the exact opposite in every way to the boy of her reveries. At her wedding, she knew only too well that she was making a mistake. Two years after the wedding she gave birth to her first child. During the pregnancy, in the autumn, she sat on the outdoor wooden staircase in her old plaid housecoat, soaking up the morning sunrays while dealing with months of all day nausea and wearing a hole in the backside of the housecoat. Because she was no longer distracted by running around and working (she had been fired from her job for getting pregnant) she had time to think and feel. Feelings became magnified as she felt she was being drawn into college classrooms along with students going back to a school far from the prairies – somewhere where large Maple trees grow with leaves turning brilliant shades of red like she had never seen in Saskatchewan. She could smell the books and see the skirts and jackets. The sensation had been particularly intense every autumn as students returned to classrooms. The phenomenon grew stronger each year but now it was as though she was living her married life on the surface, but on the inside there was an attachment to other events and another person far away.

7

Paediatrics to Teaching

[ks notebook] "Religion means what concerns me ultimately: another world to live in as a human being. Concerned for growing fully human beings, I studied emotional development of families in my postgraduate training in Paediatrics and Psychiatry at the S.U.N.Y. Upstate Medical Center in Syracuse. My research questions followed my ethic: how does a physician or parent know or recognize what the other parent, physician or child needs and is able to do?

"There I married a nursing student and we had two sons born while I studied with Ernest Becker, Ageha Bharathi, Stanley Diamond, Ron Leifer, Brad Starr, and Tom Szasz. With Tom Szasz, I learned to tell The Truth; with Brad Starr, I learned to tell stories. Our teachers taught us to interpret Madness in ways familiar from my studies of philosophy and religion. We read the myths and metaphors of Mental Illness as Moral Problems In Living to be resolved by dialogue in safe places without compulsory treatment."

THEN THERE WAS the other side of psychiatry. A female patient lay flat on her back, hands and feet strapped down, a band around her head, a gag in her mouth. People stood over her and a row of others watched from a few feet away. She was about to have shock treatment. Her frantic eyes searched the circle of strange faces. Not expecting so many onlookers, she was caught in a trap with no escape. With the gag in her mouth, she could not voice objection, nor could she get up and run. Her eyes flashed panic.

A reluctant participant, Kehn stood near the door. He was expected to learn this procedure.

After a preamble, with a crisp nurse by his side, the teaching doctor pressed a button. The patient's back arched. Her limbs stiffened. Suddenly she was motionless – unconscious.

Kehn was heard to say, "This is barbaric!" as he swiftly left the room. The heavy door closed behind him.

The teacher heard the remark. His head lurched upward angrily.

Kehn was feeling nauseous. He paused to lean against a hall wall. Minutes later he was joined by the others filing out of the room, followed by the teaching doctor, yelling, "Doctor Schramm! You're here to learn, not to criticize!"

Kehn responded, "I question the whole idea of shock treatment for anyone. We all know the treatment is a grab bag. It is not a scientific procedure with an assured outcome."

The teaching doctor shouted even louder, "You question my judgment?"

Kehn stood straight to face the doctor directly. "When I took my Hippocratic Oath to do no harm, I meant it. I think shock treatment can be harmful."

The doctor moved closer and shouted into Kehn's face, "That is a matter of opinion!"

Kehn noticed that no other person showed support. They all looked frozen as though afraid to breath.

The doctor continued shouting, "I judge this woman needed..."

Kehn turned on his heels and walked away while the doctor was in mid-sentence. Only his soft footsteps could be heard in the sudden silence as the doctor's unfinished sentence hung in the air. Kehn went out the door at the end of the hallway.

[ks notebook] "When New York State Department of Mental Hygiene objected to Tom Szasz teaching his book, The Myth of Mental Illness, in their hospital, I took a stand in support of our civil rights to academic freedom of speech, and my planned career as an academic psychiatrist unexpectedly was ended. All of us who

did not have academic tenure, as Tom Szasz did, were in various ways encouraged to leave.

"Out of gratitude to the loving families who taught me medicine, I joined them in The Civil Rights and Peace Movements. With family and friends, I explored intentional communities: a Free School for Black families in a community organization working for racially integrated housing, the experimental community of Goddard College, Rudolph Steiner's Camphill Village for mentally handicapped adults, Bruderhof Hutterites singing at dinner and making wooden toys, and a Summerhill School...

"In the 60's, the low-income families who taught me the living practice of medicine were struggling to gain access to housing and schools for their children. They welcomed me, as a physician-psychotherapist in their struggles. As a result of my participation in Saul Alinsky style community development with the civil rights and peace movements, I taught at Goddard College in Plainfield, Vermont.

"While teaching Field Studies and caring for Goddard students on "bad drug trips", I volunteered to help an injured farmer do his chores. Later Cary and Sandy Smith helped me learn dairy farming and together we developed a Farm School for students who wanted a drug-free education...

"John Dewey's philosophy influenced me more than I knew through the schools I attended and eventually drew me to teach at Goddard College. His concepts made sense of the myths of mental illness with the help of Ernest Becker's conversations and writings...

"...Myth of war as caused by mentally ill people and cured by international psychiatry (Jerome Frank) and dispelled by Stanley Diamond, Morton Fried and Marvin Harris: The Anthropology of War and Armed Conflict. I helped with the Vietnam teach-in in Syracuse, N.Y."

ANNOUNCEMENT: February 1, 1966

To Goddard Faculty:

...Kehnroth Schramm, M.D., has been appointed to the faculty. Dr. Schramm's major professional interests are in community life and individual development, and social change. He is now Curriculum Coordinator in the Manpower Development and Training Administration at Madison School, Syracuse, New York, and a graduate student in anthropology at Syracuse University.

During the spring semester he will serve as advisor to students planning to do independent studies involving field (off-campus) work in the behavioral and social sciences. He will also try to locate new off-campus educational resources.

Dr. Schramm is married and has two children. He graduated from Dartmouth with an A.B. in 1954 and from the University of Vermont with an M.D. in 1958.

His professional experience and training have included: pediatric interne and assistant resident, State University of New York, Upstate Medical Center, Syracuse, N.Y.; physician, Cornell University Infirmary, Ithaca, N.Y.; psychiatric resident, Upstate Medical Centre, Syracuse, N.Y.; assistant instructor, Department of Psychiatry Upstate Medical Center, Syracuse, N.Y.; research associate, Syracuse University, Youth Development center, and Program of eastern African Studies.

WHILE ORGANIZING AND TEACHING classes, producing reading lists for students and staff, and doing outreach work with students, Kehn also wrote three major papers:

Paper: **Dreams and Psychedelic Analysis. May 1966**

> ...This essay summarizes work for my doctoral dissertation concerned with the personal and cultural questions of human rationality raised by psychotic individuals. The existence of people in every society, who would be called schizophrenic in ours, suggests that irrationality is a universal aspect of human nature. ...

* * *

Paper: **Reason and Racism: The Anthropology of the Irrational. December 1966**

Released at the 133ʳᵈ meeting of American Association for the Advancement of Science:

...The irony of American anthropology is that our treatment of the American Indian has been suggested as a model for the future of anthropology at a time when the United States is most clearly a racist society. While the American Indian barely survived cultural genocide, he is the historian used to preserve his culture for the benefit of posterity. Anthropologists can afford to be concerned about posterity, but people of color cannot afford their scientific objectivity, their rationality.

When the United States abandoned its policy of extermination...

* * *

Paper: **The College in the World: March 1967**

...The small liberal arts college is a model of American life. If we can understand the problem of the college in the world, we may be better able to meet our responsibilities as citizens of the world. Many Americans regard The College as separated from the world of adult responsibilities. ...

* * *

Goddard College Notes:

- Continuing Course offering by Kehn Schramm: Metaphors of Man and Madness – Anthropology of the Irrational and the Individual.
...Independent study (for Senior Study).

- Economics and Anthropology of Developing Countries,
 Mondays 9:30 – 11:30 a.m. A-L Study Room

Field Notes for the Students & Faculty of Goddard College from Kehn Schramm.
These notes begin as my attempt to show you what I am doing in off-campus field studies. ...

- Greatwood Campus Faculty News and Notes.
Kehn Schramm notes for the record, as he did verbally in faculty meeting, that he is available for consultation with staff in case anyone wishes to raise questions or discuss ideas with him about psychedelics and related matters.

- Goddard College – Adult Degree Program - August 1966
The following faculty members will be available as supervisors of culminating studies: ...Kehn Schramm, Psychology...

- Greatwood Campus News and Notes – October 1966
A Faculty Colloquium is in the offing, perhaps around the theme "Human Nature and Education", or a similar topic. Kehn Schramm is getting it up and can provide information. ...

* * *

DURING THE APPOINTMENT to Goddard College, Kehn experienced a prolific few months of teaching, writing, attending conferences and meetings. In off-campus field studies, he took students into the community to learn new skills of self-sufficiency by caring for the land, growing food, and caring for others by helping those in need.

Jersey Cows with their soft brown, trusting eyes, forever found a home in Kehn's heart. It was on these work-study outings while working the fields and barns, and milking cows that the fun of singing quartets with friends became a pass time, a continuation of Kehn's love of singing with friends while at Dartmouth College.

Meanwhile, outside forces were at work...

8

Conscientious Objector Hearing

KEHN HAD REGISTERED as a Conscientious Objector to the Vietnam War. Years later a call came to attend a Hearing. Before the Hearing, an official investigation of Kehn was done by interviews of family, neighbors, schools, co-workers, and employers. Everything about him, including religious beliefs, was in question. Kehn was surprised with a copy of government research into his whole life.

In preparation for the Hearing, the research interviews were written in **Resume of the Inquiry**, dated July 13, 1966.

* * *

Resume of the Inquiry
Re: Kehnroth Schramm
Conscientious Objector

(This copy to be forwarded by Hearing Officer to the Registrant with Notice of Hearing.)

The registrant was born November 21, 1932, White Plains, New York. The registrant's parents are Congregationalists.

An official at Dartmouth College, Hanover, New Hampshire, advised the registrant entered that school as a freshman in September of 1950, and received an A.B. degree on June 13, 1954. He stated the registrant majored in philosophy and ranked 192 out of 601 students, scholastically, and there is no record of any disciplinary action ever being taken against the registrant.

A representative of the University of Vermont, College of Medicine, Burlington, Vermont, advised the records reflect the registrant entered the medical school in September of 1954 and graduated in June of 1958, receiving a Doctor of Medicine degree. He advised that the registrant's record contains no derogatory information. A professor advised that he recalled the registrant as being a "very quiet individual" who was forthright and honest. He added that on the registrant's record his religion is listed as Congregational, but he had no knowledge of the registrant's convictions concerning religion.

An official at Upstate Medical Center, Syracuse, New York, advised that the registrant came there as an intern in the Department of Pediatrics in July of 1958, and served as an intern for one year and was carried into a second year as a resident instructor in pediatrics. He advised that the registrant left his work in pediatrics at this time to take graduate work pointing toward a Doctorate in Anthropology from Cornell University from 1960 to 1961, and that subsequently, the registrant returned to Upstate Medical Center to take up a residency in the Department of Psychiatry. He advised that during the course of the registrant's work in the Department of Psychiatry, he was followed closely by faculty members charged with his instruction and developed sufficient question about the possibility of certifying him for the completion of three years work which is a necessary requirement for certification by the American Board of Psychiatry and Neurology. He advised that as far as he knew, no question had ever been raised with respect to the registrant's initial honest, character or reputation in the community, that his difficulties appeared to arise from his being unable to adjust to the demand of the training program and interaction with other faculty.

The assistant dean for Graduate Education in Sciences Basic to Medicine, Upstate Medical center advised the registrant was a young man with a good mind, but he was never able to settle down to his studies. He stated that the registrant appeared to have ideas that he could not adequately express, and was always involved with outside activities such as civil rights programs. He stated that the registrant had strong feelings of ethics and idealism regarding the practice of medicine. He described the registrant as an individual who appeared to be wasting a good mind. He advised that the position that the registrant was taking with respect to military service is no surprise to him and is consistent with the concept that the registrant left at the school. He advised that the registrant's beliefs are strong, and they possibly have been expensive to him with respect to his earning power and the fulfilment of his professional potential. He advised that this should be considered as an expression of the strength of the registrant's beliefs. He advised the registrant professed a philosophy of individualism, which philosophy apparently is consistent with his present position with the Selective Service Board. A representative of the Department of Psychiatry advised that the registrant's professed philosophy with respect to military service appears to be consistent with the concept he had at school. He advised that the registrant was more concerned with carrying out his own beliefs and ideas than with conforming to the policies of the school.

A representative of Cornell University, Ithaca, New York reported that on March 3, 1961, the "Cornell Daily Sun" newspaper contained a printing of a petition to the 87th Congress to eliminate the House Committee on Un-American Activities and the registrant's name appeared in the list of petitioners.

An employee of the Office of Dean of Graduate Admissions, Syracuse University, Syracuse, New York advised that her files reflect that the registrant is presently registered in the program and is not attending classes inasmuch as he is working on his dissertation and has given a tentative date of January, 1968, for graduation. She advised that there is no derogatory information concerning the registrant, and he is an A student.

The Chaplin at the United Camps Christian Fellowship, Syracuse University advised that he knew the registrant well for approximately one and one-half years while he was there.

The assistant director, East African Studies Program, Syracuse University advised that the registrant was connected with that program from July to December, 1965, and terminated his employment there because the program could not meet some of the demands that the registrant set forth with respect to his views as to how the program should be set up. He advised that the registrant worked as an evaluator of the Refugee Training Program for African Refugee Students, and as such, evaluated both the students and the program. He advised that he considered the registrant to be a skilled and intelligent psychiatrist, and a determined and opinionated individual. He further advised that the registrant performed quite well while connected with the program and demonstrated very definite and precise ideas as to what he wanted and how the program should be conducted. He advised the registrant was a very liberal individual who was concerned with civil rights and poverty groups, and demonstrated a strong interest in helping underdeveloped people. He advised that the registrant impressed him as being very sincere in his efforts in this area, and also as an individual who could hold his position in the face of strong opposition. The registrant demonstrated this quality while connected with the East African Studies Program. He advised the registrant was a firm believer in the rights of the individual, and the position that he is currently taking with respect to military service is consistent with the attitude he demonstrated while he knew him. He advised that he knew nothing derogatory concerning the registrant's character or moral integrity.

A representative of Camp Norway, Ely, Vermont advised that she had known the registrant's family some years ago. He, the registrant, had been hired at the camp as an odd job man in the summer of 1949. He was a counselor in the summers of 1950 and 1951. She advised she had always had a high regard for the registrant and had found him to be a very conscientious employee. He was very thoughtful, intelligent, and had very high personal standards. The registrant had never discussed his feelings with regard to military service with her. Her experience with the registrant would lead her to believe that he is sincere in any claim he might be making at this time. She added that she has not seen the registrant in several years and has had no real contact with him in the last ten years.

An employee at the Northern Westchester Hospital, Mount Kisco, New York advised the records reflect the registrant was employed there from June 23, 1955, to September 15, 1955. A representative of the Nursing Department at the hospital advised that the records show that the registrant had been assigned as an orderly. She recalled him as a very sincere, conscientious type person. She could not make any comments concerning his beliefs or sincerity.

A laboratory director at the Mount Kisco Medical Group, Mount Kisco, New York advised the registrant worked under supervision during the summer of 1956. The registrant applied himself to his duties and gave every indication of being a very serious young man. He advised that he felt that he had had very little contact with the registrant and offered no comment on the sincerity of the registrant's beliefs.

A representative of Sage Hospital, Cornell University advised the registrant was employed part-time as a Resident Doctor for about six months in 1960-61. She advised that the registrant's employment was satisfactory. She added she remembered the registrant and was not surprised to learn that he has asked for conscientious objector consideration. She stated that his manner, behavior, and general demeanor were indicative of his position in this matter. She feels he is sincere, and she has no reason to question the good faith of the claim.

An official of the City of Syracuse School District, Syracuse, New York advised the registrant was appointed to a part-time position as Curriculum Coordinator, Adult Multi-Occupational Program, in May, 1965, and resigned in February, 1966, to accept a teaching position at Goddard College, Plainfield, Vermont. He advised that during this employment there arose a certain incident when the discussion in class turned from remedial education to a profession of his opposition to the war in Vietnam and his opposition to serving in this war. He advised that the discussion almost erupted into open violence. The registrant was active to some degree in local poverty and civil rights organizations.

A representative of Goddard College, Plainfield, Vermont advised that the records of the college show the registrant has been employed as a teacher at the college since March of 1966, to the present and that his duties consist of teaching Anthropology, Student Advisor, and serving on faculty committees. She advised that during the spring of 1966 the registrant helped faculty and students to find employment related to their studies in the Goddard College area and he also taught on the campus. She added that the registrant was a consultant for one week and an eight-week course for Head Start teachers. She described the registrant as a very likeable, friendly person who stands by his convictions even in the fact of adversity. She advised that the registrant no longer studies medicine and that she has heard him say that he wishes to devote himself to keeping people healthy through the teaching of Anthropology rather than by treating them after they are ill. She advised she heard the registrant speak informally concerning his convictions and concerning the fact that he is against war and the Selective Service. She further advised that last year the college lost its physician and she had hoped that the registrant would fill the vacancy. However, the registrant refused to do so because he did not agree with present day medical treatment. She stated the registrant's work is satisfactory and that he belongs to no campus organizations, and she believes the registrant is sincere in his desire to be classified as a conscientious objector. The dean advised that he has been acquainted with the registrant since he began employment at the college in March of 1966 and that he is very popular with many of the students at the college. He advised that the registrant believes that every individual has the right to develop his own ideas and that the registrant is teaching in Goddard College because the college allows him to put his philosophy and teaching to practice. He further advised that the registrant feels that present day medical and psychiatric treatments are far removed from his convictions. The registrant feels that society causes mental illness and that by teaching Anthropology and not practicing medicine can the registrant help society. He advised the registrant is a pacifist and does not believe in war or violence. He advised that the registrant's request to be classified as a conscientious objector fits his character and convictions. He further advised that he knows nothing derogatory concerning the registrant and that he has no doubt the registrant is sincere in his request to be classified as a conscientious objector.

A neighbor of Poundridge, New York advised that she had known the registrant's family for a number of years and moved about five years ago. She stated she has not seen the registrant since he went to college and never discussed his feelings in regard to military service during the period she had contact with him. She added the registrant gave the impression of being a very serious young man. He was a good student at school and was active in church affairs with his family and had strong moral views. She advised that the registrant had appeared to be a very sincere person and she considered him to be a person of great integrity and for this reason, although the registrant had never discussed his views as a conscientious objector with her, she would be inclined to consider that any such claim made by the registrant would have been made in good faith on his part.

Another neighbor of this area advised that the registrant was a very philosophical type person when he was young and inclined to discuss matters of a serious nature. She stated she was acquainted with the registrant during the period of time he was in high school and occasionally saw him while he was in college. She advised that she is not surprised to learn that he is claiming to be a conscientious objector as she felt that it was very much in character for him. She believed that he would be totally sincere in making such a claim.

A neighbor of Plainfield, Vermont advised that she has known the registrant for about a year and described him as a very agreeable and intelligent person. She stated the registrant volunteered to help out on her farm when her son had hurt himself. She advised that she does not know what his beliefs are, but she does know he is a conscientious objector. She advised that she has heard others say that the registrant is a conscientious objector and feels that he is doing more benefit by teaching at Goddard College. She stated that she has no reason to doubt the registrant's request to be classified as a conscientious objector and the sincerity of this request.

Another neighbor in this area advised that the registrant and his family resided there for over a year. She advised that she met the registrant and his wife and is aware that they have two young children. As she has learned from other people, she stated the registrant is a medical doctor and that his wife is employed as a nurse at Goddard College. She stated the registrant does not practice medicine although he is an MD and mentioned that she cannot understand why he does not practice medicine after spending years in medical school. She advised that they have been satisfactory neighbors and does not know if they attend church or what their religious affiliation might be.

Another neighbor advised that she would describe the registrant as "just a trifle odd." She stated that there was nothing specific in his behavior that makes her feel this way, but due to numerous small things such as his lack of association with neighbors, his frequent absences from the neighborhood and the fact that he has done no work on his yard and has allowed weeds to grow, she feels he is somewhat different from other people in the neighborhood. She advised that she had heard that the registrant is Jewish but added that she was aware of no information concerning his religious affiliation or beliefs.

The registrant's wife, a reference, advised that they have been married since 1961 and that the registrant is currently working on his dissertation for his Doctor of Philosophy degree in Anthropology from the University of Syracuse. She advised that her husband has been a pacifist ever since she has known him and that he has often spoken on the subject of Selective Service. She stated that the registrant does not believe in war and violence and that he feels that they are not the means of solving the world's problems and that he wants no part of military service. She advised that the registrant does not believe anyone should be forced to kill or take part in military service when it is against his will and added that the registrant does not believe in the draft. She advised that her husband had taken part in a teach-in at Syracuse University while attending there and that he participated in the Peace March on Washington two years ago. She added that she is sure the registrant is sincere in his desire to be classified as a conscientious objector and that the thought of his serving in the military would be completely against his convictions. She advised that the registrant felt he was more benefit to society by teaching Anthropology than by practicing medicine.

Another reference advised that as a professor at Upstate Medical Center he knew the registrant was a student of the school. He advised that he has not seen the registrant since he left the school and has little correspondence with him since that time and this correspondence has been in connection with the registrant's Selective Service involvement. He advised that he has written a letter to the Selective Service Board at the request of the registrant, setting forth his views with respect to the registrant's claims and sincerity as a conscientious objector. He advised that the registrant is sound with respect to character, integrity, morals and sincerity. He described the registrant as an individual in the strictest sense of the word, and for this reason he feels that the registrant is sincere in his claim as a conscientious objector. He stated that the registrant is a person with strong personal beliefs and convictions, and a staunch defender of individual liberties and freedom. He further advised that for these reasons the registrant would possibly be rebellious with respect to compulsion of any form. He stated that although he personally does not sympathize with the registrant's views with respect to military service, if the Selective Service System must have a conscientious objector classification, he feels that the registrant should qualify. He advised that it was his understanding that the registrant was active, to some degree, with local poverty and civil rights groups. He advised that he had never discussed military service or the Selective Service System with the registrant.

Another reference, who is a reverend and chaplain at the Christian Fellowship at Syracuse University advised that he has known the registrant well for approximately one and one-half years while the registrant was attending the university. He stated the registrant was a thoughtful individual who was well trained to help people to become whole individuals. He feels that the registrant is sincere in the expression of his views opposing war, and these views are consistent with the beliefs the registrant demonstrated while he was associated with him. He further stated that he had attended meetings where the registrant explained his position as a conscientious objector and also his opposition to the present war in Vietnam. He further advised that the registrant professed a strong feeling for individual freedoms and was a worthwhile and sincere person dedicated in his efforts to develop whole individuals through teaching. He stated that he has the highest regard for the registrant and considers him to be a sincere and worthwhile person.

Another reference a member of the faculty of Goddard College advised he has known the registrant for about two years. He advised that he has had many discussions with the registrant and served on panels with him and as a result is familiar with his ideas. He advised the registrant's convictions form a pattern which involves a repugnance for all forms of violence. He stated the registrant believes that people should carry on their processes of life in as non-coercive a fashion as possible. He further advised the registrant has a strong disinclination toward being a part of a mass organization and particularly any organization created or formed for the purposes of violence. He advised that membership as such would be morally and philosophically repugnant to him and he would be sincere and genuine in this. He advised the registrant's beliefs are not based in any one religious tradition, but on his consistent philosophical and moral approach to life, and in this, is most sincere. He advised he would describe the registrant as a "Libertarian", that is, one who believes that the only way for people to grow is by freedom from authority and any form of coercion. He advised the registrant not only lives out his moral and philosophical beliefs but is firmly committed to them. He stated that while he can sometimes question the registrant's approach, he is convinced the registrant is quite honest and sincere in every respect. He also regarded the registrant to be in good character.

Credit and criminal records are negative.

Prepared: July 13, 1966

* * *

KEN WROTE the following letter dated July 14, 1966

Local Board #12,

Peekskill, New York

Gentlemen:

This letter is to call to your attention to certain facts, relevant to my reclassification which emerged as I reviewed my Selective Service record on July 12, 1966. I will file this letter with you when I am interviewed on July 20, 1966, by Local Board #12 in Montpelier, Vermont. With respect to this interview, you have asked the Montpelier Board for advice regarding the status of my conscientious objection, but not my deferment as a teacher. This request for 11-A was made by me over the telephone directly to Mrs. Levine, and led to President Pitkin's letter requesting that I be deferred as a full-time teacher.

The letter from Mr. Getty Page, of the Vermont State Medical Society, indicating that he believed I was not essential to patient care in Vermont, seems to be the only additional information, relevant to my request for 11-A. It seems to me that the Montpelier board should advise you on both the request for 11-A and for I-0, in that order. These requests for deferment are related, as I have tried to explain in previous letters to you this year describing my employment situation. I am simultaneously employed in writing my dissertation in anthropology for Syracuse University, teaching students at Goddard College, and obeying the dictates of my conscience.

On January 18, 1952, when I completed your questionnaire regarding my draft classification, I indicated that I believed I ought to be classified I-0. I did not sign section XIV, requesting form 150, because I did not know anyone who was a C.O. at the time. Therefore, I erroneously thought my beliefs completely separate from those of religious pacifists. I am now fourteen years older, with a much clearer understanding of what I meant when I classified myself as I-0, "conscientious objector opposed to both combatant and noncombatant military duty and available for assignment to civilian work. I then wrote: "I believe that I will be of more value to my country as a doctor than as a soldier". This statement is <u>not</u> different from the way I described my teaching at Goddard, when you classified me I-A in February, 1966. 'Doctor' has always meant teacher to me, as it does in Latin. My present teaching position would not be possible without the philosophic, medical, pediatric, psychiatric, and anthropological education which I bring to my daily work with students and colleagues. I am licensed to practice medicine in New York and Vermont. Students working with me are contributing to the medical care of individuals through their efforts in: social science research, community development, pre-school teaching, dance therapy, psychodrama, and psychotherapy with emotionally disturbed children. Indirectly and directly my teaching is contributing to the health and knowledge of civilians.

It is my belief that if more teachers and students were permitted by Selective Service to engage in activities such as these, we would be able to create a genuinely democratic society here in the United States. Without such radical education, on the scale and with the skill necessary, we provide inadequate human services, by too few sensitive professionals, for too many persons, rich and poor. As I have said before: I am conscientiously opposed to the violence done individuals by compulsory childbearing, compulsory education, compulsory employment, compulsory military service, and compulsory professional services. Without the development of voluntary alternatives to these compulsions, we increase the likelihood of coercion and violence, while diminishing the possibilities for freedom and love in the world, here and now. This cycle of compulsion and violence leads us ever closer to the suicide of mankind. Unless individuals, like myself, oppose this compulsory genocide by individuals like myself, there will not be another generation of humans on this earth, nor, possibly, in this universe. This is the basis of my request for reclassification as a teacher, a conscientious objector, and a free man in an unfree world.

Kehnroth Schramm, M.D.

* * *

Hearing before Local Board #13, Montpelier, Vermont
Recorded from memory by Registrant #30-12-506, on July 20, 1966

The registrant appeared at Local Board #12 in Montpelier, Vermont at 7:00 p.m., Wednesday, July 20, 1966. The registrant's wife was denied entrance to the hearing as a witness, by the Clerk of the Board, who told her to remain seated in the hallway while the registrant entered the hearing room. The Clerk introduced three board members, who were seated at the table. The registrant asked where he should sit and was told by Judge McLeod he could take either of the two empty chairs.

The Clerk stated the purpose of the meeting so quietly and quickly the registrant was unable to hear it. Immediately, Judge McLeod asked: what are **you** doing teaching at <u>Goddard</u> College, when you are a <u>surgeon</u> from New York? Mr. Wheeler said quickly: Yes, why are you teaching at <u>Goddard</u>?

The registrant stated that before he answered any questions, he would like to get clear the purpose of the meeting. Then Mr. Lyle Ford entered and upon being introduced by the Clerk, shook hands with the registrant. Judge McLeod repeated his question. The registrant repeated his request for clarification about the purpose of the meeting, stating he believed it unusual for a Vermont board to be asked to advise on a registrant from New York, regarding the status of his conscientious objection. To advise regarding a teaching deferment, he believed to be more unusual. The Clerk repeated more slowly and loudly, that the purpose of the hearing was to advise the registrant's local board regarding his conscientious objection.

Mr. Lamorey asked registrant whether registrant was associated with a college newsletter called Apulse. He brandished a copy from his coat pocket and asked if registrant recognized this. A drawing of a male reproductive organ was on the part of the newsletter toward the

registrant. Judge McLeod said he didn't believe a Dartmouth graduate and graduate of University of Vermont Medical School would be associated with such a thing. Registrant stated he was not associated with the newsletter, as Mr. Lamorey checked the names listed in the newsletter. He asked did registrant know Frank Adams. Registrant said yes. In this context the registrant was unable to discuss beliefs he had published in Apulse, which are relevant to his conscientious objection.

Mr. Wheeler wondered why a physician would teach at Goddard. Registrant attempted to explain that he was teaching students working in the Vermont State Hospital, Head Start Programs and with emotionally disturbed children. Thus he was using his previous experience in Vermont and his professional training. He had first sought to find a teaching position last fall while at Syracuse where he was studying anthropology. Goddard offered him in January an opportunity unique in this country, to relieve the shortage of professional services by teaching students working in local communities, agencies, and hospitals. Registrant reminded Mr. Wheeler that he had only been working at Goddard since March 1st. Registrant's work with Head Start, Adult Degree Program, Winooski Valley Family Consultation Service, and the Vermont State Hospital had just barely begun, when the Selective Service System requested this meeting. Registrant had tried to convey this to his local board when he was classified I-A in February. He told Judge McLeod and the board that it was impossible to explain his work as a teacher in numbers (of classes or students or hours of teaching), because he worked with individuals, as individuals, and not with classes. He met with, wrote to, or talked with students by phone whenever necessary. Many students are now away from campus and some adults are just beginning their studies this week.

During this period of direct questioning by Judge McLeod, working with pre-arranged questions to which he wrote answers on the paper before him, there seemed to be disagreements among the board members regarding the interpretation of the registrant's status.

Mr. Ford said: You are employed full time as a teacher. You deserve an occupational deferment, why do you need an I-o? The registrant said he was a full-time teacher and a conscientious objector. The Clerk of the Board quietly reminded Mr. Ford, who was sitting next to her, that the board was to advise only about the registrant's conscientious objection, not about occupational deferment. Mr. Lamorey, Mr. Wheeler, and Judge McLeod indicated they felt registrant ought to be caring for the troops in Vietnam with malaria. Registrant replied he was not an expert in malaria; he was expert in human development. Then at 7:30, Judge McLeod stated: "We believe you ought to be in Vietnam right now, but that is your local board's decision to make, and we will write them a letter to let them know you've had a hearing. Unless you have anything further to say the meeting is ended." Registrant said he believed it was the job of some people to go to war, and others to prevent war, and he believed he belonged in the second category. Although, there was a great deal left to say, the registrant could find no way to discuss this with the board. Therefore, he asked to have their names and thanked them for listening.

Mr. Carroll Coburn, a Local Board #12 member and former trustee of Goddard College, was absent during the entire meeting. No explanation for his absence was provided the registrant, who had been given the names of board members by the Clerk during the previous week.

The attached letter from the Radical Education Project is included here, because the registrant was unable to discuss the relevant question of his alternative service as a conscientious objector, with Local Board #12 of Montpelier, Vermont, to whom this letter was addressed.

9

Canada

[*ks notebook*] "In 1967 when the Doctor Draft threatened to send me to Vietnam after I had applied to be classified a conscientious objector, friends in the Montreal peace movement suggested I apply to fill a sudden vacancy to teach cultural anthropology and a culture of poverty seminar at McGill University."

IT WAS TIME for another heart to heart talk with mother. She was on her hands and knees transplanting flowers in the garden. Kehn paused to watch for a few minutes, wanting an indelible memory of her to be printed on him. Her short curly blond hair had strands of white glistening silver in the sunlight. He approached and kneeled beside her.

"Oh, Kehn, I didn't hear you come. What a nice surprise!" Her voice skipped along happily. "What brings you here in the middle of the day?"

After some light conversation, Kehn mentioned his problems. "Mom, they don't want to accept me as a Conscientious Objector. They insist I'll have to go to war in Vietnam."

There was silence. Then she asked, "What's the alternative?"

"I'll take my family to Canada and continue my objection from there. I have been hired to teach anthropology at McGill University in Montreal."

"Oh!" she sighed and paused... then brightened, "Well, that's not so far away. Just a couple of hours and you can visit often on weekends."

"I can't come back to this country. You will have to visit me. I will be arrested if I come back."

Her eyes darkened, "Oh, God! What has happened to this country? My son arrested after all our family history here? ...Because he wants peace? ...Because he does not believe in violence? ...Because he..." Her voice trailed off as she transplanted another flower with vigor.

"Mom, we will be leaving in the next few days."

She kept her head down to avoid showing watery eyes. A tear dropped into the earth.

Kehn laid a hand on her shoulder. "Mom, I'm sorry. I will have to go away one way or another. It's either war or peace. I choose peace. I cannot support this war. If the situation changes, of course we will visit. Hopefully we will come back here to live one day sooner than later."

"What about medicine? Will you continue?"

"I don't know. To be a practicing physician in Canada, I'll have to qualify all over again. I will be teaching anthropology for the next while. There were problems in Psychiatry. I cannot go along with certain procedures that I consider barbaric... like shock treatment and some of the drugs they are now using and experimenting with on unsuspecting people. They also wanted to keep us from studying certain texts authored by good teachers. I believe we should have the right to study and discuss, and then make decisions based on knowledge, and not to be kept in the dark. There are people who want control of our thinking by blacking out knowledge and curtailing discussion of ideas. There is tyranny in medicine by some old guard. As doctors, I believe our human rights are being violated where knowledge is concerned and that will have a dangerous impact on society. It does now. I want to continue teaching and encouraging people to *think* so that we can build a better world."

"Good. You are an idealist. You always were," she said.

"Probably. I am concerned about ethics... ethics about how to treat human beings, not just patients. Having good ethics does not start or stop in the hospital." Kehn stood up to pace. "I made a scene about a woman having shock treatment. It did not go over well."

His mother looked up at him and stood to have a face-to-face talk. "Did that woman choose to have shock treatment? Maybe that is where you need to compromise."

"Compromise on what! ...The Hippocratic Oath? Harm people because I am told to do so? Shock treatment is inhumane. If she chose to have that sort of treatment, someone advised her. That is where the responsibility lays. I took an oath that I will not harm anyone. I did not take that oath on the promise that I will pick and choose the person I harm or take chances with. Shock treatment is unpredictable."

"You were just watching, weren't you?"

"I was there so I was equally responsible."

"Remember when you tried to convince your Uncle Ted that he was not responsible for the bombing of Japanese people. The same goes for you now."

Kehn listened carefully to his mother.

"You always were a determined boy when you put your mind to something. I'm pleased you are still that way. I am proud of you but you can probably expect a life of trouble when you won't compromise on your principles. The world is made up of many unprincipled people in all walks of life and you will be running into more of them."

"I've decided to work outside of hospitals for a while. Maybe I can make a difference by continuing to teach. I've been preparing a Dissertation for my PhD in Anthropology but I'm going to have to leave it behind for now."

"You have been working very long hours in hospitals for at least eight years and have diplomas in pediatrics and in psychiatry. Actually, it's longer if you count your job as an orderly and working in the science lab. You may need a temporary change. Hopefully it's just temporary." She paused, furling her brow with memory. "I remember when you were only nine years old, you stood up to me and told me that you will take on those doctors who do harm to people."

"I remember. I have and I will. I've been fortunate in my choice of schools. I've had some great teachers. My troubles seemed to have started in the specialties I chose."

Mother kneeled to continue planting. "Kehn, teaching runs in this family, too. Besides being a physician, your great grandfather was also a great teacher."

"Yes, I know." Kehn knelt and handed his mother plants from the cardboard box. "Most of the doctors I've met have been good people but there are bad apples among the good. There are those who just don't think but do things because it is a technique they learned. They don't think! They took the Hippocratic Oath but don't know the difference between doing harm and not doing harm... or they forget, somehow thinking the Oath is theirs by osmosis and they don't have to do anything to live up to it. Then there is the 'old guard', as we call the ones who are guarding allopathic medicine with all its idiosyncrasies as though they own it. They refuse to look at alternative or other culture medicine, or other ways of thinking as though they also own thinking or non-thinking. In medical school, we joked about taping a message on our foreheads saying that this one certain surgeon was not allowed near us even in an emergency or imminent death."

Mother laughed and sighed at once, letting out pent up emotions.

Kehn went on, "Then there is administration staff telling physicians what they can or cannot study; they want to tell us how to think and do our work. But they have not taken the Hippocratic Oath and don't have the need to live by it. They wield tremendous power because they control money."

"I see your point. Where is Carolyn? Gone on another visit with her family?"

"I guess she needs the break... I suspect she may be seeing someone else."

Mother looked surprised. "Oh? What makes you think that? Who?"

"I don't know for sure. Old boyfriend, I suspect. Regardless, for the sake of the children, I don't intend to do anything to disrupt my marriage. I'm just grateful for her support through the problems. She is willing to move to Canada with me."

"Well, marriage is for a lifetime. Adultery is not worth a divorce. You do have two babies now. She'll get over it and when you are my age, it will be behind you. Your wife is your wife no matter what she does. Do you suppose your wife is lonely because you have been working so hard?"

"That's who I am. She married a doctor. She was a student nurse. She knew what to expect. She knew doctors spend most of their time working. I intend to be home more in my new job."

Dropping her tools in the plant box, Mother suggested, "I think we're finished planting for today, let's have lunch."

"I'll remember this conversation with you by my green knees. ...I helped to organize the Peace movement."

"Oh! Well, you be careful. Some of the demonstrations have turned ugly."

"I intend to spend my life teaching people that peace is a better way to go. In Canada we can get on with our lives as a family and I can continue to do my work for peace. I hope my sons will grow up knowing they do not have to be inducted into war but will have a chance to make their own choice. I need to talk with Dad."

WITH PROFOUND SADNESS, Kehn left the United States where he had deep family roots in shaping the United States of America. His sons slept in the back seat of the car and his wife was beside him. Passing through miles of his green New England, Kehn was deep in thought – Declaration of Independence... Constitution of the United States... United States Bill of Rights, Amendment 1, states that: 'Congress shall make no law respecting an establishment of religion, or prohibiting the free exercise thereof; or abridging the freedom of speech, or of the press; or the right of the people peaceably to assemble, and to petition the Government for a redress of grievances.'

Kehn thought about the discussion of People's Rights that resulted in a near brawl in his classroom. In a college classroom where discussion of ideas should happen, some students quickly became polarized and quarrelsome, wanting to start a classroom war over the question of duty to the country versus Vietnam War issues that others objected to. In a microcosm, it became clearly evident on that day that there are people who are ready and willing to have physical combat and wield anger without discussion, while others would like to have a discussion of the issues and try to avoid the war... and there are people in the middle willing to do both... or nothing.

THE DECISION TO LEAVE the United States of America had followed three milestone events where individuals in powerful places tried to force their will on a man who defended himself and was unwilling to compromise his morals for the benefit of a career. There had been the attempted sexual abuse by a physician who was determined to have his way by wielding a threat to block Kehn from becoming a registered pediatrician. This man caused Kehn to leave pediatrics rather than be submissive. There was Kehn standing alone in psychiatry to defend people being abused in the name of science; followed by an actual block because of Kehn's determination to read certain books. Then when Kehn found work that he loved at Goddard College there came the orders to serve in a war that he did not believe in, instead of following his calling to be a teacher and physician for citizens dealing with daily war on the home front.

[ks notebook] "...I am related through my mother's family to the Pilgrims who landed at Plymouth Rock in Massachusetts in 1620 and through them to Henry Wadsworth Longfellow and the Iroquois, to Charles Sumner, and to John Whipple who signed the Declaration of Independence. North America is my only home shared with aboriginals and other immigrants like myself who left the religious intolerance, political repression and economic deprivation of Scotland, Old World Eurasia, and Africa to build a New World. ..."

WELCOME TO CANADA. The big sign made it stunningly real. Wheels carried the family across the border, leaving behind family, friends, work, and all familiar things and places. They were leaving their beloved New England country and lifestyle. Kehn took a deep breath – Today is the start of a new life.

[ks notebook] "When my Draft Board Chairman, a Quaker, would not accept my application as a Conscientious Objector and threatened to send me to Vietnam, I moved my young family to Montreal in 1967 where I taught Cultural Anthropology at McGill University while we worked to build a Peace Co-operative.

"After teaching one year there, the Draft Board declared me "over age" and I was able to visit home again. I met Hans Huessy, only son of Rosenstock-Huessy and Chairman of the University of Vermont Department of Psychiatry. I decided not to accept a position as Chief Resident Physician with him because my predecessor had just had a heart attack and I feared I would, too.

"I accepted a tenured position as Associate Professor of Social Studies at Regina Campus in the newly formed Human Ecology Program with an architect, a psychologist, and a philosopher. I taught courses in anthropology and human ecology, developed an integrated undergraduate and graduate curriculum and worked for two years to develop a human ecology field station at Matador Co-op Farm at Kyle, Saskatchewan, north of Swift Current to supplement an ecological field station on one section of virgin prairie. I moved my still young family there.

"I invited my Vermont farmer friends to see and maybe join the Farm. Sandy said she never saw so much nowhere in her life! At that time a share in the Farm cost $100,000 and my friends decided to stay on their family farm in Vermont."

10

Crossing Paths 1969 to 1976

IN JULY OF 1969, Ken was teaching at the Regina Campus in Saskatchewan, Canada. He was now known as Ken; the letter 'h' in his name had been misplaced. As much as he loved the prairies, he felt misplaced in a new country.

That summer, Ken crossed paths with Daisy, the girl from the prairies who was now living on the West Coast. They came from opposite coasts of North America to meet at the centre of the continent in the sun drenched green and golden flat, windy prairie land of the northern country.

Daisy was a five-foot-three, slender, thirty-one year old with long brown hair and green eyes rimmed with long lashes that were blond. After being called "bedroom eyes" by a young man when she was fourteen, she has worn black mascara ever since to change the look. In public, she was usually mistaken for a teenager, but in actuality was a single parent of five children aged one to eleven. Often the idea of getting older seemed appealing to her because of the assumed wisdom and more respect from the public. She had run away from her first husband in Regina to Toronto with her three children. The father of her youngest two children, the photographer, had run off with another woman nearly two years earlier. To escape his emotional games while six and a half months pregnant with her fifth child, Daisy had packed up clothing, books, children's toys and some bedding, leaving furniture behind, and boarded her children onto a train, heading west, from Toronto to Vancouver.

Going through Regina in the middle of the night, the train sat in the station for the longest hour while she prayed her children would not wake up because if they did, she knew they would want to see their grandparents. It was an awful feeling to be sitting in a railway car and not see her parents but though she was ashamed of another failure, she was most afraid of getting stuck in Regina and in the past if they got off the train. The destination was to make a new start and give her children nature – beaches and forests on a nil budget and no car to transport a family around.

Her large extended family was living in Regina and surrounding farms. Daisy's reason for being back there in the summer of 1969 was that she had accepted an invitation to accompany Saul, a new boyfriend, to Montreal where his family lived and then to go on to Vermont where he had left his red canvas canoe. Saul held an Anthropology PhD from McGill University and briefly taught at the Regina campus. His planned trip around the world came to a sudden halt when he stopped in Vancouver and was introduced to Daisy by common friends that had also come from Regina.

Daisy's children had been dropped off with her parents in Regina while she made the longer trip east.

One short afternoon in the green of Vermont gave a lasting peaceful impression. Daisy had not met Ken yet but the trip home followed Ken's travel route from Vermont to Montreal and then to Regina, where Daisy and Ken's paths would cross. And then Ken would make his way to the West Coast, following Daisy's route. Like a game of tag with providence at play, they followed each other's pathways, touching and retouching until one day their lives would change forever.

MEANWHILE, ARRIVING in Montreal, Saul's parents accepted Daisy into their home grudgingly. They were upset on three or more counts – the first one being that she was taking their youngest and prized son away, all the way to Vancouver. The second grudge being that they were convinced their PhD son should do much better than take up with a mother of five children. They were convinced Daisy must be after their money, or his money that in reality he did not have since he was unemployed after losing his job in Regina. Then the third grudge was a most important factor. Daisy was not Jewish. Not only that but somehow they knew that she had roots in a family that emigrated from Germany in the early 1900s. This caused Saul's parents a lot of raw emotion because their families had been victims of World War II. It did not matter to them that Daisy's family bloodlines were mixed with other European ancestry.

Saul's father paced the floor relentlessly, falling into tears of anguish while verbally reminiscing about next of kin, especially his sister, lost to the Nazi death camps. Saul's mother had grown up in France and was extremely attentive to her husband and son while giving Daisy the silent treatment coupled with icy bourgeois arrogance. Eating breakfast with Saul and his mother was so silent and awkward that the sound of every bite of her bagel and every swallow of her throat was echoed through the kitchen.

Daisy was in the awkward position of knowing her presence was causing pain. She was sympathetic to nice people and felt their pain. At the same time she was aware of being closely watched to make sure she was not packing up the family silver.

Then it happened! It was time to leave. Saul's mother had gone out somewhere, having said her goodbye to Saul privately. As Saul and his father were outside packing luggage into the car and there was no one in the house, Daisy dared to fulfill a yearning to play their piano for five minutes because she had not been close enough to a piano to play one for years. She played a few simple tunes and marveled that it came back so easily. Then she left the house.

On her arrival outside, Saul's father went into the house and came right out in a hurry, waving his arms in excitement. "The lamp from the piano is missing!"

She was stunned. She stayed outside as Saul went into the house with his father.

Saul came out a few minutes later. Looking straight ahead and not speaking, he started the car.

"What happened?"

"I found the lamp behind the piano," he answered. "The housekeeper must have dropped it there."

The experience brought back childhood memories of swastikas drawn on the street sidewalk at the front gate of Daisy's home by someone in the night. Her father stood comfortingly beside her in the Regina sunshine, explaining that the war was not her fault. Then he erased the swastikas.

SHE HAD NO BATHING SUIT. In a moment of abandonment, she threw off her shirt in the wilderness and paddled the red canvas canoe in her pink lace bra, experiencing a new daring and wonderful freedom on Lake Superior. Times were changing.

Back in Saskatchewan while visiting farming relatives, Daisy discovered times were also changing. That summer she was surprised that many Saskatchewan farms were finally getting electricity from a main grid that changed prairie life forever. Telephones were no longer party lines in big wooden boxes on the wall. Most farmhouse windows were no longer dotting the prairies at night by the light of dim coal-oil lanterns. Nor were the lanterns swinging their way to outhouses. Instead, bright electric yard lights dotted the landscape. The outhouse was mostly no longer in use, giving way to newly built indoor bathrooms.

In fact, many houses within the city of Regina were new to indoor plumbing. It had only been twelve years earlier when newly married that Daisy lived in a tiny house in Regina with no indoor plumbing. The horse drawn 'honey wagons' that emptied outdoor toilet buckets were gone. Refrigerators replaced wagons delivering ice to houses that could afford the ice, and kids could no longer hang onto the rear of the wagons to eat ice that often had straw in it. The horses pulling wagons to deliver milk were gone. Daisy and her toddler would pet the horses in the mornings on her way to the babysitter and her work only ten years ago.

Society in general was going through a major change at the end of the '60s in many pockets of Canada.

Only two years prior, as a founding member of a meditation centre by Kinmount, Ontario, Daisy and her children had lived in a log house with no running water, only a single light bulb for electricity and a woodstove for cooking and another for heat.

The family emerged from the countryside of Ontario to find the hippy movement had taken hold with zest. Women wore either short skirts or long colourful cotton skirts and bared their breasts by throwing away bras. They began the fight to breastfeed babies in public. The women's movement was taking hold with a few determined women at the helm. Young women threw away bobby pins. Hair grew long and free on both men and women.

Men threw off ties, unbuttoned their shirts to bare a chest showing off an array of beads. Eyeglasses were often rose or mauve coloured. Beaded headbands emerged along with ponytails and earrings worn by men.

Music was driving society, causing changes from attitudes to hairstyles. Musicians dared to call for change by expressing opinions about war, mind-altering substances and the material society. Music festivals sprung up in large fields, attracting thousands of freedom seekers and music lovers alike. The young were crying out for peace, love, and no more war.

Vehicles had changed from the comfort of a sedan to the small housekeeping and sleeping units of the van decorated on the outside with brightly painted flowers and peace signs. They moved across the country with children in their teens and twenties running away from parents' suburban lifestyles and purse strings that somehow represented establishment, to a life believed to be superior with freedom. The young explored Eastern concepts of religion.

Black and white television had only come to prairie homes a mere ten to fifteen years earlier and colour television was in its infancy. Computers at home were not even a dream. In business, computers were monstrosities of limited use and had not yet taken over as society controllers. In the early '60's, only a few short years ago, Daisy had been a government employee and had witnessed the first computers, the size of an outhouse, roll past her desk for installation.

Except for agents of the United States government prowling Canada looking for boys and young men who had crossed the border in a bid for freedom from conscription into the Vietnam War that they did not believe in, freedom from daily government control in Canada was a reality, in keeping with the freedom of braless breasts.

Daisy and a friend had walked into a Kitsilano office that was advertised as a place to meet and talk. Soon after taking a seat, the friendly office worker walked across the floor. He was a tall man wearing ordinary shoes but Daisy saw his high boots. She saw his legs clearly in Royal Canadian Mounted Police boots. She knew he was an undercover policeman trying to get information on drugs in the area. She and her friend had no business there and left.

BACK IN REGINA, it was time for a few days of visiting with old friends from the university crowd and the artist community before heading back to the west coast. Daisy and Saul were invited to supper, without children, at the home of his former colleague Professor Bill and his wife, Marianne. Bill was a short, blond, opinionated, gabby, fun kind of guy. Marianne was a dancer with free flowing hair that matched her free flowing clothing; she reminded Daisy of the dancer, Isadora Duncan. They were a likeable, middle-aged couple that had left the United States for life in Regina. They had two young sons not present for this childless supper.

Excluding children was not Daisy's way and she was critical in thinking – she would have invited Bill and Marianne's children to her home. But as the four sat around a small kitchen nook eating spaghetti with a red sauce and sipping on red wine, she realized her five children would not fit around the nook built for only four people. Making light talk, she said, "It's nice being home, visiting my family and our friends."

Bill answered, "Your sister's boys and our boys chum together and are in the same classes at school. It's a small world."

"Regina is small for me," Marianne stated. "I gave up my dancing career in the States when the campus here offered Bill a job. Coffee? Anyone?"

The telephone rang. Bill jumped up and galloped to the hallway. He could be heard extending an invitation. "Oh, sure. Come on over."

Bill came back, announcing, "Ken Schramm is coming over with his wife and kids. They're coming back from a trip... to the States, I think. They're stopping here for a visit before going back to the farm."

Daisy's senses had perked at the sound of the name 'Ken Schramm'. "Who is Ken Schramm?" she asked, wondering why the sound of a name should resonate in her body.

"He was hired to replace you, Saul," Bill answered. "We gave Ken tenure to lure him from McGill to teach here. He's a strong-minded individual. He has his students involved in a co-op farm, building on what he was doing in Vermont. His wife is giving him problems. The university is probably not going to continue funding the farm project he is working on, even though it's a good one. Let's go to the living room."

Before they managed to get up from their chairs, Bill had run ahead to play the piano with booming gusto. They followed the sound.

The sound of the black grand piano filled all spaces of the combination dining room and living room furnished with only four hard, straight-back, armless wooden chairs standing at attention in a line on a shiny, golden coloured hardwood floor. The space was stunning sparseness.

From their wooden chairs, they listened to Bill zestfully pound out well-known classical music with no need for music sheets. Barefooted under a long flowing skirt, Marianne began to dance, gracefully exhibiting a well-trained body, and yes, she danced like Isadora.

The impromptu show was in contrast to Daisy's inward thoughts – the hardness of the chair was a reminder of when she was punished as a child and made to sit on a hard wooden chair on a wooden floor to think about her misdemeanor (of which there were many), but she understood now why there was no furniture except for the grand piano and bench, and why there was only seating for four around a kitchen nook.

The ring of the doorbell caused Daisy's heart to leap. Bill abruptly stopped playing. Still full of energy, he leapt across the room to open the door.

People filed through the open door in a row – Carolyn and her voice first, beautiful blond boys aged about four and five, and Ken at the rear. Daisy noted that he was wearing a sport coat over a clean white shirt open at the neck and looking every bit the university professor. Immediately and unexpectedly Daisy was somehow caring deeply for him. She could sense a quiet, tired sadness about him as he trailed his family into the house.

Without a backward glance, Carolyn rushed to a chair in the living room, leaving Ken to look after the boys who wanted to explore. There was no place for them to sit anyway. Clearly in protection mode, Ken wandered around with the boys.

The conversation with Carolyn and the others took off like a racing car, loudly bouncing off the bare walls.

Reluctantly, Daisy sat down again. From her chair, Daisy watched Ken for a few minutes. Knowing she was in the wrong place, she left her chair and the babble of loud mouths.

Entranced, Daisy was drawn to Ken like a magnet. There was something familiar about him, as though she had known him forever. She wanted to talk with him and got closer. Shy and not wanting to intrude on him, she kept a respectable distance but hoped he would acknowledge her.

Ken concentrated on his boys to keep them out of trouble. He was aware of her but was in no mood for what might be a flirtation. In the background, Carolyn's voice was a pitch louder than anyone else and he was tired.

What really bothered Daisy was that the hosts did not offer a cup of tea or even a drink of water to these guests even though this family had been traveling and still had many miles to go that night. It was unfamiliar behavior to prairie-born people like Daisy.

ABOUT AN HOUR LATER, out on the road in the dusk of the evening, the group assembled to say goodbye to Ken and his family. As Carolyn headed for the car, she passed within inches of Daisy's face without acknowledging her. For some unknown reason, at that moment, every detail about Carolyn became imprinted on Daisy's memory – the sound of her voice, her walk, the way she dressed and combed her hair. Daisy had no idea why she felt such an entanglement, maybe even a hint of jealousy. She noted that Carolyn dressed in a plain grey, calf-length skirt with a grey cardigan over a white blouse and plain low-heeled shoes. Carolyn's light brownish, almost blond hair was rather plain in its near shoulder length and she wore no make-up, giving her a matronly look. But the overall impression was of a self-assured, socially outgoing person needing no special primping – a woman who had just stepped out of a schoolroom rather than traveling.

Impressed and a little envious, Daisy thought Carolyn must feel really secure with her husband and children. She became aware of her differences to this woman as she stood on the street in her blue jeans and embroidered denim shirt, and long hair. She felt especially young, or perhaps it was merely that she lacked the self-confident worldliness that this other woman exuded; but more than that, she recognized her own comparative quietness.

After putting his children in the car, Ken walked quietly to his car door. As he opened it, he turned around to look at everyone and then at last, at Daisy. His face was sad. The visit had not gone well for him.

Then the car started slowly. He looked through the rear view mirror one last look. Daisy felt extremely sad and confused while watching the car go down the road. Her world seemed to have shrunk to Ken leaving, her feeling of loss and sudden loneliness, and for a few minutes she was oblivious of her surroundings.

As the car disappeared around a corner, she became aware of feeling resentment toward these people she was still in the company of for letting Ken go on another leg of his journey without offering nourishment to this tired man.

Daisy hurt for Ken. The vivid memory of him was indelibly imprinted on her that evening.

LEAVING REGINA in the summer of 1969, on the way back to Vancouver, Daisy found herself in a campground in the Rocky Mountains. It was a warm evening, the same July evening that men were walking on the moon for the first time in history. Radios were loud in all the adjacent camping spots. People listened intently. Still in her jeans and embroidered shirt, and glad that everyone around the world was distracted by the moon that was not visible from under the canopy of evergreen trees in dense forest surrounded by mountains where Daisy sat, she found solitude. Sitting on a log, she listened for her children but not to what was happening on the moon. Instead, she wondered where Ken was walking this evening... where was he leaving his footprints?

THE FOLLOWING SPRING, Professor Bill came to Vancouver and chose to spend the whole of Easter day in Saul and Daisy's home. They had moved to a cedar and glass home with a lawn that banked Seymour River. The home was extremely comfortable but to Daisy it felt too ostentatious; she constantly thought about people around the world who had nothing. She felt guilty for suddenly having too much. But in this home she found herself cooking Easter dinner to include Bill from the Regina Campus. His presence brought up intense memories of Ken.

As she pulled the bronzed turkey out of the oven she needed to deal with lingering resentment toward Bill for not giving Ken at least a glass of water that summer evening. It was that Easter day that Daisy realized her continuing intense thoughts about Ken were coming from an unconscious knowledge of something... somewhere that she could not explain.

After dinner more ex-Regina people dropped by. Professor Bill had come with a mission. During the evening, the friend who had introduced Saul to Daisy was given the good news that, regardless of disagreements, she was being bestowed with a Masters Degree in Psychology after all.

But where was Ken? Daisy's memory of him was intensified now.

AFTER ARRIVING back at the farm that July of 1969, a farmer had invited Ken to walk with him to the edge of a field.

"You have to take your family out of here," he told Ken. "Men are complaining that your wife flirts when you are teaching in the city. Men don't want problems in their homes. There is unrest..." the farmer paused, kicking up a little dirt with his shoe before saying, "I'm sorry to tell you this."

Ken hurt. He had wanted to stay a long time. He gazed over the shield of prairie land with the big sky to the horizon. He would miss it. He nodded his head sadly toward his friend in the moment of realization that this part of his life was probably over. He wondered what to do next.

ON AN EVENING after that talk in the field, thinking that Professor Bill was his friend, Ken confided with him by telephone. "I have a problem. I'm having to decide what to do from here on."

Bill asked, "What's the trouble?"

"I got notice from the farmers that I have to move my family off the farm. My wife has taken off to visit her parents. I have good reason to believe she is not being faithful to me on her trip!"

"Where are the kids?" Bill asked.

"The children are here with me."

"Take the kids and run!" Bill shouted.

"And take the boys away from their mother?"

"Yes. You don't need that kind of trouble in your life, especially in your own home. That's the best advice I can give you."

[ks notebook] "When faculty support for my field studies ended, I took a research leave to study intentional communities in the Kootenay and Slocan valleys. I moved my family to a Quaker community in Argenta, B.C., where my wife and I separated in 1970 and later divorced."

ARGENTA, BRITISH COLUMBIA. Ken told his wife that if the other man would not leave, he would leave because "enough is enough".

Declining the invitation to live as a threesome with his wife and her lover, Ken took his young sons down to the bank of the nearby lake to talk. Explaining that he has to leave the boys with their mother prompted a parting gift of a swift kick in the groin causing an injury. The memory of that kick and the heartache of leaving his children would be with Ken for the rest of his life.

In pain, physically and emotionally, Ken limped up and down long, dirt, mountain roads with a backpack on his back for many days. Intermittent tears ran down his face. At night he slept under trees near the side of the road. He hitchhiked whenever possible and stopped into bars and cafes. His curly hair grew longer. His usually clean-shaven face sported a new beard.

Stopping at a phone booth with trucks and cars roaring by, he called his mother in New England. "Mom, I'm so homesick! I don't know where I'm going! I've been on the road for a couple of weeks wandering from town to town. I only know I'm headed toward the Pacific Ocean."

"Come home. We miss you. Come home!"

"I can't! I have to stay in Canada... in British Columbia for the kids. I have to be close to them. I can't abandon them here."

[ks notebook] "I continued my field studies of intentional communities in B.C. by hitchhiking and camping in the Slocan Valley. From a Fall article by Alan Edmons in Macleans Magazine, I learned about the healthiest group of people he had seen living in such communities. I went there to Sidera's Place on Lasqueti Island and later Calvert Island to study the health of these people and I became family physician to our Coast Range Ranch Co. I was able to help a family care for their mother who died of cancer at home with us. Soon after her death, I was asked to resolve a leadership conflict by committing a dissident to Riverview mental hospital. Finding I could no longer work there, I left Calvert Island on H.M.S. Thomas Crosby, United Church mission ship, with the woman who had helped me in my practice. I was determined to find a better way to support family home care.

"We married in 1972, and after brief visits with our families in Alberta and Vermont, we left to work at United Church Mission Hospital in Bella Bella. A few months later we learned our community (Sideras) could not remain on Crown land. They moved farther north and later to The South Seas. In May I passed my medical licensing examinations and worked at Riverview Outpatient Clinic to help form the new Community Mental Health Teams. ...In Spring 1973 we moved to Calgary where I completed my training in family psychiatry and psychotherapy. ...Returning from Calgary to Vancouver, ...I worked at Crease Clinic until I began consulting and making home visits with social workers of Children's Aid Society, becoming the Vancouver Resources Board. In private practice, I worked with the Unified Family Courts of Delta, Surrey and Richmond; Vancouver and North Vancouver Health Departments to help families care for their members as Dr. Chamberlain's Toronto Clinic were doing."

IT HAD BEEN SEVEN YEARS since Ken Schramm and Daisy met in Regina. Over the years she thought about him constantly, usually at dinnertime when she was quiet within herself, enjoying feeling grounded amid the smells of creating a meal for her family. She would wonder about Ken and then wonder why, after all these years, she still daydreamed about him almost daily.

On a sunny spring day, outside her townhouse in False Creek, Vancouver, Daisy watered flowers of many colours in planters that she had built with a saw and hammer on the patios. She looked up to see Ken walking by. He was following a woman with red hair. They were clearly a couple but not walking together. Ken noticed Daisy. He smiled a warm greeting. She smiled back. The meeting felt gentle. Again it would be memorized as a milestone.

Paths crossed again. They were living as neighbours, only a few feet between their houses. He needed to walk right past Daisy's home to get to his car. She watered her flowers daily. They quietly acknowledge each other. He mostly wore a three-piece suit and tie, she noted. He walked with a purpose whenever she saw him. And once again in the passing – the look – there was an invisible connection. She wanted to reach out and touch his soft curls that flowed neatly to his earlobes.

At this time, Daisy was having an extremely full life and had been living common-law with Saul since that summer of 1969. They were busy with family, friends and lots of music. But this man Ken entered and stayed in a most secret place – Daisy's mind.

As Daisy was watchful of Ken, she realized he did not appear to be losing sleep over her. Most of the time he seemed deep in thought. Daisy noticed that the woman he was with never smiled, nor did she acknowledge anyone in her path. Daisy had a feeling that all was not well with the couple.

Ken had become the mystery in Daisy's life. Why? Now he walked by her home daily. She lingered and reminisced over each passing, every acknowledgement, and every silent smile. She knew that he was different in her life than any man she had ever known. There was no secret crush, no lust, no sexual fantasy; it was somehow simpler and more real than that. There was no expectation of anything, only the awareness of innocent deep caring for this man.

Their parking spots were side by side. Meeting in the car garage, Ken got into his small white BMW car while Daisy watched from the large Dodge van. She watched as his left shoe, holding a beloved foot, disappeared into the car before the door closed. This was the event that surprised her with the realization of deep love for this man... a love with no agenda, just unconditional love. He drove off not knowing that she was caught up in the revelation of loving his foot... loving him.

When he drove away, she was angry with Saul for sometimes selfishly parking the van too far over so that Ken could not use his own parking spot. Often Ken had to use an inconvenient spot against a wall that was not a real parking spot. He simply moved over without complaining as though he had better things to do than to complain about a parking spot.

THEN HE WAS GONE AGAIN! Daisy's busy life went on while Ken continued to enter her reveries. She wondered where he was as she had done for years. She was drawn to him somewhere in time and space as she prepared the evening meals for her family.

11

Meeting Again in 1981

ON A WARM EVENING in August of 1980, Daisy dressed for a party at a cooperative farm in nearby Langley. She wore her own creation, a red dress. Saul wore the red shirt she had spent many hours sewing and embroidering a paisley pattern with flowers and birds across the chest. As she walked behind Saul toward the door, he suddenly stopped in the open doorway. Half in and half out, he turned to face her to exclaim that he had been having an affair with another woman for months.

Shocked, she asked, "Why are you telling me right this minute?" He did not answer. Then in a gut reaction she blurted, "Well then, why don't you leave and live with her!"

Immediately she was sorry to have blurted that because she had just given him permission to leave. He jumped on it instead of giving a response she was hoping for. Within seconds her life changed.

Daisy had not seen this coming. Not true! She remembered her own private prediction that he would stay twelve years and leave. It had been a journey of twelve years to this point. In an ironic thought, she worried about how another woman would care for the shirt he was wearing or would she just ruin it, and what about the buckskin suit she had sewn for him?

The next morning, two old friends, married psychologists from the Regina University, knocked at Daisy's door. In previous days, they had hung around having dinner together several times followed by walks on the beach. Daisy had cooked dinner for them just the night before the big news and then walked in the park at which time the wife had confided information about her own affairs, shattering Daisy's belief that the couple was wildly in love because they had divorced their spouses in order to be together.

Daisy refused to answer their knock because now she was suspicious that the couple knew of Saul's affair. Hating being an underdog, she slipped out the patio door to disappear into the park and wandered the beaches, ending up at Spanish Banks and avoiding contact with all people. At sundown she dismissed a lifeguard who became concerned about the woman spending all day lying in the sand beside the water. She was heartbroken and did not want to face anyone, including her children.

Now certain things were making sense. Saul's parents had been visiting recently and suddenly, without a word to Daisy to even say goodbye, they had packed their bags and disappeared to stay in a hotel. And there was the woman's scarf left on the passenger seat in the van. And one day, there was the broken bed in the back of the van.

Saul did not leave right away. He lingered another month with a looming threat that he would eventually leave. She did not know when. During that month, with Daisy's youngest children they attended her family's reunion in Alberta as usual, where they pretended nothing had changed. They attended an aboriginal wedding on the Blood reservation in Alberta.

After that, Saul took Daisy for a trip to Ladysmith on the island. It was like a honeymoon in a cosy cabin, all meals served, canoeing the ocean and bicycling the dirt road. Near the last day of the *honeymoon*, on one of the bicycle rides – actually riding like mad to keep up with him, she was tired of the suspense and called out, "Saul, why did you have an affair for many months behind my back?"

He called back over his shoulder, "I needed to cover my ass. Besides she owns a house."

She had expected an explanation but not what she got.

AFTER LOITERING a whole month, he suddenly got out of bed before dawn and left with a few clothes in a small bag.

Then he returned often to pick up one thing or another, always unannounced. Often he would sit down to dinner unexpectedly and uninvited, as though he still lived in the house.

From friends, Daisy was slowly learning that Saul had been attending their social functions with his new girlfriend instead of inviting Daisy for many months, or seeing her when Daisy thought he was working. Daisy had been the underdog all along and the so-called friends had watched without saying anything.

Having heard somewhere that statistics show men who leave their families usually try to return within three to six months, Daisy felt justified in having brief affairs with him during the months of separation while he was living with the other woman, in hopes that he would change his mind and come back.

Having gotten through autumn with a trip together to Winnipeg to visit Daisy's daughter at the Royal Winnipeg Ballet School and staying together in a hotel room, then attending a few Vancouver concerts as they had been in the habit of doing before the separation, winter settled in. Saul hung around again like a puppy-dog during the Christmas season.

With a new spring season beginning, Daisy answered the telephone at work in her usual business salutation. Saul wasted no time asking, "If I live separately, can I have you both?"

In one fell swoop it was over! Daisy finally blew her cork, yelling at the top of her lungs, "There can never be reconciliation under those or any circumstances! I will never be up for a shared man, and especially not for a sexually transmitted disease!"

Her answer carried through every paper-thin wall, vibrating through the whole, old wooden building. She was aware that the office next door went into complete silence.

The realization sunk in that she was truly finished with Saul and had been for some time.

After that communication, she felt anger, relief, exhilaration, desperation, strong, weak, up, down, all at the same time. She wanted to laugh and cry. She wished she could yell at Saul all over again and really get all of this out of her system. She was embarrassed at what others may have heard through the walls. The silence was deafening throughout the building. There was not a whisper, nor the sound of a typewriter, not even a footstep for a long time. She guessed they were hoping not to miss more.

She just wanted someone to talk with about her mixed feelings and knew she needed to talk with another adult. Her children were not an option. Her boss was a friend but he was away on a trip.

She sought immediate conversation with her doctor whose office happened to be right across the street from where she worked. He had been physician to her family for a couple of years, even though she questioned the quality of his care. Her doctor had little time but made a referral to a psychiatrist and gave her the slip of paper with a name on it. She shoved the paper into her pocket without looking at it.

Back at the office, she called the number on the paper to set up an appointment, making no connection to the name. Uppermost in her mind was remembering the arrangement Saul had just proposed. The gentle voice of the man on the other end of the telephone sounded soothing, resonating deep within her. She felt inwardly calm for the first time in many months and looked forward to meeting with him.

A day later, dressed in her usual bright colours: a gold coloured wool coat, that she had sewn and embroidered with an orange and white border, and her favorite flowered knee-length rust coloured skirt, and a silky form fitting yellow turtle-neck sweater, she found herself sitting in a common waiting area of a large building in the famous West End Robson Street corridor. With her back to the appointed office door, she surveyed the surroundings made of shiny grey and white marble that echoed every sound.

Daisy heard the sound of the door opening. Without turning around, she listened carefully to the sound of soft footsteps. A strange excitement grew inside her chest as she felt the person approaching. She was aware of something between the person and herself that was in the unseen realm of communication... something that transcended the five senses, reaching deep to her primal core. She turned around.

There he was! The familiar man, who had been in her life, her dreams and her reveries for twelve whole years, was approaching her! His face was strong yet soft. A kind soul was looking at her through blue eyes. He was smiling softly. His head was haloed in a golden glow from the sunlight pouring through the skylights onto golden-brown softly wavy hair, graying a little at the temples. He was dressed casually in a cotton shirt of soft pastel stripes open at his throat, beige cotton pants and soft-soled beige shoes. This man with a body she wanted to hug and relax into was now coming closer. She was aware of a magnetic pull toward him. She felt at once relaxed and excited. She was aware of a bond to this man across the eons, from a place in the realm of life that is at the same time familiar and unknown, unexplainable in language, larger than this moment in their lives, and deeper than these bodies, deeper than their souls. In this destined meeting, they transcended time and space. On the other hand, she had no real idea if she was in a one-sided fantasy. After all, he had never given her any reason to feel or dream such a connection.

"Daisy?" he smiled gently.

"Yes. Hello."

"Come in."

She followed him into the bright, spacious room with several armchairs and a daybed with bright cushions. A stack of large, plump, rose and gold coloured cushions was on the floor at the end of the room beside the largest most beautiful round woven grass basket Daisy had ever seen. The room felt serene.

"Please have a seat," he offered.

She moved toward the rocking chair.

"That's usually my chair," he said, "but if you prefer it..."

"Oh!" She quickly moved to another armchair, embarrassed that she wanted to sit in his space. It should have been obvious that the rocking chair would be his.

Ken casually sat in his rocker.

The only desk in the room was far away against the wall. This was the first office Daisy had ever entered where there were no barriers between people. Instead, the chairs were arranged in a circle with space in the middle to be filled with communication.

After some moments of just drinking in his presence and enjoying how he looked in his rocking chair, she exclaimed, "I didn't know you are a doctor!"

Giving a little nod, he answered, "Yes."

She continued, "We met when you were teaching at Regina University. Then we were neighbors in False Creek. Then I didn't see you for years. Somehow, I didn't put the name together with you when I was referred to you because I thought of you as a professor... in a university setting. I never expected to see *you* today. The referral said Kehnroth Schramm, M.D. and I only knew you as Ken Schramm. I...Oh, my God, it's you!"

He nodded again.

Silently, they looked at each other for a long moment.

Breaking the silence again, she flustered, "You're a psychiatrist! I didn't even know that you are a medical doctor!"

"I've been a physician all along, close to thirty years now. I like teaching. I taught for a few years."

"You took over my ex-husband's, I mean common-law... you took over his job in Regina."

"Yes. They hired me to take his place and gave me tenure to teach in Regina. Before that I taught anthropology at McGill in Montreal. Before McGill I taught in Vermont. I graduated medicine in Vermont and specialized in Pediatrics and Psychiatry in Syracuse, New York; then completed Psychiatry in Canada. I was senior resident physician in Psychiatry in Calgary at the Foot Hills Hospital."

"You must have had to re-write and do extra work to qualify in Canada!"

"Yes I did. Those are my credentials in very short form." He smiled gently and waited.

This was the first time they were together in stillness that allowed Daisy to just look at him, drinking him in, face to face... and where he was not otherwise preoccupied. They were alone... together.

She liked the way he held his hands with fingers of one hand gently supporting fingers of the other hand and thumbs just touching each other. She liked his hands.

Silence... stillness... fullness... just looking and relaxing... not talking.

In a calm tone that was in keeping with the quiet, he offered, "How can I help you?"

"Oh, yes." She had almost forgotten why she had come. Those tumultuous emotions over Saul had gone so far away that they no longer mattered. In fact, in the company of this man she felt happiness. She said, "Because we have met before, we know so many of the same people." She did not know why that mattered right now or why she would say it.

"Confidentiality is always kept. I will never break that promise."

That was comforting.

Her story started to escape her mouth. "After twelve years, Saul left me a few months ago for another woman. He had been having an affair for months. He traveled around the province in his work so I didn't know."

In the midst of the story, Daisy's attention was diverted to a large framed picture behind Ken on a distant wall – a poster of a young boy and girl walking hand in hand along a path through the forest into the light together. The picture suddenly took on another meaning. Transcending present time in the room, she saw this man Ken and herself as children of the universe in that picture, holding each other's hands in a connection beyond this life... into a previous deep connection and into the future.

He asked, "What about your children?"

The story she had come to tell was no longer important but his question brought back the reason for this appointment.

"As you know, I have five children now ranging in age from thirteen to twenty-three. Not all living at home anymore. The boys moved back home to help out until I found a job. Now they are in their own place again. They are all in shock. They're all musicians and dancers. The music has stopped in my home... except for my fourteen year old but she has been away studying with the Royal Winnipeg Ballet School. I used to play the piano and my daughters would sing. That has stopped. My youngest, who I thought was a budding opera singer no longer sings, in fact I caught her smoking with friends in the park. Saul took her out for an ice-cream cone and told her I would not let him see her any more, which was not true. I believe he did that in retaliation because I told him to stop showing up for dinner unannounced. He had been in the habit of just walking in and sitting down for dinner as though he had never left. The last time he did that I experienced the phenomenon of my hands disappearing because of the stress. He was acting like he lived there but after dinner he would leave again. I had to put a stop to his behavior."

"There is a medical name for your hands seeming to disappear temporarily under stress." Ken explained it carefully and then added, "I prefer to work with whole families rather than only one person in a family. I can come to your home and visit with the children."

"I'm not sure."

"To help only one person when others in the family are also affected can be counterproductive."

She had not counted on that. "I might be embarrassed... talking about myself in front of my children."

"We can work without embarrassing any one of you. People only share what they want to share in a family meeting. You can also see me on your own for privacy. Anyone who wants to talk privately can do so. Confidentiality is always respected."

The telephone rang. Ken walked across the room to answer. A female voice resonated with tension out of the telephone into the room. Ken was clearly concerned but calmly answered, "Yes, I'll pick up dinner... Okay. I'll be there as soon as I can be."

On coming back to his chair, Daisy asked, "That's your wife?"

He nodded. "Yes. I need to look after my son."

They sat in silence, looking at each other. Ken was in no hurry to break the silence, waiting until Daisy was ready. She realized there was a lesson here. This man had no need to fill each moment with noise. He was comfortable with silence – the minutes between conversation. Also, she was learning that he had patience. There was timelessness in his presence.

After a while of the world coming to a stop, she said, "I am just so surprised to see you."

Ken nodded with a quiet smile.

In the quiet timelessness as the sunlight that was coming through the window began to dim, true recognition entered. Ken, the man facing her was the boy she yearned for as a child... and then, he was the young man she went to college with in her imagination. She knows him! She knows his face! She knows the feel of him!

The knowledge was profound that they were two souls living apart on earth but know each other in another realm reaching deep where their souls are drawn together transcending the present era.

A quiet inner peace began to wash over Ken. He felt a peacefulness that had eluded him for many years.

FOLLOWING THE MEETING, Daisy felt a strong urge to visit a well-known psychic because her world had topsy-turvied again.

She chose to see a young man unknown to her but with a reputation of speaking uncanny proven truths. In his living room on the North Shore he told her that her Uncle John, her mother's brother was present with her son at his side. Since this man had not been told anything, the opening message was a complete surprise. How in the world did he know of her baby boy who was born too early but lived four hours before he died, and whose body was buried in Regina. She had kept his memory in her heart and had not spoken about him to anyone, not even her children since losing him sixteen years earlier. And, Uncle John was in fact her mother's brother who played with her until he went into the army and away to war. Telling Daisy many things about her life, the psychic told her that her mother was ill. In fact, her mother had been confiding in Daisy about her health concerns but Daisy had not told anyone.

The psychic claimed his messages were coming from her uncle John. He told Daisy that she should learn to drive a car. She wondered how on earth he knew that she never learned how to drive when it seemed every adult in the country could drive a car. He adamantly warned Daisy not to move from her townhouse but to stay put regardless of outside forces. He concluded the session with a statement from Uncle John who wanted Daisy to know that a half-married man was coming into her life and to be careful.

"Half-married?" she wondered out loud, "I wonder who that refers to... my ex or someone new?"

The psychic assured her the half-married man was not her ex anything.

She rushed home to type out pages of what she heard so as not to forget and to examine the information over and over, wondering about the half-married man mystery.

IT HAD SNOWED heavily and unexpectedly. Even though it melted later that day, her next appointment with Ken was cancelled, causing a surprisingly horrible feeling of immense loss. Then the day arrived to see Ken for another appointment. Anticipation and excitement gave way to determination after deep thought for a week.

That morning, having taken time off work, she visited a flower shop on 4th Avenue to pick out flowers from the outdoor display. She chose flowers from all the colours for a rainbow bouquet.

Entering Ken's office, she shoved the bouquet of flowers at him, along with a poem written the night before for him... about him, on subtly flowered stationery to match the bouquet. He fumbled with the bouquet and the poem, not knowing what to do. He took the easy way by laying them on the desk. She realized he had no vase, so they lay there, waiting – poem unread. She wondered if he would take the flowers home or if they might end up wilted in the garbage.

Taking chairs and looking long in silence at each other, she then explained. "I have come to say goodbye. This is a giant mistake."

Ken was clearly surprised.

Before he could respond, she continued, "I should have recognized your name and not been referred to you because I have been in love with you for twelve years since our meeting in Regina... and I can't do this. *You* can't do this! I mean... *we* can't do this!"

Ken was quiet.

She went quiet, letting her reality stay in the air. It felt good to get it out. Then she continued, "For some very strange reason, it is as though I needed to have amnesia about your name."

...Another silent pause...

"After we met in Regina, Saul and I traveled with the kids back to B.C. I remember being in a campground that evening in July of '69 while American astronauts landed on the moon. The campground was buzzing with radios... but I sat on a log as men walked on the moon and I thought only about you... wondering what you would be doing... wondering why I was so drawn to you. I have always wondered what the connection is because your face has been interrupting my thoughts for twelve whole years. That picture on the wall behind you... I see you and me."

Ken turned to look long at the picture. His face was solemn when he turned back to Daisy. In his soft voice, he questioned, "You have had a relationship during those twelve years with Saul."

"In some ways it was twelve years of a good relationship. We never fought. To the outside world, we were an ideal family. But always hanging over my head was the fact that he had not intended to stay with me. He was on his way around the world when I met him but he just never got around to leaving. He told my children not to call him 'Dad'. And me? I enjoyed much that we had together but I was also aware of a lonely spot... something unfulfilled ...With you, all the loneliness goes away... but," her voice softened to a whisper, "you are married."

"Yes, I am married."

"The red-haired woman you were with in False Creek?"

Ken nodded. "We have a two year old son."

"I have just seen a psychic who told me a lot of things that ring true. I mean, they are true and he had no way of knowing... and he says a half-married man is around me."

Ken listened with steady eyes but did not say anything. After more silence, Daisy rambled in an attempt to justify seeing a psychic, "I have had a lifetime of experiences outside the norm." She rambled on for a few minutes and finished with, "It's all very normal in my life."

"You are fortunate that you were referred to me because some other psychiatrists might like to cure you of what they would consider a condition."

"I know! And nobody should try to rid me of my visions or ways of knowing. They would be in for a fight! There is more to reality than most people are willing to know. I also know you understand... I just know. I don't tell my stories to just anybody. In fact, I don't tell most people, even friends... but I have also sat on their chairs after they left my home and unintentionally read the secret thoughts that they had while sitting on the chair, from the energy left behind temporarily. I learned as a child to be quiet about certain things. I like myself the way I am."

"You don't need to change. You are probably the healthiest person I know right now."

Standing up to leave, she said, "I have to leave now and never return."

Ken silently stood up in his sure-footedness and walked a half circle to stand nearer to the window, the opposite direction of the door. Now she was between him and the door.

Instead of moving toward the door, she moved toward him, clasping his hands in hers. Face to face, the closest they had ever been, they looked into each other's eyes. He was swimming in pools of green. He could smell her rose perfume. There was deep magnetism between them, evident in each other's eyes, running through their bodies, binding them together on the inside, but on the outside Ken made no move.

She could see that he was using great strength not to yield or buckle, exactly what she expected of him.

Painfully, determinately Daisy looked into his eyes and said quietly but clearly, "I do love you. That's why I have to leave. I won't bother you again."

"I'm sorry. I can't..." Ken's soft voice drifted off.

Tenderly she said, "Bye. Take care of yourself." With that she let go, turned and walked out of the office.

Ken stood motionless, looking at the door as it swung shut, hearing the sound of the lock clicking, footsteps across marble leaving and fading out... then silence...

WEEKS HAD GONE BY since Daisy last saw Ken. She stood on a small hill overlooking the ocean. A chilly wind came off the blue-green water with white frilly ripples on the waves that glistened in the sunshine. She wrapped her yellow trench coat a little tighter around her body. She mused that she is like a heroine in a book with the wind fresh on her face and gently blowing her long dark hair, remembering the love she now knows like none other she has ever known in the past. This heroine can never see her love again.

The heroine disappeared. This was reality!

She knew it was right to leave him alone. She hoped he is well and happy. It was easy to imagine him with his child... happy with his life. On a whim, she had bought a silver music box for his child even though the child would never receive it; she wondered now why she did that except that any child of his, she also loves. Better to have known Ken and loved him than never to have known such depths of true love. "I know... I know..." her words were caught up in the wind and blown to wherever, "I know there will never be another love like him."

ACROSS THE CITY, Ken was deep in thought... sadly... as he locked the door of his office at the day's end and headed for home. He was feeling the same chilly, fresh wind on his forlorn face as he walked down the street to catch a bus.

He was thinking of the pregnancy. He had brief happy thoughts about taking the private dance classes with his wife as prenatal exercise with two lovely older ladies who taught with an Eastern flair. In years of difficulties with this second wife, the pregnancy had provided a respite. He thought about not being welcome at the birth. But then the perfect, golden-haired boy that had an aura of a god on earth was born.

The birth had been quickly followed by the unexpected urgent advice by attending physicians that Ken must hire a nanny right away.

As Ken walked toward the bus stop, he thought about the two years filled with a baby crying and not sleeping, a nanny who filled in daily to care for his child and his wife when he was working, and him having to do his medical practice during the married nanny's available hours.

Ken was on his way home to where he felt like an outsider, being pushed out the door not only by his wife but also her girlfriends. The women had been law students together and now the three women seemed bonded in a case to get rid of him.

As the blocks went by under his feet, Ken remembered his parents' hasty retreat from his home after traveling clear across the country from Vermont to see their new grandson. Under the circumstances, Ken had been relieved to see them go but as his worried mother went out the door, she strongly warned him about his wife.

On a bus that raced over a bridge and past the beaches before heading inland and up the Point Grey hill, Ken looked out over Kitsilano Beach toward the island peaks across the water. He was reminded of the various therapies he arranged for himself and his wife in hopes of solving problems. Finally, in therapy on an island just north of the peaks that he could see from the bus, he had come to the realization that he and his wife were on separate life paths.

Wanting to work from home had been blocked. He wanted an office in the basement where clients could see him until his older boys could come and live in it while attending university. The house was in an upscale neighborhood close to the university and could accommodate his workspace easily without disturbing the family upstairs. Blocked by his wife in this plan, he was forced to rent expensive shared office space downtown, and forced to leave home, then having to rush home to care for his son instead of being at home within easy reach of his son.

Ken had always planned for his two older sons to live with him when they were old enough for university. Their visits were tolerated but his wife was clear that his sons would never be welcome to live with her in her home. His sons were growing up. A serious dilemma was looming.

He thought about the nanny's excellent job of taking care of his wife and his baby, but he was finding no way to overcome the difficulties in a marriage where his wife would not talk with him. All too often, he was told to get out and find sex elsewhere.

[ks notebook] "...My wife became pregnant while studying law at U.B.C. For me this pregnancy was the happiest time of our married life; ...our son was born in June of 1979... I could not find any way in two years to heal my own family without becoming a Scapegoat and leaving them. My marriage had broken and I could not fix it..."

12

Surprises

"In order to do my best, my calling, I need to live and work with others who know that life is love and love is knowing each other in love as the gift of life. I need to be growing and learning, breaking out of the boundaries of myself, my limitations..."
Kehnroth Schramm. M.D.

ALONE IN THE OFFICE at her place of work in the music centre, Daisy had set up a music tape and turned up the volume in the library of tall shelves filled with music scores. She was amusing herself by typing letters to the rhythm of music.

On the 4th Avenue sidewalk in front of the small two-storey office building, Ken paused to look up at the windows over the street shops. He checked his feelings – kind of scary but exciting anticipation. He entered through a door and started up the long wooden staircase to find Daisy. At the top there were two open doors. He glanced into the first office and headed down the hall to the second doorway. He saw her! A bit shy and afraid of rejection, he stood in the doorway.

"Hello."

She looked up to see his smiling face. Standing before her was a miracle of all miracles.

"Ken!" In a surprising moment her world became complete.

"I thought I'd drop in and see how you are doing."

"I am so glad to see you! It's been so-o long!"

"My wife and I have separated earlier today. Would you like to talk?"

These were words she never dreamt of hearing. "Yes! I'm so happy to see you! I have to finish the day here. Can we meet later? I would like to invite you to have dinner with my family tonight. My daughter is home on a spring break from the ballet school and we planned a dinner. She will be meeting me after work to shop for the groceries. Would you like to join us?"

Visibly relieved at his reception, Ken answered, "Yes, I would like that. May I use your washroom?"

"Yes, just down the hallway."

She watched as he walked softly and then in a moment of delight he skipped and clicks his heels together at the end of the long hallway.

He had no idea she had seen that.

SHOPPING FOR GROCERIES together was a surprise that neither one had expected to do today. Each paused in secret moments over vegetable stands to feel the presence of the other and take comfort in the warmth of each other's aura.

They carried the bags of groceries along the railway tracks, a route chosen deliberately away from traffic routes. It felt good to reminisce together about their childhood dreams. It turned out as they grew up they shared a common romantic dream about trains and railroads carrying each to the love of their lives. While walking among the weeds and wild flowers growing between and alongside the wooden ties, fifteen-year-old Lana in her red skirt and waist length brown hair swinging from side to side, skipped alongside, bending occasionally to pick wild flowers.

Daisy explained, "Since she was old enough to walk, she picked bouquets of flowers for me and at least once got into trouble. Along with her and a bouquet, an irate neighbor showed up because Lana had plucked her flower garden. Now she is picking flowers for the dinner table. She is such a romantic."

They carried the dinner across an untamed field, taking the long but fun route to Daisy's home. She still lived in the housing co-op.

Daisy mused, "Lana is always dancing. I had to hold her up by the waist so that she could dance before she could even walk." She paused, not quite knowing how to express herself. "The world is perfect right now. Us... You and me in a field of wild flowers... and my daughter is home."

"Yes, I'm with a Daisy in a field of wild flowers and with her flower child. Perfect."

"The kids are all coming to have dinner. I hope you are up for them."

"I'm looking forward to this evening."

COOKING DINNER TOGETHER turned into a challenge. Not only was the kitchen small, really meant for one person at a time, but their nutritional needs were different.

"I can't have salt in my food," Ken informed Daisy as they started to prepare a spinach salad. "I have high blood pressure and my doctor says I can't have salt... he doesn't want me to eat eggs also."

Daisy had no idea how to make a spinach salad taste good without salt or boiled eggs and wished she had thought of something else to make.

She made small talk. "We call this supper on the prairies. It's dinner on the west coast. I like the word *supper* better. Dinner is supposed to be at noon and a lunch is in between, like a... a lunch."

"Yes, lunch on the prairies is in a lunch kit. Farmers eat dinner at noon in the kitchen, or because they are working in the field, they have lunch kits brought to them."

Talking was fun and easy.

Daisy's evening ritual always had been to set the table with lighted candles, tablecloth, napkins and her favorite long stemmed red tinted wine glasses all around even when there was no wine, just milk or water. Daisy had decided long ago that children should enjoy a family meal and be in the habit of good manners around food. It had always been a family tradition that unless impossible because of classes, all family members were to sit down together at least once a day to share food and talk. For years it had been a time when there was to be no complaining to each other, no giving children heck for anything, no arguing, but instead to simply have positive communication.

The table setting to include a guest was the same as every day. Large dishes of food were always placed in the centre of the table and then passed around from one person to another, allowing each person to decide the size of their own stomach. Daisy took pride in knowing her children were healthy and there were no over or underweight people in the family. The family filled all the spaces at the table. Background classical music, as usual, could be heard from the stereo in another room. Sons Marcel and Antony, daughters Faith, Loraine, and Lana sat around the table.

Daisy was keenly aware that Ken was sitting at her side and wondering if for him, it was strange and somewhat scary. After all, she thought, as she looked at all the faces, some of her children were now young adults.

For Ken, it was strange and scary under the circumstances.

"I remember you," Marcel remarked. "You were our neighbor."

"Yes, I was a neighbor. I moved away because our townhouse was leaking badly. Running water was coming from the ceiling."

"I remember that," Daisy butted in. "The guy above you was moving out, disgruntled, so he deliberately broke pipes under his kitchen sink. He had asked me to be his witness as an Ombudsperson, expecting I would side with him. When I went there, I could see that he had done the damage on purpose and the floor over your head was a lake running down the edges into your walls as fast as it could."

"It was enough to cause us to look for a house of our own. I was not going to wait around for mold to set in."

Daisy asked, "Will you all tell Ken what you're doing now?"

Each one told a brief story and each one told a story that included music or dance. Ken listened carefully.

Daisy explained, "My parents taught me that music is a universal language, so I have encouraged music and dance. I love all the noise. To me, it means *health* and healthy thinking. I don't know of any musicians who make war, just the opposite. They try to make peace. In our last house, we had a ballet bar in the dining room. At Christmas, my brother Bill and the girls would do a fun rendition of the Nutcracker Suite in our living room." Daisy got wistful. "All the different music sounds coming from all the rooms... I'd play the piano with my girls singing."

Ken said softly, "I hope we will sing together. I would like that."

Daisy liked the soft way Ken was with her children. He did not pry but listened carefully to their conversations with him and each other.

Daisy felt a need to tell all before Ken disappeared again or was it really because it was an opportunity to once again remind her children about their roots. "I was brought up in a musical home." Daisy reminisced, "My father was not formally trained, but he played a harmonica *all the time*. He brought home a parlor organ. He would play music for us to fall asleep with when he wasn't working on Sunday nights. He sang and danced and played music all the time, and gave me a sense of a world without trouble through music. Anyway, my parents are the reason I've gone out of my way to give my children music and dance."

With a blush, Lana changed the conversation, "Mom says you have teen-aged sons."

"Yes, I do. They live in the Kootenays with their mother."

There was visible excitement among the girls.

THE DINNER had gone well and after the bustle of cleanup shared by all as usual, the family had gone out in different directions for the evening.

In the suddenly silent house, Ken and Daisy stood in the hallway beside the staircase, facing each other in surprise. It was their first time alone in the privacy of a home. His eyes were soft, full of wonder, and a little unsure of what to do as she gazed past the blue of his eyes, deep into his soul.

Blue eyes had been a family trait and both wives had blue eyes followed by blue-eyed sons. He now swam in green.

She moved her body close to his body, feeling his warmth and he hers. They became electrified in blending auras. She felt sure of herself in the most natural way of anything ever in her life. "All the kids have gone out for the evening. We're alone at last."

He nodded.

She put her arms around him fully for the first time, drawing closer so no space was between them, bellies touching, and kissed him fully on the lips. He responded.

"I want to make love with you," she told him.

A flicker of uncertainty flashed in his eyes. A solemn look came over his face as he sat down on the staircase, motioning with his hand to the back of his neck.

"Put your hand here, please."

She put her hand on the back of his neck to feel a large round scar against the whole of her palm. Holding it calmly, she felt the warmth of Ken's neck, inwardly grateful that he was allowing her to touch him and share his scar, and wishing to heal him of anything and everything that hurt him. She felt sorrow for how this must have happened to him and grateful that he lived through it.

Ken looked up into her eyes a long moment – searching. He felt completely naked – trusting. "I was born with Spina Bifida. I've always been afraid of passing on a genetic defect to my children."

She understood and gently took his hand, leading him up the stairs...

As the dew came up, perfume washed over them in the night air from roses Daisy grew on the patio by the bedroom's open door on the third floor and from the wild roses growing beside the nearby park pond where frogs sang their serenade to them all night long through the small open window above their heads...

13

Promises

FEAR FLED during the night. Peace of mind had washed over Ken in knowing he had found a place of feeling safe for the first time in many years. He could feel his heart relax in anticipation of continuing what he found.

In the early morning Ken rose while Daisy slept. He paused to look at the surprise of her. But, as usual, his child concerned him; he always had been there for him in the morning. Finding the telephone downstairs in the dining room, he called to check up on the wellbeing of his two-year old son. The call was a stinging reminder of his troubled life.

He needed to walk – and walk. Along the seawall in the May sunshine, he sorted out why he was here now, back in False Creek with Daisy and her family instead of in the more luxurious house on the hill with his wife and child. The farther he walked, the clearer it was again... he could not force himself onto a woman who clearly did not want him. He thought about how he must protect and take care of his child in divorce... how he must provide support for the mother of his child in her new life... how he must get over the hurt of another failed marriage measured against believing that he is giving her what she wants... after all she told him to find someone else to have sex with... he will not cause hurt to mother and child by separating them but instead he will take care of them to be together... he trusts the nanny will help... he must go back immediately but only to personally make it clear to Jane that he wants a divorce.

It was a long walk, several miles along the seashore and then up hill but the walk helped to think it all through.

AFTER TALKING with Jane, the fresh air of late morning felt like a new beginning.

Ken walked to the jewelry store on the hill. He was sure of what to do there.

The night had been a little uncomfortable sleeping with Daisy on the narrow foam mattress on the floor. She had gotten rid of her big bed that was from her past relationship. If Daisy continued to want him around, he thought, it will be necessary to consider a double bed of some sort so that neither one falls out of bed in the night. But in the meantime, Ken realized he must look for an apartment to live in, perhaps later today. First, he needed to see Daisy again. He thought she must be wondering.

DAISY WAS UNSURE of where Ken had gone or if he would return. She was happy anyway. Any time spent with Ken was a special gift.

The children were unaware that Ken had stayed the night. She had taken the day off from work and was having brunch with her two youngest daughters. She was standing by the table when Ken surprised her by coming through the door and reached for her hand. He opened his other hand for her to see a gold ring in the middle of his palm.

"I feel married to you. My wish is to marry you by Christmas," he said.

Ken then turned to the daughters seated at the table, whose mouths were open. "My wish is to marry your mother if you will have me."

Too surprised to speak, the wide-eyed girls nodded.

Daisy wanted to hug him but because daughters were watching, she simply said, "I feel married to you, too."

He held the ring for Daisy to see it clearly. "I need to explain the ring. It is a bamboo design."

"How unique! How did you know? I spent weeks learning to paint bamboo in a Chinese painting class... meditating on bamboo. I planted bamboo on the balcony upstairs outside my bedroom window." There she was rambling, wanting him to know her.

He continued, "Instead of an enclosed solid circle, it has two arms lying side by side, together, supportive of each other but not controlling each other. This is a symbol of how I would like us to be with each other because of our children and previous commitments and responsibilities."

"I understand... a perfect ring for us."

Ken slipped the ring on her finger. "Bamboo represents longevity. Bamboo is an evergreen that survives difficult conditions and renews itself. This ring is a symbol of strength and forever."

"Ken, I feel like we've known each other forever. I want you to stay here with me and my family starting today."

"Another stray that you are willing to take in?"

"Well, I don't think of you as another stray. I've been waiting for you to come home."

In a moment of humor and truth, they smiled with each other. Ken was fascinated by this woman who was open to including and care for lots of people. Daisy's mind raced with the truth Ken had so wisely and clearly identified. She had been taking in stray after stray over the years, most recently several stray teenagers. Her kids had a habit of bringing their troubled friends home. The cat was a stray that came to stay and the dog came to save his life. Before all that, she was taking care of people who had followed her to Vancouver from the meditation centre in Ontario, and even from Regina. And before that, she had been a caretaker on the meditation centre and looked after hundreds of people, including strays that arrived needing extra care.

Then she remembered something. "I have to tell you, though... my mother and sister and brother-in-law are coming next week for their usual spring holiday. You're going to be in a crowded house here for a while... lots of family... maybe more than you are bargaining for. My life and home is always spilling over with people and animals, and lots of activity and noise. This is normal life for me. I wish we could have more time to ourselves before more family arrives, but they are coming."

It was more or less what Ken expected of Daisy.

The girls witnessed adults wanting to be together but promising to look after children and family first.

After twelve years of pining over this man, Daisy felt like the luckiest person on earth. This was the perfect surprise that she had dared not dream.

Or was it? Maybe the magnetic attraction between Ken and Daisy could be explained by physics Quantum Entanglement. Two separate objects (in their case, two human beings) behave as one, each particle able to tell what the other is doing through a connection regardless of distance. Also, the Theory of Strings in physics is that strings made up of particles too small to see with the eye, move through time and space, connecting everything. The fact that there had been a lifelong connection between Ken and Daisy that manifested in longings, unexplained feelings, faint visions, even unexplained knowledge of where the other person was located in the world that caused each to want to go in that direction and eventually drawing them together regardless of distance, time, or space is a testament to an unseen force at work. It was no accident that Ken and Daisy were drawn to a meeting place in the middle of a continent, then circled each other over twelve years, drawing closer and closer until – SMACK – they got close enough for the magnetic force to unite them as one with the knowledge of coming home.

Ken wrote a String Theory poem:

the elegant thing
with theory of everything
made of strings
is
we are made to be played

THAT EVENING as the sun lowered over the ocean, Ken and Daisy found a log on the beach where they could sit and have a private talk. Lighted merchant cargo ships were anchored in the bay while smaller sailboats lazily made their way home in the blue waters topped with small red and pink rippling waves. People were strolling around, some hand in hand or arm in arm, while some were settling down on the sand or onto benches to watch the sunset. Others were gathering sandy children to leave.

Daisy felt the need to ask, "Why did you come to me?"

"I came where there is love."

That answer drew a smile followed by more curiosity. "You had no love in your life?"

"That's right... I should qualify that. I have love with my children."

"Ahh. I know what you mean. Me, too. But that's so sad."

"I wish I knew the name of the truck that hit me. Jane won't talk to me about it. I had taken her to therapists for individual and couple counseling but no one was able to help us. My own parents were here on a visit and were forced to leave in a hurry. As my mother left, she warned me about my wife. I thought maybe Jane and her friends wanted to get rid of me so they could live together. The morning I walked out, I went back a couple of hours later, trying to find a way to stay. I asked her if she ever loved me. Her answer was that she is angry because her life is changing."

"Angry because her life is changing? No love?"

"Jane has told me numerous times to get out and find sex elsewhere."

"Even though you were married?"

"Yes. I'm not the kind of guy who has one-night stands. I'm much too serious for that. I had to court her with expensive dinners out and pay for any intimacy. There were always strings attached. She made it obvious she didn't want me."

"That's sad. I can't imagine... oh, my God!" Daisy felt sorrow for Ken, but realized the implications of this giant opening and her luck in being able to walk right in. She really wanted to jump up and down for joy and grab Ken and hug and kiss him and assure him that she has enormous love for him and that they will be happy together and she has so much to offer that he will never be unhappy again and... As her mind raced, she wondered about how lucky could she get. Outwardly she did not make a move, trying to be cool, reserving outright pleasure so she would not scare him about being too happy for another woman's loss because underneath it all she knew how it felt to have her life changed; she did have sympathy for Jane. She contained an urge to shout the words *I am happiness!* Instead she asked, "What happened to your marriage to Jane? She wouldn't say she *ever* loved you?"

"She would *not* say she ever loved me in past or present. I was trying to stay. She told me love and sex are separate. It has become clear to me she wants neither one with me. I believe she just wants the security and prestige of being married to a doctor."

"You mean she doesn't want you, the man? She just wants a captive trophy, enslaved to her?" While looking at the grains of sand below her feet, Daisy mused, "So you are the half-married man!"

"Yes, I have been a half-married man."

"I grew up in Regina with girls who went into nursing just to catch a doctor. There is expected prestige and money in marrying doctors. Actually in Regina, the first best catch was a doctor, then a Mounted Policeman because Regina was where the Mounties trained and there were lots of those red uniforms around. Third was a hockey player. I tagged along with my girlfriends to the Mounties' summer concerts in the pavilion in the park on Sundays and to hockey games in winter. My girlfriends hoped to marry one of those guys. I wasn't interested and I didn't want to be a nurse. My mother always told me *not* to marry for money and *not* be a social climber because love is more important. That moral was fed to me like food to grow on. I believed my mother."

"I was never aware of myself being a catch because I'm a doctor. I was always too busy to know any of that."

"How did Jane become a lawyer?"

"After we married she went to university. We had discussed that she would study something to do with medicine so that we could work together. She chose law. She told me, 'It's a way to print money'."

"A way to print money! Whew!" That had an impact that brought Daisy a better understanding of what went wrong in Ken's life over the last few years.

They got up from the log and walked along the water's edge. As the tide receded, there was smooth wet sand and a fresh crop of empty seashells, and fresh footprints trailed behind. They paused to look at them, amazed that they were now making footprints together. They walked in silence for a while.

"What happened to your first marriage? Did she love you?"

"After that summer of meeting you, I was told to take my wife and leave the farm where I was working because of her flirting. They did not want trouble with wives. I moved my family to Argenta. There I came home to find another man in my house. I asked Carolyn to ask him to leave. She refused. I felt I had no choice but to leave by myself. Adultery was one thing. I was not going to live as a threesome. By then I was fed up after years of those kinds of troubles. ...The hard part was leaving my sons. Back in Regina, my friend Bill Lavant had told me to take the boys and run when she went on one of her trips."

"Why didn't you? I mean, did you?"

"In those days, fathers rarely were awarded custody of children. I decided that adultery did not make her an unfit mother, just an unfit wife. With a new husband, I believed she could provide a good home for the boys. I took the boys down to the lake to talk to them about my leaving. They were angry and hurt and I received a swift kick between the legs. I was in a lot of pain that lasted a long time. I wandered with no real destination, hitchhiking along the roads for a few weeks. I slept under the sky. I was homeless. It was a desolate time. In a café, I read an article that pointed me to exploring an alternative community on an island. I went there and became their physician. That's where I met Jane."

"Oh." A feeling of jealousy washed over Daisy. "I wish we had gotten together in 1969 and saved ourselves from some troubles. Twelve years with the wrong people... people who did not appreciate us... both you and me. Why didn't you talk to me in Regina that night at Bill and Marianne's house? I have always wondered that. I followed you around, wanting to get to know you."

"Because you were with Saul. I was determined not to be interested in any girlfriend he might have. Besides, I was upset with Carolyn that night for flirting with Saul and ignoring her own kids."

"Yeah, I remember but I didn't care. I was more interested in you."

"If your children had been with you, I would have been more interested in knowing you. As it was, I only thought of you as

Saul's girlfriend, possibly just another university student... maybe a hippie."

Daisy was a little startled at being called a hippie. "I've always denied being a hippie but I think I'd rather be a freedom lover than some other things. ...Darn! We sure missed it! I was told not to bring my children; otherwise they would have been with me. I didn't know it then but Saul was secretly planning to drive my kids and me back to Vancouver and dump me because that's what his mother wanted. And your marriage was on the rocks. I feel really sad about that. ...Anyway, how did you meet Jane?"

"I found the community on the island and went for a walk in the forest where I saw a red-haired woman with a child on her back. I was taken with her agility and beauty in the ambience of the forest. The child made her look especially attractive."

"Oh."

"It turned out the child was not her own. As a member of the community, she was assigned to taking care of another couple's child."

"So you got together?"

"I still had unfinished business with Carolyn. I invited Carolyn and my sons to visit me on the island. I hoped to reconcile for the sake of our sons. Carolyn refused to come. My parents came all the way from Vermont and brought my sons to visit me. Carolyn and I divorced and she married the other guy. I thought he would want to adopt my sons and be a family."

"You would have given up your sons to him?"

"I thought that if Carolyn and he wanted so much to be a family that it would be a healthier situation for the boys than a broken family."

"That was really big of you."

"It did not turn out that way. My sons were angry that I left and they were not forgiving. They refused to have the guy adopt them, insisting on keeping the Schramm name. It all ended anyway. I was told he was a bigamist."

"She divorced you for a bigamist? He had another wife?"

"I was told he did."

"How did you meet Carolyn?"

"She was a student nurse."

"Oh, that makes sense."

"I have always wondered why she chose to marry me. She had been dating an Engineer."

"Why did you marry her?"

"She was bright and fun. She climbed in my dorm window. I liked her spirit. I asked, Why me? I don't remember getting an answer. She won me over and I married her."

Daisy laughed, "Romeo and Juliet in reverse."

"Yes, but at our wedding, while we were getting our picture taken, she told me, 'If it doesn't work out, we can get a divorce anyway.' That's how we started married life... not the once in a lifetime marriage I had intended. I have never quite figured out why she wanted to marry me, why she gave up her relationship with her former boyfriend to marry me and then tell me we could easily get a divorce right after the marriage ceremony. On the day of our wedding, the Berlin Wall went up. It was symbolic of my own experience."

"That would be shattering. What happened with Jane? Why did you marry her?"

"We met in a spiritual community where the emphasis was on living simply. Being in the commune was a time of learning, meditation, being mindful, sharing, being thankful. The leader of the commune warned me that Jane was not what she projected and that I should be careful. I was enjoying the commune. After what I had just been through with Carolyn, I felt like I belonged, so I ignored the warnings and started a relationship with her. Later when the men in the commune were under suspicion of rustling cattle and they wanted me to commit a guy who was a dissident, I left. I don't take orders like that. I refused to be a party to any of that. Jane came with me."

"Of course. I bet you were the best catch she had seen. You mean you did not really invite her?"

"I let it happen. I then took a job as physician to a coastal native community and because I was hired by the church, we had to get married if she was to come along."

"You got married because of a job?"

"I did. By then, I thought she was my best friend."

"Ken, I think I see a pattern here. Women choose you and they also tell you when to leave."

"In some cultures it is the women who decide who to mate with and when to mate. In traditional Lakota culture, the women could either move another man into the home or put the man's moccasins outside the door to let the man know it is time to leave. The women continue to raise the children. I never want to force myself on a woman. I would rather she tell me when it is right to be together and when it is time to leave."

"Wow! I never thought of it that way."

"Differences between Jane and myself became apparent when we moved back to the city and found out we were complete opposites in our values and our material needs."

"How?"

"We met in a commune where we lived in tents with natural light shining through the plastic. We ate our meals communally and slept when it got dark. When we left, she refused to discuss the communal life and the teachings we had experienced. When we visited my family in Vermont, she kicked me under the table, attempting to control me in what I could discuss with my family about our communal life. I got the picture."

"Well, I bet she was in the commune to be taken care of. On the meditation centre where I lived, often people were sent to me from the city just because they needed to be taken care of physically or emotionally for a while."

After minutes of silence, Ken continued, "You and I have been caretakers. We are both eldest children – five in your family and five in mine. Your doctor told me you are mother earth."

"Oh?" Daisy somehow felt insulted by being called mother earth; she wanted to be seen as a young woman of romance right now, not mother earth. "Right! But as a doctor, you are a caretaker in a bigger way than I have ever been. Anyway, back to Jane..."

"Yes, back to Jane. I was a convenience, then an inconvenience. I think she loved the life she had with a doctor but not with me. Our differences became apparent when we came to live in the city. She needed all the things I never wanted... a big house in a prestigious area, gardeners, a financial advisor, a nanny. ...I told her she was killing me with all her expensive needs.

I have always wanted a simple life. I wanted to practice medicine in the basement room of the house so that I could be at home with my family but she wouldn't allow that. I was forced to rent an office. That's where you found me, in an office I shared with another therapist. We had major conflicts about my older sons. I had always hoped my sons would live with us so I could support them through university from my home but she made it plain they could not. She refused to have my baby. Then in law school she and her two school friends all got pregnant around the same time. For me, the pregnancy was the best time... hope for our future. But that didn't last. After the birth, she rejected me and was unable to cope with a baby. The doctors advised me to get a nanny so I was both father and nanny until I found a nanny for the hours I needed to work. I met Jane when she was looking after someone else's child. I never expected what happened. Now she and her girl friends all have children about the same age and are all divorcing together. They are the same two friends who helped Jane drive me out of the house."

"Sounds to me like those women all took a law class about what a child is worth in long-term security. What do you suppose Jane will do now?"

"I expect she'll move the two friends into our house and she'll practice law. She'll be fine so long as I provide a nanny."

"Women need to have a balanced perspective in order to raise sons or daughters. Sons grow up to be men. Some women don't get that."

They paused to look at scenery. The sky had turned red as the sun sat on the horizon. In the distance, the sound of bagpipes came from the open air Kitsilano Showboat stage. The shimmering surface of pink and blue water seemed to dance in time to the sound.

"I am extremely homesick for Vermont." Ken became wistful looking over the ocean into the distance. "I have tried to fix my marriage but I can't fix it. I am convinced she's out to kill me one way or another."

"Really? You mean really kill you?"

"I have had the worry that she would commit suicide and frame me for her murder, or that she would kill me. She will not talk to me. I left her to save my life. It was because of the way she treated me!"

As Daisy watched Ken's face, she could see his pain. "I am so sorry! That's really scary! Do you think she was looking for a plan?"

"I don't know. All I know is that I felt unsafe with her."

"That's a lot of disappointment and heartache."

"All I ever wanted in life was to be a pediatrician in Vermont, marry one wife for the rest of my life and have children and grandchildren. I wanted to make a safe world for families to bring up their children. After a first failed marriage, I thought I married my best friend when I married Jane. I don't know what happened, but I am afraid of her. I can't trust her. ...I am troubled about leaving my child with her. I need the nanny to take care of him and see that he is okay when I'm not there."

"What about taking custody of him?"

"I hope to keep him safe by being available for both of them as much as I can be, to take care of them, and have the nanny working as much as possible to take care of Andy. I want to share in parenting Andy. Now that I am out of the house, I am hopeful that she will feel better. My goal is to help Jane, not to hurt or cause her more grief. I want to help her get on her feet to pursue her own life as a lawyer and hopefully she'll be so busy that I'll have Andy most of the time anyway."

"I understand. For years, I thought my marriage was good. It was common-law but lasted twelve years. Our relationship was barely beginning when I met you in Regina. On top of his plan to dump me, on the way home he hatched a different plan; if he found a job right away, he would stay and if not, he would go. I was unaware that my fate was in strange hands. Ironically, a professor at Simon Fraser University had read his PhD thesis and came to my home within the first week that we were back to offer him a job. I didn't even have a phone in the house, so the guy had to come in person, unannounced. Suddenly Saul had a job and for the next twelve years we became a family."

With surrounding sounds of the evening, they were deep in thought, digesting stories they had shared.

Daisy broke their silence. "During the last few months, it was just odd for him to tell me to get other friends when we had always shared friends. So I took another evening course and tried my hand at writing prose for a friend's book. He would visit our friends when I was busy. But when I suggested we visit them together, he would always make excuses and I would let it go. I found out after he left that he had been telling our friends that I was having an affair. A total lie! He was obviously planning his exit and wanted to look justified while I was clueless. You know, I fell into that relationship and I tend to stick with things even though I should have gotten out right away. ...Here's an odd part of the story. On my birthday just before he left me, he took me to the Island for my birthday. I insisted on bringing my youngest daughter along because I did not want to leave her. One evening he took us to a park in the middle of Victoria that has a cliff. We were looking out over the city and I could feel him pressing his body against me from behind. I had a sudden sharp awareness that he wanted me out of his life. Sometimes, reading a person's mind is an awful experience. I was really scared of him in that moment because I was standing very close to the rim. I stepped sideways away from him to stand with my daughter. I was suddenly glad I brought her along. It was only a week later that he told me he was having an affair and was leaving me. I don't think he would have deliberately caused me to fall. He's not that kind of guy. It was his unusual behavior that was a prelude as though he could not figure out what to do. When I discovered a woman's scarf on my seat in the van and the broken bed in our van, he challenged me about what I thought happened. I didn't have an answer so I didn't say anything. He was leaving hints of what was on his mind and it was up to me to figure out what the hints meant. Years before that, Eric and I were on our way to Toronto because of his numerous affairs in Regina. We were swimming in a lake with my kids. He swam up to me from underwater and grabbed my feet. He was pulling me down. I saw him clearly. I was a strong swimmer and got free. I thought he was playing too rough. When he surfaced, I asked him why he did that. He adamantly denied being near me. That was when I got really scared. I never trusted him after that. He too, gave me fair warning. I was newly pregnant and stayed with him, hoping for the best. So... Ken... I can really relate to your fear of your wife.

People think their feelings are hidden while they put clues out in ways that can be picked up on. It's awful when you can't trust the person you sleep with."

Looking to the horizon, Daisy said, "I spent the last twelve years thinking about you... year in and year out... day and night... Ken, we really should have gotten together in Regina. That summer in 1969 was a turning point in both of our lives. As a result, we each had relationships with other people that in my view, wasted years of our time when we should have been together. They stole our young years and copped out of the getting old years."

Walking for a few minutes and then finding another log to sit on, they continue sharing stories of their lives.

Ken had been telling Daisy about the Pediatrician who wanted a homosexual relationship. "He told me that I would never get registered as a Pediatrician unless I allowed him to have sex with me."

"Why didn't you press charges or at least make a complaint?"

"Who would have believed me? Not in those days! He was a person in a powerful position, able to block me. I thought it better to change my career rather than to enter into that kind of war. I could not win that war and I was not willing to have sex with the guy. I became concerned about why he perceived me to be homosexual. I was interested in women, not men. I thought I had better get any false perception straightened out. I then concentrated more on girl friends and had eight marriage proposals before I met Carolyn and did get married."

"So you went into psychiatry?"

"Yes. I had been told I was the slowest doctor on the ward, so I decided that in psychiatry, I could spend more time with people than I could in other specialties."

"Why don't you prescribe drugs to your patients?"

I studied medicine before drugging people became the billion-dollar industry that the pharmaceutical companies control and now are controlling how physicians are trained to think. I have studied the use of drugs. I have my personal reasons why I don't use them. One of my best friends in Vermont committed suicide after he had been given a new antidepressant drug to try."

"Oh, God! You must have wished to help him."

"Yes, but I was already in western Canada. Then my own father became disoriented on a pharmaceutical drug given to him for depression by his doctor. He was on a new drug and he was hallucinating to the extent that he lost touch with reality entirely. His life became a nightmare of visual horrors and distorted beliefs. I went home to see my father and saw him in that state. His doctor hospitalized him. Then they gave him shock treatment and fried his brain. He never recovered. He became permanently disabled and remains in hospital even now."

"That's awful!"

"My father told me that if he had been making fifty dollars a day instead of spending fifty dollars a day for medical care, none of this would have happened. His brother and partner in business was run over and killed while changing a tire on the highway. He lost his brother and business at once. As a result, my father was depressed. My personal burden is that I have been unable to help my own father. His doctors were in charge and he was convinced that his doctors would help him with medicine and then shock treatment... against my objections! I was unable to convince him not to allow it. He really believed them that it would help. Instead it completely ruined his life and cheated our whole family."

"How is your mother fairing?"

"His problems propelled her to work harder. She did make her million in business despite the difficulties, just as her father predicted but the money is being spent on my father's hospital care. My mother is determined to keep her family together no matter what we are all going through, and she does! To her, we are the Schrammily. She tells my father that if he ever forgets who she is, she will bop him. He never forgets. She had always been the person I could talk with. I'm very homesick for Vermont and I miss the discussions with my mother that I have never been able to have with my wives, or with my children. I left home as a teenager for high school and lived with another family. My sisters are a lot younger than me and grew up differently than I did. I had to work my way through school from very young. I asked my grandfather for financial help when I went to medical school. He refused, telling me it would be more beneficial for me to work and earn my own way. My grandmother snuck me a few dollars from her apron pocket as I left. Later in life, my grandfather married his secretary and when he died, he left his money to charity."

"Gee. What a story! You are obviously here and not in Vermont because you have children here."

"Yes. I have wanted to go home. I am homesick but I can't leave my sons. I can't leave Andy alone with Jane and I am committed to helping my sons through university."

The sun set and a cooler breeze came from the water.

"I almost gave birth to my youngest child on this beach," Daisy reminisced. "I had left Toronto, running away from Eric's games. He had left me on the meditation centre when I was newly pregnant. I moved to Toronto where Eric was busy flaunting girl friends in my face. I sold my negative retouching machine to afford train fare and piled my children on a train to Vancouver. I was six and a half months pregnant then. I had promised my children that as soon as we found an apartment, I would take them to the beach. After a three-day train trip, we spent a couple of days in a hotel by the train station while I telephoned every advertised place for rent and got turned down. No one wanted my children. I tried phoning every agency I could think of for help and was told by everyone that because I had enough money for one month's rent, there was no help available. They didn't bother to figure out that I needed to feed my children, too. Finally, one man told me to come right over and he would rent a suite to me. He did rent us an apartment in the east end... top floor of a house. He even helped me pick up our luggage from the train station. Later, I learned he housed stray women and their children, and never, ever bothered them. He was a true guardian angel of women and children in need. He is one person in my life that was a brief encounter and we lost touch when the house was sold, but I would like to find him again to let him know how much he helped. I had walked the Granville Bridge four times that day with my children, looking for his address because I didn't know Vancouver. The fourth time, midway on the bridge, I felt something give... kind of like something broke and that night I started into light labor. We had absolutely no furniture. The only furniture in the place was a stove and fridge, so we slept on the wood floor with only blankets and pillows. I denied to myself that I was in labor, so the next morning

I went to the store to buy the makings for a picnic lunch and then I took my children across town on the bus to Kitsilano Beach. We spent the day here on this beach under that tree over there for shade."

Daisy paused, pointing to the tree. "If you walk up to it, it has a face naturally imprinted on the trunk. There had been forty days without rain, so it was hot and dry in mid August. I had come across the country to the end of the earth and unknown circumstances, and now I was afraid to go with my children to the Showboat only a few feet from my spot or to any other part of the beach. Showboat was on that evening and my boys were asking me to go with them. I couldn't. I spent my time looking for tiny seashells right in front of the tree and feeling the sand around my bare toes, and looking after my sleeping baby under the tree and keeping a watchful eye on all my children."

Ken waited silently while she paused to relive the time. She continued, "At about nine o'clock, with the sun setting just like now, I had to admit to myself that I really was in full labor and it wasn't going to go away. I took my children by bus across town to our apartment, not knowing how I would arrange their care so that I could go to the hospital. The only option I could think of was to call Social Services for help because I couldn't leave my children alone, but that was a horrifying prospect. In those days, Social Workers were taking children away from single parents with little excuse. When we got back to the house, like magic the woman in the lower suite opened her door and offered to take care of my children. She was also pregnant. Her husband was a longshoreman. I felt like another angel had been sent to take care of us. We were so lucky! So there are three people who acted as our guardian angels and protected my children. I was out of money and gave them my last ten dollar bill for the care of my children."

"In hard labor, I took another bus to the hospital. The doctor commented with amusement that I was all sandy. My tiny daughter was born two and a half months premature very soon after I arrived there – about twenty minutes after ten and she was whisked away. I was told my baby might not live – only fifty-fifty chance. I saw her the next day. I was looking through the window of the Intensive Care nursery because in those days mothers were not allowed to touch their premature babies. She was so tiny with tubes in her but I saw her energy in her hands and knew she would live. I named her Faith right then. I am extremely grateful to the pediatrician Doctor Smith, a young intern at the time. He was the only doctor to take the time to talk with me about my baby. I was ignored otherwise."

"In those days, they had unmarried mothers' wards. Because I had admitted that my husband was no longer with me – that is where they put me – a ward with rows of beds filled with mothers giving their babies up for adoption. A Social Worker, who looked like an army captain, visited my bed daily, trying hard to convince me to give my baby up for adoption. She told me that because I already had four children, I didn't need another one since I had no husband.

"And then I walked home because I had no bus money. The baby was in the hospital for a couple of months until she gained from her birth weight of 2½ pounds to 5 pounds. I had no spare money so I had to walk back and forth to the hospital just to view her through a window. Then the same social worker came to my house just before Faith was to be released from the hospital. She was standing on the top step of a long staircase when I opened the door. This time I was not in a hospital bed. Even though she was bigger and taller than me, she was standing on a stair step below me and I was at even height to her and very determined. Once again she told me she wanted my baby for adoption. I threatened to push her down the stairs if she did not leave my baby and me alone. She left and I never heard from her again. In hindsight, it was my good fortune that she did nothing about me threatening her. So that was how I came to Vancouver. I really felt like some higher power was looking after us.

"Here is the stupid part of my story. I had just brought my baby home from the hospital. My daughter Loraine was about to turn six and wanted Eric to be present for her birthday. He was the only father she remembered. I had no way to contact him. I was at the West End beach with my children and another woman from the house and her children. I wrote my wish for Eric to come for the birthday on the seawall with some charcoal found on the beach. My wish was a silent but very loud call into the universe.

"At home, I lit a birthday candle and made a wish for him to come for my daughter. During the night, I was woken by a male voice clearly saying, 'He will come.'

"Eric surprised us by coming to Vancouver in time for the birthday but he brought a girlfriend, the same one he had when I left Toronto. Not only that, they rented a room in a house just a block straight up the hill from where I had written my wish on the seawall. There was a lesson in that. I learned that when we wish for something we should be very specific. I had forgotten some important details. Very soon after arriving, he abandoned the girlfriend on my doorstep for me to take care of while he took off to India on my brother's money. I looked after his girlfriend for a couple of years while she continued to steal things from me – clothing, money. I was fresh from the meditation centre and in a frame of mind to be able to take care of her regardless of the situation.

"When Eric wrote a letter while stranded in Europe months later, wanting me to buy his ticket home and he promised to start again with me by taking my son on a motorcycle trip to Mexico, I refused to answer. I was truly free of him emotionally and I abandoned him to Europe, not caring if or when he ever got back. His former girl friend was furious with me. Meanwhile she had become pregnant. Her new boyfriend went to jail for selling marijuana. I supported her emotionally all through her pregnancy – the same woman who was partly the cause of me leaving Toronto while I was pregnant. Her parents finally came from Ontario to take her and her baby off my hands."

LEAVING THE BEACH, Ken and Daisy decided to go to a local Greek restaurant. On the walk up the hill, they exchanged more thoughts and memories.

As they passed block-long rows of apartment buildings, Daisy said, "I've been involved in local issues, trying to make a better world for children. I marched in the first peace march here. Then I was very active in trying to protect housing in this neighborhood for families with children and to keep the highrises out. We won the battle but lost the war. Instead, they built these block long three-storey apartment buildings and got rid of family housing anyway. The beach has changed. It used to be filled with children. Now it is filled with swinging singles lounging like walruses and smelling of coconut. Adults live within walking distance to the beach while families with children must pay parking for a car or bus fare to get here. I have prayed for years that I would find something, some way, to help people in a meaningful way."

Ken explained his story. "I took part in the first peace march in Vermont. I guess we were on the same wavelength. I'm a registered conscientious objector to the Vietnam War. That's why I came to Canada. My wife thought that if we were based in Germany, she could ski the Alps. I think we might still be married if I had done what she wanted, so I am probably to blame for the divorce. While I was teaching at McGill, I received a letter stating that I was too old for the induction so I was able to visit home again."

Daisy reminisced, "There were lots of draft dodgers in Vancouver who were refusing to go to Vietnam. It's a roundabout kind of fate but it has allowed us to meet. As a child, the only place on earth that I imagined going to in a train was to New York, not because of New York City but for something else. I would look down at my feet and picture buckled shoes on green grass in New York State. And that's where you were. This happened all through my childhood. I only heard of people wanting to go to California but the New York countryside was drawing me. At night I would listen to the trains going by; they were only two blocks away, and I'd imagine they would take me to meet a person who looked like you. The only boys I was attracted to as a young girl had your colouring and looked like you. I feel I have been yearning for you all my life as though I have been destined to be with you."

"I can relate to that. I was drawn to the prairies where you were. I would watch the trains and imagine heading west to the prairies. When I did arrive, I thought I was seeing heaven with all that open sky and golden fields."

ON FOURTH AVENUE, a line of people waited to get into the popular restaurant. From inside, lively Greek music wafted over the waiting line outside. Ken took Daisy in his arms. They danced a slow spot dance, bodies together feeling each other's warmth in a world of their own.

A woman's voice rose from the line of people behind them. "I am so jealous. I never had romance."

WHILE EATING SOUVLAKI, savoring spices of oregano and black pepper, enjoying the olive oil and lemon, and the saltiness of feta cheese with cucumbers, tomatoes and onions, Ken told Daisy, "You will write my story."

"You want me to write your story?"

"I don't know how I know, but you will."

Stunned, she held her breath for a moment and then responded, "How can I write your story? You're a physician... a university teacher... from Vermont. I'm from the Prairies. You know so much I have no idea about." Then she saw humor in the moment. Laughing, she said, "I always wanted to be a writer. I did months of research on Louis Riel and actually wrote a book but burned it in a bonfire at the meditation centre in a moment of cleansing because I was living in a rustic log cabin with no running water and I realized that I had no real knowledge of homesteading on the prairies when I wrote the story. I took courses in all the different kinds of writing." She laughed again. "I even took a course in how to be a clown just so I could know how to write about a clown. After being bruised from head to toe by doing somersaults and trying to ride a unicycle, I never did write the story. The moral of this story is that I never thought I would be writing about a physician or medicine. So I haven't prepared for this."

"I want you to work with me. I will teach you."

"How can I write without giving away confidentiality?"

"You would write about what I do. You can write about how I work which is different than most other psychiatrists."

Daisy was confused. "Writing about you is a big job. You are so large in your beliefs, what you have done..." she paused, "...your losses. How about writing it yourself?"

"I'm asking you to write my story."

"When I prayed to be able to help people, I got a big one."

"I'm always in trouble of one kind or another. Life with me won't be easy. Be careful about what you ask for."

"I'm up for absolutely anything!"

They were both aware of a connection that could not be explained. Though he would never admit to being psychic or intuitive, she would soon learn he sometimes knows things without knowing why or how – just knowing.

They held hands across the table. Physical surroundings disappeared as they blended together in a world transformed by love. They were starting a new life – together.

Her hand in his, Daisy knew a deep knowledge of knowing him from beyond this life... and now she had come home.

Daisy took up the gauntlet. Somehow she will write his story.

14

Daisy's Story

THE MYSTERIOUS WEB of life works in wondrous ways. The doctor who Ken and Daisy had each chosen as their family physician, and each had known for several years was one and the same; he had uncannily brought together two old acquaintances after they had lost touch.

It was Ken's compelling honesty that made a trip together necessary to meet face to face with the doctor. He wanted to explain that he and Daisy planned to marry as soon as the divorce from Jane was final.

What the meeting taught Daisy about Ken was that he bravely faced problems head on to clear up any issues. Ken's courageousness and the doctor's reaction were burned into Daisy's watchful memory.

The doctor was clearly surprised and cheerful. "Well, while you are here, we should check your blood pressure."

Ken reluctantly complied, distressed at the process.

With the cuff still on Ken's arm, the doctor spouted numbers that were unfamiliar to Daisy but one was close to 100, and one close to 200. "The medicine doesn't seem to be helping. Your blood pressure is extremely high, as usual... too high." He removed the cuff and opened a file over an inch thick and recorded the measurements while offering no alternative treatment.

Ken's breathing had become labored. He was extremely upset. Now Daisy saw his fear.

Ken had been under this doctor's care since 1975 and taken his prescriptions of medicine for high blood pressure for six years. Daisy wondered why, if the medicine had not helped, a different treatment was not offered. Daisy had just learned that Ken's heart was a ticking time bomb. She was scared.

OUT ON THE STREET after leaving the doctor's office, Ken explained, "It runs in my family to have high blood pressure. My mother has it and my grandparents had it. It's common to have elevated blood pressure measurements at the mere thought of having the cuff on. Unfortunately, the medication I am on has terrible side effects. It is numbing externally and hard on my internal organs. I don't know which is worse, the possibility of my heart failing or the side effects of a medicine that is slowly killing me. I hope that by living with you, you will help me to heal."

ON A WALK along the seawall in the evening, Daisy made a confession to Ken. "I still have to divorce my first husband. We have not laid eyes on each other in almost twenty years but we aren't divorced."

Ken was taken aback. "Why have you not divorced?"

"I tried to get a divorce. Regina was a small city and I knew through the grapevine that my lawyer was having an affair with a younger woman but still living with his wife and kids. Whenever I would consult with him, he would just stare at his wife's picture on his desk and then send another meaningless letter and a fifty-dollar charge. I worked for the government. That was my weekly salary and I had children to support. In those days, divorcing for any reason was extremely difficult. So I just left town and disappeared with a new boyfriend for protection because I was afraid of my husband. I ran away and changed my name. I lived my life from then on as though I was not ever married. I had decided common-law would be better because I could believe the other person to be committed to the relationship so long as we were together and to have the freedom to quit without lawyers if it didn't work out. In other words, so long as the other person was present, I could fool myself by believing everything was okay. I guess my theory was wrong."

"My divorce is in the works," Ken replied. "I have already informed Jane that I want to marry you at Christmas time. I have told your children that I will marry you. I hope you will get the divorce."

Daisy was suddenly confronted with fear and guilt. More than anything she wanted to marry this man. She had never before known love like she felt for Ken but she had unwittingly betrayed him already by having unfinished business not mentioned until now. The past marriage had been so far out of her mind that it had become unreal. She became aware of feeling like the elephant stuck to a post after the rope had been taken away because it was business she had ignored and now the invisible tie had come up to haunt her. She had to examine why so much fear. On reflection, it was the legal process that caused fear.

Her life began to flash in front of her. She remembered, as a child, having a premonition of her future. She had accompanied her mother to a movie theatre when word came that her brother was in the new clip. In those days, black and white movie news clips shown as extras in theatres before the main movie were the only way to actually see what was going on around the world. Her mother's brother, Daisy's uncle John, who she had been close to since birth, was a Canadian soldier stationed in war-torn Sicily and was doing maintenance on a large tank in the clip. As uncle John looked up in the film, his suntanned face flashed his familiar brilliant smile. In that moment Daisy had intuition that she would marry a German boy who was growing up in the same war that she was viewing on the screen. When the movie finished and the lights came on, while walking up the aisle in the theatre, she wondered about the intense knowing.

At age fourteen, Daisy had gone with a girlfriend to ride horses at Regina Beach as they had been doing all summer. After many Sundays when the girls would disappear, traveling by greyhound bus to the farm, Daisy's father got concerned. He was sure they were just going to meet boys. He followed one Sunday to investigate, only to find they were just riding horses.

He decided not to interfere again. After all, his family was farmers and he always had his own horse. His children had always played around the horses and he had often sat the small children on his horse's back. His white horse, Tony, had been his pal and they loved to race across the pastures. His mother would hurry to the doorway of the house and with hands in her white apron, called, "Wendal! Stop!" in fear that his horse would stumble in a gopher hole. It had been the darkest day of his life when his parents had told him they sold his Tony to the glue factory. He cried hard, even in front of his children. Then he had gone to the horseracing track at the Regina Exhibition and discovered his horse was there in the race. He went to the barn and had a brief reunion. He could understand his daughter's love of horses.

It was the next Sunday that Daisy met Karl, nicknamed Cisco Kid. He was all decked out in a fancy black cowboy outfit like in the movies, matching her fantasy of meeting someone completely different than all the prairie boys she had ever met. Newly arrived from Germany, he was eighteen and spoke with a charming accent. Being partly German with an Italian grandparent gave him a flawless olive skin, slick black hair combed into a flawless ducktail under the cowboy hat, and stunning deep blue eyes rimmed with black eyelashes and perfectly shaped dark eyebrows.

For weeks Daisy and her girlfriend had been practicing to ride like jockeys. They asked for the lightest English saddles and pulled their stirrups up high. They would race each other around the fields. Then with ankles rubbed raw with open wounds from the metal stirrups because they had no riding boots, they had to walk the overheated, foaming horses to cool them down.

Walking horses that particular Sunday was a prelude to Daisy's future. The girls had stayed long enough to meet Cisco Kid, also a Sunday rider because he worked as a well-trained tailor the rest of the week.

He was hungry, so Daisy walked the mile to the fish and chips stand in the tiny beach village and with money she had earned by babysitting, brought food back for him.

They sat in the tall grass by a fence. As he ate, he realized she had just won his interest even though he had a girlfriend back in Germany.

She was just as hungry, not for food but for something different.

They rode horses together, sometimes on one horse.

She came from a family that danced every weekend. Her father, who absolutely loved dancing, had taught her the dances familiar to the prairies. Karl brought a new element of dance – Latin dancing. She had always been drawn to playing Latin rhythms on the organ. It was a thrill to actually learn to dance them. He jived like in the movies. She flew in all directions over and around him. It had been fun, far better than doing simple jives with girlfriends.

Those were the days of big bands and ballrooms with tables ringing a large, shiny dance floor and a balcony with tables overlooking the dancers. People dressed up. Women wore dresses special for the occasion and high-heeled shoes. Men wore suits and ties. Saturday nights at the ballroom was where Daisy and her boyfriend danced along with her parents and their friends. Her father was the smoothest dancer of all and would always take a turn at floating Daisy around the floor. Then in the middle of the dances nearly every Saturday night, Karl would inevitably be asked to sing a set of songs and many women swooned.

Occasionally, they attended Saturday night dances or celebrations in the town hall of her grandparents in the town of Vibank. Remembering those days she thought, if she and Karl had been able to just dance, they might still be together. But life is not like that.

At the age of eighteen, after four years of dating, Daisy knew that caring for this man was like sisterly love and she would like to move on. He was still as handsomely dashing as ever. He had an eye for beautiful women and they for him, so he could move on rapidly. Knowing that, she decided to quit the relationship by not hurting his feelings. To let him out easily, she proposed marriage one evening while sitting in the car in the midst of a field of weeds beside the railway track. She expected he would say "no" and it would all end amicably.

He said, "Yes!"

At that moment, panic set in and she felt herself sink. Trapped! And she had done it to herself! When she arrived home to tell her parents, her father suggested that since his father, her grandfather, had died only a couple of weeks ago, she should wait at least six months to marry. Her father said that unless she agreed to wait, no family member would attend. Her parents had embraced Karl as another son but were vying for time because they knew he was not ready for marriage. Being her father's child, stubborn had met stubborn. She privately went along with a date to marry Karl that he had suggested even though there was no pregnancy or urgency.

She went to a dress shop to find a wedding gown. There was only one formal wedding gown in the whole shop, just her exact size and it cost only thirty-five dollars, a week's salary, the exact amount she had with her. She hid the wedding gown under her bed.

On the appointed day, Daisy came down the stairs in the white lace-wedding gown and a glittering tiara with a short veil. She stood for a minute in the living room in front of a family of gaping mouths and shocked parents, and then left the house alone, walking out into the cold, crisp snow of February.

She married the young man who was a casualty of war. Whenever he had a pencil and paper, he would draw airplane fighters and lines that shot at each other. He could not escape his own life experience and was suffering post war syndrome – in those days unrecognized as a syndrome. Those who lived it had no name for it – it was just life that hurt and gave nightmares day and night. On Christmas Eve when Karl was just a boy, news came that his father, a handsome German soldier had been killed. Fatherless, Karl tried to help his pregnant mother and three small brothers. He was the oldest and felt responsible for all. He was forever carrying scars and nightmarish boyhood memories of the family's trek by foot across Germany, running from the Russians, from east to their family home in the west. His baby brother died of starvation at a few months old on the dusty road and was buried in a strange town where they left his baby carriage beside his grave. Karl had been helpless at a train station as Huns on a rampage raped women. A woman giving birth behind a bush was attacked by the Huns and died along with her baby. Karl's mother had been helping the woman and narrowly escaped with her own life. His younger brother was blown up when he picked up a grenade while Karl was supposed to be looking after him. His grandfather, a concert violinist before the war, committed suicide in the forest over the sudden worthlessness of the German Mark; he had become a destitute man over night, unable to help his family. Karl scrounged for food to bring home to the family. He had been inducted into the Hitler Youth as a young boy and was at war with the Russians, trying to save his own family. He had not been able to accept his widowed mother making friends with American soldiers in return for food to feed her remaining family; Karl remained faithful to his father's memory. After the war, food of any kind was hard to come by, so the boy would go to farms and beg for food for his family. It was on those farms that he met with ferocious large dogs protecting their properties, causing a lifelong fear of dogs.

War had caused severe damage. This young man had no idea of how to be a married man with a family and turned to alcohol and gambling to hide the pain – and to advice from his friends who had also left war-torn Germany. Those men advised Karl at his wedding, "Beat her if she doesn't behave." When Daisy heard this, she realized she was in real trouble.

Her parents knew unconditional love for their children. The wedding that they missed was never again mentioned. Life continued as one big family that included a son-in-law. It was the unconditional caring of her family that gave her strength and grounding through the years to come.

In the privacy of Daisy's married life she was barely out of her teen years and had no idea about how to deal with her husband's problems, have babies, work to support her family, all at the same time. She had no prior experience with any of his vices that cost him all his income, but especially in the deep-seated root of his problems – he was a casualty of war. She had no idea why Christmas, her favourite time of year, caused her husband to get angry and refuse to celebrate, including refusal to have a Christmas tree in the house. Reaching out, she was disappointed in the failure to find adequate counselling. There simply was no professional help available. She tried the Lutheran church minister, the same man who married them, with no luck; his statement that he would beat her, too, struck a fear that there was no hope. She called police. In keeping with the times, they told her they would not interfere in domestic matters.

It was okay with Karl to leave, with no notice, several times with no promise to return, but not okay for Daisy to leave. In desperation, Daisy had run away several times with one, then two, then three babies, to her parents' home and finally to rent an apartment. When her husband continued to come after her and reunions failed, she jumped into the arms of another man just to make sure she could never return to her marriage. He was a photographer she met at her work in the government office.

At work, she was busy typing but suddenly was aware that a man she had never seen before was leaning over a filing cabinet gazing at her. Her first impression was that she did not like him. He explained that he was the government photographer. His studio was beside her office and he had been watching her for some time. She had been unaware of him. Now he wanted to do her portrait and he was inviting her on a day excursion to photograph prairie crocuses with him. It sounded like fun and a change in pace. Instead of listening to her gut, she accepted the invitations and entered a new relationship to escape her marriage.

With her new common-law partner Eric, who was a former Air Force photographer, Daisy was learning new things. He taught her how to be a professional photographer and how to camp in the bush Air Force style. Their friends were artists and the university crowd. They built and ran the first bohemian style coffee house in Regina while she took a new job at the Saskatchewan Arts Board to support it. They explored the esoteric. The idea of Heaven and Hell was being torn down and replaced with countless questions. Encountering ideas from the Far East caused uncomfortable feelings. Daisy's grounding during this period was in remembering that her mother and father seemed comfortable with 'knowing' and questioning, talking and reading about these things. And Daisy remembered that she had seen spirits as a toddler. It was the idea of reincarnation that spooked her.

Alan Watts came to town. In his lecture he asked the question, "If you peel an onion, what are you left with in the centre after all the layers are peeled away?"

That one lecture had a profound effect on Daisy, opening the door to years of questioning and research.

After Eric's unfaithfulness in Regina, he wanted to start over by moving to Toronto. To prove Daisy's spirituality, Eric asked her to give the gift of her walnut dining room suite to the woman he had been unfaithful with. Daisy agreed – kicking herself later for not giving it to her own sister.

On moving to Toronto, Daisy and Eric gravitated toward Buddhism when her youngest sister invited them to meet a Buddhist monk newly arrived in town. From that meeting, they became founding members of the Dharma Centre in Kinmount, Ontario.

On a first trip with the teacher, Ananda Bodhi, to the acreage that would become the meditation centre, Daisy sat down on the ground beside a grove of trees to meditate for a few minutes and the intense knowledge came to her that this place would have a profound effect on her life. Within a few weeks, Daisy found herself living there in the old log cabin with a new baby and three children, and no modern conveniences. She had become the cook, dishwasher and caretaker of hundreds of people who came and went, some of whom were monks and teachers from near and far.

While living there, Daisy had been given some second-hand clothing by a female guest. Daisy had been wearing the rust colored corduroy jeans for only a few minutes when she knew Eric had sex with the woman who had worn the pants.

Asking them both about it the same day, they admitted it to be true. It was then Daisy realized that the many indications in the past had been correct. Eric had been continually unfaithful. She also realized that wearing other people's clothing was too dangerous for her. She needed to protect herself from the intense vibrations of others.

Finality seemed to follow when a few men were sitting around meditating and Daisy joined them. Her meditation experience seemed normal to her as she expanded into the powerful, giant being as she had done before. She was aware of being timeless and watching her hand move and seeing it in all positions at the same time. Suddenly all the men, including Eric, jumped up at once as though in pain and complained that Daisy was too powerful in the same room as them and that they felt her mind was overpowering their minds. Daisy left the room and from the kitchen she could hear them telling her to stop. The last thing she wanted was to invade their minds and did not think she was doing that. She worked at shrinking to feel less aware and less powerful.

She already had one baby with Eric and was newly pregnant with another. It was a cold, snow covered winter day when Eric walked out the door to find work in Toronto because they were broke and still feeding many visitors. As she watched his red plaid jacket go out the door, she was suddenly hit with the strong realization that she had seen this scene before in some far reaches of her being and it accompanied the knowledge that he would never come back.

A few evenings later, while sitting with a monk by the fire in the pot bellied wood stove, she dozed off only to be startled awake with the distinct knowledge that Eric was at that very moment having sex with another of the women from the group. It was as though she had just been there and seen. This knowledge bore out to be absolute truth.

With two questions in mind, Daisy traveled to Toronto to confront the teacher about the behaviour of many people. She had also come with the question about her throat. While meditating the day before, she had opened the lower chakras but when the energy rose to her throat, it was like the finger of a flame that wagged around in her throat chakra but would not open it. Instead, it had caused a hot, sore throat.

Ananda Bodhi listened carefully and then disappeared into his kitchen for a few minutes while she sat and waited. He came back offering her a cup of hot broth. He was holding a mug with little purple violets painted on it; Daisy knew this meant he was friendly toward her.

"Drink this," he said as his taller than six-foot frame towered over her.

Looking at the steaming, cream coloured pool centring the flowers, she exclaimed, "But it's too hot!" She saw the humour in sounding like the three bears story.

"Drink it." His words were stern.

Daisy drank. The broth burned her mouth.

"It burned my mouth," she complained.

"Yes, your karma has been in your throat. This will clear it up. Regarding your question about the behaviour of certain people, I came to teach the sinners."

That answer seemed enough. Her throat cleared up immediately, allowing the throat chakra to open the next time she meditated.

Daisy imagined staying on the meditation centre but a move back to Toronto followed a dream where she found herself with her children in a car that was driving down a country road. They were stopped by a giant crack across the road. As a result, she knew her time at the meditation centre was over.

In Toronto, Eric continued playing with her emotions, flaunting girlfriends in her face while Daisy's belly was growing with his child. He denied the child was his while at the same time he informed Daisy that she was not as spiritually advanced as he and their friends because she would not sleep around.

There was a sudden rainstorm that flooded a staircase in her apartment. Slipping in water and falling down the whole flight of stairs while pregnant was a defining moment. Desperate to save self from emotional abuse, she ran away with her four children while six and a half months pregnant with her fifth; this time selling her negative retouching machine for the price of train tickets, piling a few belongings and the children on a train to go clear across the country to Vancouver. After debating the east coast or Montreal, the west coastal city was chosen because it promised easy access to nature with its beaches and mountains ringing the city – a place to bring up children and not need a car – she hoped.

A young woman on the train advised Daisy to live in Kitsilano. Within a few months Daisy was able to leave the eastside apartment for a run-down but liveable house near the beach in Kitsilano, a place where she found acceptance and a feeling of safety from judgment. No longer did she have to pretend that her husband was just away on a trip, but she could live freely as a single parent among the hippies and the U.S. war evaders. It seemed that the west coast people were far more accepting of people seeking freedom, or just needing a place of safety, than people were in other parts of the country.

People from Regina found her. She soon found her home had a large fishing boat under renovation in the backyard and Regina people crashing in her house. Amused, she thought if Edgar Cayce's predictions do happen, then at least she had a boat to float and save her children.

The people from Toronto and the meditation centre also came. They filled her house for a time. Her teacher, who had become a Tibetan Llama named Namgyal Rinpoche on a trip to the East, had also come several times, holding teaching sessions in her home.

During that time, she continued to learn to draw in her energy that seemed to want to expand way out and large. She just wanted to live a normal life and take care of her children.

Her living room was furnished with only cushions she had scrounged, a worn Persian rug she had bought from the Salvation Army for two dollars, and a lamp she had made with paper mache.

Her ten-dollar guitar that she was learning to play hung on the wall. Daisy had been vacuuming the room when the vacuum cord had made a perfect treble clef in the middle of the rug. She stopped to stare at it and listen to the newest intuition. Music! Yes, *music* would be multiplying and a *doctor* would come to live with her.

The streets of Kitsilano were filled with people making music. Flutes and guitars could be heard from small grassy knolls filled with people not bothered by cars driving by. They sang about peace, love and social justice. Fourth Avenue was flourishing with small businesses like the beginnings of the organic food stores, a health food restaurant, a bookstore filled with books on eastern philosophies and esoteric subjects that the western world was just waking up to in a big way. There were the stages in small bistros lining the street where people gathered to listen to musicians.

Daisy was discovering herself as a separate entity, a person defined by her own self – the person she had not known since before her first marriage. She had been lost. The defining moment came to her while she was skipping across the benches above the outdoor stage of Kitsilano Showboat overlooking the ocean. Now she was found.

Later Daisy would decide that the three years spent with her common-law partner, father of her two youngest children, had been productive; they had been explorers together and neither life would be the same again even though they would never meet again.

ON AN AFTERNOON in October of 1968, Daisy was walking along 4th Avenue, pushing her youngest two babies in a white baby carriage bought at the Salvation Army store. Her oldest three children were in school. Feeling whole and good inside herself with the warm autumn sun on her face, happy to be living in Vancouver, she had come from a walk on the beach to shop for groceries. Actually, the walk on the beach had included a few minutes of lying in the sand and meditating on a grain of sand and the truth that one can get completely entranced in one grain of sand.

A beat up old car stopped beside her. The driver behind the wheel with a big smile on her face was her old friend from the university crowd of Regina. She and Daisy had recently rekindled their old friendship after finding each other in Vancouver for similar reasons. Beside her friend was a tall, dark-haired man with shining eyes. He had seen Daisy walking and expressed a wish to meet her. Introductions were made through the car window and they drove off.

At the time, Daisy had decided that in no way was there the need to go searching for another man to enter her life. She was content in the belief that opportunity would knock on her door when the time was right. There had been many knocks on the door over the months by men wanting a relationship. Often she would feed them some soup and play her guitar to entertain herself when they hung around too long but she had refused them all. No one had appealed to her, although she had been amazed and amused at the number of men who claimed to want a relationship with her and a ready-made family of five children. A couple of nineteen-year olds tried to convince Daisy they were sexually a best match for a thirty-year old woman like her. She was amused but not interested.

That evening she had made a very garlicky snack out of a wheat cereal, eaten it, and was surely stinking to high heaven when there was a knock on the door.

To her surprise, the man met earlier that day was at the door. She invited him in. His story was that he had gotten his PhD in Anthropology from McGill, taught at Regina University the past few months, and was now starting his travels around the world. They simply talked for a couple of hours and then he left. She thought he had gone out of her life for good.

Instead of traveling the world, he went back to Montreal and headed west again in his Peugeot station-wagon packed with his belongings, to knock on Daisy's door a second time.

Saul held the title of doctor because of his doctorate in Anthropology, and he immediately started to learn to play the flute, standing daily exactly in the spot of the treble clef to practice his flute. His first gift to Daisy was a piano, followed by fulfilling her wish for a pedal harp, and he replaced her cheap guitar with a great sounding new one.

Daisy was convinced he was the doctor of her premonition – not realizing another doctor, the love of her life, would come into her life much later.

Never the less that was the beginning of the next twelve years that Saul's mother never forgave Daisy for. On their seventh Christmas together, his parents were guests in the Vancouver home. As Daisy was setting the Christmas Eve dinner table, Saul's mother brushed up beside her, saying, "My friends tell me that because you have not gone away in seven years, I might as well accept you."

Daisy said nothing, just smiled. She always knew that the mother played a major influential role in Saul's life. His mother missed the social events the two had enjoyed together all through his university years. Daisy also surmised that her own days with Saul were numbered and it would only be a matter of time before the mother won her boy back.

Then as the twelfth year came around, Daisy had a dream: Saul's mother handed her a small glass box with a large crack across the top and said, "It is time." Daisy woke up knowing her time with Saul was ending. Within a couple of weeks, it did.

GETTING A DIVORCE would be a new freedom from a discarded and forgotten first marriage that happened long before all these changes. Daisy's first step was the need for legal advice. She chose to save money and call on the free clinic with law students from the university to answer initial questions about how to do it. She had an evening appointment but the street door was locked.

Daisy had felt critical of Carolyn for divorcing Ken to marry a bigamist, but as she stood on the street wondering what to do, she realized that on some level she had also been a bigamist, or trigramist, or whatever it might be called. The difference was that she had not signed legal papers for a second or third marriage. Feeling discouraged while looking at another blockage, she wondered about knowing the difference between the present and premonitions of the future that can sometimes be elusive in meaning. The realization hit that she may be trouble and she began to worry about fallout on Ken.

THINKING ABOUT THE PAST caused Daisy to think about what was different. Why was loving Ken different? There was magnetism between her and Ken that was a feeling of coming home. She had never before had that feeling. The love for Ken surpassed all surface infatuation, it was deeper than fleeting romantic fantasy; it would be sustainable through whatever should happen in life and no matter what age they would be.

She thought about what made Ken different. The other men had little to offer in deep communication; she always felt separate and unexplored. She had craved to be known. Ken fulfilled the need to communicate deeply. Ken wanted and satisfied deep intimacy. He explored her as she explored him, bringing up the question about where do we come from and where do we go and what are these intimate relationships that make us know we have come home in the other person where love is complete and unconditional. There was great satisfaction in exploring and knowing each other naked inside and out, backward and forward. Knowing was important to Ken and – he was different.

A NEW DAY DAWNED with Ken and Daisy wrapped in each other's arms while sleeping.

A nightmare woke Daisy. Breaking their embrace by springing upright very suddenly, Ken woke up wondering what happened.

She looked down at his sleepy gaze. "Ken, I was just being attacked by a large, rabid, red-haired dog. I know what it means. Jane has red hair. She is angry and is going to try to get revenge on us... or me... or you!

15

To the Kootenays

TO ATTEND his oldest son's high school graduation, Ken asked Daisy to accompany him to the Kootenays. Having no car because he had given his car to Jane, and Daisy did not own one or know how to drive, he rented a car. It was morning when they started the long drive from the coast to the interior of British Columbia.

Every morning Ken had been talking with Jane or the nanny on the telephone regarding his son and concern about Jane's health. It had been excruciatingly tough for Ken since his separation because Jane was denying him access to see Andy. He had not seen his son since that morning in May. He was being punished but so was the child being punished. His wife seemed unconcerned about the fallout on their son. It was taking a toll on Ken. This morning, Ken had talked with her before getting into the car but continued talking about Andy and Jane during the first half hour of leaving town.

Realizing increasing discomfort, Daisy blurted, "I think there are three of us in this car. Jane has come along."

On cue, the car shrugged and shook as though answering. They limped into a Langley service station near the highway. The car was diagnosed a lemon; another had to be delivered.

A couple of hours later and a fresh start to the trip, Ken decided he must contain his worries better and not constantly wear them loudly on his sleeve. Ken missed his son every moment and Daisy could not change that or make it better. More than that, he was plain homesick to be with his son. Getting together twelve years after meeting in 1969 was too late because other people had come between them. The dilemma was invisible – feelings woven into the threads of life and players unable to reweave the cloth of life to fix mistakes made.

The saying that if you weave a mistake into a rug, the rug becomes perfect popped into Daisy's mind. She wondered how that could be true in lives lived or if ever a life had been lived without mistakes. It was obvious that this man beside her was suffering a terrible loss and even if he managed to be quiet about it, the loss was constant – his pain was constant and she could not fix it.

LATE IN THE AFTERNOON, they arrived deep in the forested Kootenay mountains to a large home made of golden coloured logs sitting on a ridge high above a blue lake. Ken was tired after hours of driving. It was a relief that Carolyn invited them inside for tea.

While drinking tea around the kitchen table, his teenaged boys wandered in briefly and went out again. It was immediately apparent that no love was lost on Carolyn's part for Ken. She was polite but her way of speaking seemed crusty, or maybe it was just the brusque, bossy way of talking that Daisy thought typical of some nurses.

Ken, on the other hand, was clearly softer in nature and in speaking. If Daisy had not seen this man and this woman together twelve years earlier with small children, she would never have guessed they were ever man and wife - nor that they could ever be intimate together to make children. The match eluded her.

Seated beside a window and wanting to find something easy to talk about, Daisy tried a compliment, "You have such a beautiful view of the lake from here," but her voice sounded childish to her own ears.

Carolyn ignored her. Instead, she faced directly at Ken from across the table and spoke bluntly with no light inflections in her voice, "I want you to take the boys to live with you. Stephen is graduating now and Peter is going to graduate next year. It's time for them to think about college, so it's your turn."

"What do the boys want?" Ken asked.

"It's what I want," Carolyn droned. "Also, you owe me money."

Ken was surprised. "I've paid you maintenance. What do I owe money for this time?"

Again with no tonal inflections, Carolyn answered, "Stephen smashed up my car."

"I did not give him your car to drive," Ken answered.

Unfazed, Carolyn's voice was still monotone, matter-of-factly droning on, "I want four hundred dollars for the damage your son did to my car. You can take your sons after you give me money for my car."

This woman's way of thinking stunned Daisy and what she found out by listening is that what little Ken told her about Carolyn's behavior toward him over the past years had to be true.

Ken was less surprised. He had been down this road before. "Stephen crashed it. I didn't. I had nothing to do with it. You want me to take the boys but you want money I don't owe you in order to take them. How does that figure?"

"You are their father." Carolyn was more agitated now. A spark lit her voice. "This is the third time he has wrecked my car!"

"Maybe he is wrecking your car for a reason. Have you thought of that?" Ken posed an important question and at the same time remained calm.

Instead of answering to Ken, she directed herself at Daisy. "By the way, there is a tent set up outside for you to sleep in." It was obvious that Carolyn wanted Daisy out of the way.

"Thank you." Daisy got up to leave the house. She was surprised at being invited to stay and not have to go miles into town to a hotel but now she was uneasy about leaving Ken to fend for himself with Carolyn, not that she could help anyway.

For what seemed like an eternity, Daisy stayed in the tent, not feeling welcome enough to wander around. She knew only too well that Ken chose not to escape but bravely stayed to talk with his family. One thing seemed clear – Ken was soft and Carolyn was anything but soft and he was not frightened of her. Daisy pondered Ken's lack of fear of his first wife versus his extreme fear of his second wife who on the surface seemed softer.

Tired after the trip, she dozed off while analyzing Ken's fear of Jane and no fear of Carolyn. She was wakened by the sound of the family, including Ken, getting into a car and driving off to the graduation. The sound of the car grew quiet in the distance – then nothing.

It was quiet in the Kootenay mountains. She waited with only the sound of crickets to keep her company. A porch light was on but other than a few feet of dim light, the surroundings turned black. A serene treat happened as the sky filled with twinkling stars and planets like nothing seen in Vancouver. It looked like the winter nights on the prairies of her childhood.

Finally there was the sound of the car coming back; then the sound of people getting out of the car, followed by the sound of Ken's soft footsteps across the grass, coming closer.

Ken entered the tent and laid down fully clothed beside Daisy. She reached for his hand. He did not respond. He was completely still on his back, inconsolable, eyes staring at the top of the darkened tent, hands across his chest. She withdrew her hand. She had never before seen him like this.

Breaking the silence, she asked, "How was the graduation?"

"Okay, I guess." His speech was stilted.

"I didn't get to see much of your sons. How are they doing?"

"My sons are estranged from me... angry that I left them." He was breathing hard.

"How can they blame you?"

"It hardly matters who is to blame. Every time I come near that woman to see my kids, she extorts money from me. The boys think only about money. They have none of my values... only hers."

"She wants you to take the boys to the city. Are you going to pay her for the car?"

"Yes, I'll relieve the tension by paying her. The boys can come when they are ready. They've made it clear to me they don't want to leave here for the city."

Daisy reached once more for Ken. This time he allowed her to take his hand. They were silent, listening to the sound of the crickets.

Ken broke the silence. "I'll have to rent an apartment big enough for my boys for a while. I need to take care of them, re-educate them... teach them that there is more to life than money. They will wreck havoc on your family. I can't allow that."

"I really want us to be one big family in one house. I'm up for it."

"You don't know those guys. They won't let it happen."

"I won't come between you and your kids. We did promise to let each other be free to look after our children. I understand."

Understand? What did Daisy understand? She was not convinced that any job was too big. She felt strong and capable of a larger family. On the other hand, in one day she had come face to face with the realization that her best efforts to make this man happy and fill his life with love and what she believes to be the gift of her wonderful family, may not be enough. The hole in his life, where there had been his hopes and dreams in his children, could never be filled. Even if all three sons would come to live with them, Ken would still have a hole where there had been years of unfulfilled fatherhood and all the associated problems of children alienated from him. It was not just the loss of Jane and Andy, it was also Peter and Stephen and all the lost years.

Ken wondered what he has done to this woman beside him. The last thing he wanted to do was disappoint a third woman, especially one who was reaching out to him so completely open and honest. He had asked her to marry him and now he realized that his children must come first. Responsibilities and promises made were overwhelming in all directions.

ALONG THE DIRT ROAD before coming to the highway, they made a joint decision that instead of heading home, they would drop in on Daisy's sister Marilyn and her husband at their ranch outside of Calgary. Somehow, the idea of going in the opposite direction gave them the needed break away from all responsibilities and troubles for a few hours – a time for breathing.

Arriving at the exciting time when cows and their calves were being rounded up for transfer to foothill pastures of the Rocky Mountains for the summer, Daisy was invited to take a horse and help with the roundup. She was happy to participate in an innocent roundup – no animals being hurt. She disliked saddles and the bouncing on a horses back that most riders did. Bareback had always been her favorite way to ride. Surprising everyone, she hopped onto the horse with only a bridle. She and the horse became one as she melded with his body, feeling each muscle of the horse and working together. She and her sister's cowboy husband worked the cattle together, much to his surprise. He kept grinning in admiration at her agility. She worked the sides of the field, jockeying the perimeters, gathering up strays. With the wind in her hair and a horse to ride, she found bliss.

Ken watched in surprise and fascination from the fence along with Daisy's sister.

Finished and exhilarated, Daisy rode up to Ken, stopping the horse in front of him.

She had never seen him looking so freely excited. She did find a way to make him truly happy in the moment after all.

"You are amazing!" he exclaimed. "I've never seen anyone do that without a saddle. Can I ride with you?"

"Sure, hop on behind me. You can step on the fence to boost yourself up." She sidestepped the horse to meet Ken.

Once behind her, she could feel his excited warm body against hers, his breath on her neck and his arms firmly around her waist.

He spoke softly into her neck. "You are the person I have wanted to be with all my life. You are full of surprises."

"And you are my dream come true... to ride with you through life," she answered.

They had found an eon of peace in this small space of time with a horse, the smell of a farm, the immense sky, fresh warm air on their faces, and the joy of being together... bodies close and sincere sweet words being exchanged.

16

Timing

BACK IN VANCOUVER, Ken and Daisy were happily lounging in the sunlit bedroom on the third floor of the False Creek townhouse, reading to each other from a large book.

Daisy paused to look at Ken. "Chagall is my favorite painter. Thank you so much for this book. He paints like I experience the world. Life is not linear. Many things happen all at once. And after living in the far North where earth seems not to be separate from space, I came to understand his way of painting things in all directions. I saw Inuit people read upside down as well as right side up. They seem to see things more circularly, like Chagall."

"I want to paint with you. You can teach me how to paint."

"I want to paint with you, too."

"And I want to sing with you. We can finally enjoy life together. I am really Ferdinand the Bull."

Daisy laughed, "I thought you were a workaholic and here you are lying under the tree with me, smelling the flowers."

Turning a page, she exclaimed, "Look, here's the print I have in the living room. It's Chagall's self-portrait. I need to tell you a story. ...Well, when I was sleeping on the sofa by myself and wondering where sex had gone, I woke up to see a giant penis on the wall above me. Chagall painted himself as a big penis. See the droopy one in the corner and the giant upright one across the whole picture. I never saw it in the painting before that moment even though it had hung on my wall for years and when I ask people about the painting, they don't see it either until I tell them."

There was sudden interruption by thunder on the staircase. Ballerinas! It had always been a joke that dancers can walk like elephants. Loraine and Lana bounced into the room.

Loraine excitedly announced, "Mom! Ken! We want to go and pick up Stephen and Peter today."

"I don't think they are ready," Ken cautioned.

"But we are anxious to meet our prospective new brothers," Loraine argued.

Lana agreed, "Yes, we want to meet them."

"I don't believe they want to come," Ken responded again.

"We'll find that out when we are there," Lana laughed.

Ken's caution was ignored. Daisy did nothing to intervene as the girls left immediately in Loraine's small, old, red car.

Ken became visibly alarmed. "Daisy, I tried to tell you the boys are not ready. We should wait until they want to come."

JUNE 30th, 1981. Ken and Daisy were preparing dinner as the girls arrived home with Stephen and Peter who were reluctantly cordial as they came through the door.

Loraine was excited about a broken car. "My steering broke just a couple of blocks from here. I can't believe it. What luck!"

"Turn that around!" Daisy told her. "You are lucky! You drove through mountain passes – not once but twice – there and back, driving on the edge of steep cliffs, and your steering broke only two blocks from home where you could safely walk home. I'd call that good luck."

EVERYONE WAS SEATED around the dining table and starting to eat when Peter spoke up, "This spaghetti sauce is too lumpy. My mother makes a smooth sauce." He was genuinely distressed.

Daisy was surprised. This was the first complaint ever about the meal she always cooked when expecting unexpected guests as often happened in her household, so that there was always enough to go around. It was lumpy with fresh tomatoes and other vegetables, lots of meat, and deliberately not like the canned versions sold in stores. She assumed her family was well nourished because they always ate her sauce with gusto. Daisy's oldest son had affectionately nicknamed spaghetti and pizza "good old Canadian food" because of her habit of experimenting with cooking food from different cultures and not always to his liking. Ringing of the telephone interrupted her thoughts. Even though the telephone was situated near the dinner table, Daisy got up to face away.

Carolyn spoke loudly in her ear. "How's everything?"

"We're fine. They got here safely and are eating dinner now."

"Good. I want to tell you that no one should tell the boys anything about why Ken and I divorced."

Daisy was at first stunned, then miffed at orders that were obviously at Ken's expense. In those orders, it was clearly understood that Carolyn had spun her own yarn to her boys. Disgusted, Daisy managed to politely answer, "No one has. You can speak with them." She handed the telephone to the boys.

OUT ON THE SEAWALL, the usual evening stroll gave Daisy an opportunity to fill Ken in.

"Carolyn told me that no one should tell the boys why you and she divorced."

"I have never told them about her adultery. I figured they could talk to her about the divorce if they wanted to know. It was obvious that there was another man around that she did marry."

"But they are angry and blame you."

"Yes. It has been my choice not to talk with them about their mother."

"Ken, the girls tell me that when they arrived at Carolyn's place, she was naked in the garden. She has teenaged sons."

"I can't do anything about that."

"The boys don't seem very happy to be here. I wonder why they came."

"They are angry and are rejecting your family. They are rejecting your daughters in fear that they want something from them. I tried to tell you the boys are not ready to be here. No one would listen to me. Now I need to rent an apartment to take care of them."

"Yes, you did tell me. Hopefully they will come around and things will be alright."

"You don't know them. They might destroy your family. I can't let that happen. As their father, I'm obligated to care for them and their education but they aren't ready to live with your family."

IT HAD BEEN SIX WEEKS since Ken and Daisy started a relationship together. A lot had happened. Ken had been in increasing distress over his children. Daisy completed a month's notice at her previous job and had been working with Ken for two weeks. Ken's older sons arrived and were living with Daisy's family, at least temporarily in a bright, shared bedroom – the best one in the house with big windows overlooking the park and inlet waters.

Ken had not been allowed to see his youngest son since the day he left Jane even though he had called daily to talk with Jane, continued financial support, and continued to have productive conferences with the nanny. Now on the same day as his two teenaged sons were angry at being brought to Vancouver, Ken had unexpectedly been told by Jane that he would be allowed to take his youngest son out the next day. Daisy could not help wondering if this sudden change was in competition with the older sons, to keep attention in her direction.

JULY 1ST, STARTED EARLY as Ken arrived at Jane's house to pick up his son. It appeared to be going all right until he was carrying his son to the car. On the public street Jane suddenly started a loud scene about taking her son away. Ken was shaken.

It was a no win situation. Ken could not turn his back on his traumatized child and walk away. He could not stay where he was not wanted. His sympathy for Jane was overridden by the child's apparent need to spend time with him. But Ken already knew that what lay waiting for him in False Creek was two sons who had large chips on their shoulders.

Daisy wondered about the public scene that Jane made. Was it staged? On the other hand, she was sympathetic about a mother whose child was leaving for a visit with another woman. She remembered how her own stomach ached when she was leaving work and standing on a street corner to see the van go by with Saul taking her daughters to meet his new girl friend. Never the less, Daisy was more concerned about Ken and his small child.

On arrival in False Creek, Ken took Andy out to play in the park to unwind and to concentrate on this small boy who he loved with his life and needed to re-establish a relationship with.

It was Canada Day. Living in the midst of a large park on the waterfront, celebrations were happening in the public areas and on the water right in front of the townhouse.

Ken and the blond, curly haired two-year-old could be seen from the front patio of the townhouse as they played ball. Ken had sadness about him.

Daisy was in the kitchen when friends dropped in. They were a middle-aged, married couple Daisy had known for many years and who had adopted sons from two different countries. Ken's sons came into the room to see what was going on.

Making introductions, Daisy proudly announced, "Peter and Stephen are Ken's sons, and going to be my step-sons."

The boys glared dirty looks all around and walked away.

The visitors were visibly embarrassed. They made excuses to leave immediately to attend the park celebrations.

Daisy felt humiliated. She had been slapped hard in front of friends with the realization that these boys felt strongly about never joining her family.

Out on the patio, Lana and Loraine had several friends visiting and were introducing Stephen and Peter.

Loraine explained, "These guys are going to be our new brothers."

Stephen and Peter scowled in disgust.

Peter grunted, "My father is a jerk." Then he muttered, "Look at him with that kid."

Stephen said, "Our mother told us he is supposed to have lots of money like our friend's father who is a psychiatrist, too. She says it is our turn to get it."

The girls and friends listened with open mouths.

Peter continued, "But he doesn't give it to us. He went off and had another kid. I don't even like the way he dresses. Our friend's father wears a suit."

Sorting books in the bookshelves near the open patio doors, Daisy could hear clearly what was being said. She stopped to look past the teenagers to watch Ken in his comfortable navy blue jogging suit and running shoes, playing ball with his two-year old child.

In an exasperated response, she decided to take this on. She walked over to the doorway and invited the boys in.

They slowly follow her into the room, leaving gaping teenagers on the balcony.

"You are insulting your father in public."

Peter fought back. "He's a jerk! He left us and had another kid!"

Daisy warned, "I expect you both to treat your father with respect and do not insult him in front of other people. Understood?"

The boys did not answer.

In her steam, Daisy marched out to see Ken, interrupting him with his youngest son. "Ken, your sons are saying insulting things about you to the girls' friends."

Ken looked at her as he caught a ball. "I know. What did you expect?" He was curt. "I'm busy." He turned away and continued to play with his son.

Ken had never before spoken to her in that manner. It was not what he said but the desperate sadness in his words and the tiredness of his face that really stopped her in her tracks. The extent of the blunder to let her daughters forge ahead regardless of Ken's cautionary warning was obvious. Timing! In their zeal to include Ken and his sons, Daisy and her daughters had forgotten that timing is important.

AS EVENING FELL, Andy had to be returned to his mother along with a plate of food for her that the child asked for. Following this, Ken and Daisy strolled along the seawall on their usual evening walk. The lights of the city shone on the smooth water. Ken was hurt and unusually silent.

She broke the silence. "I thought we could be like the Brady Bunch as one big happy family."

"Brady Bunch?"

"Yes. You know, that family sitcom on television."

"I don't watch much television. The boys won't blend if they can help it. Jane made it clear that when college days come, the boys would not be allowed to live in her house. You are my only hope for a family. I don't want your family to suffer because of my kids. My sons are afraid of your daughters. They need more education in real life, not just college, before they are ready for your family. My responsibility is to take care of them now. I need to rent an apartment and live with them. Marriage will have to wait until they are ready."

"My kids are willing to include them. I feel really upset that our marriage has to be on hold but I understand."

Ken stopped walking to look at the water mirroring all the city lights. "Tonight," he said, "all the colour has disappeared from my vision." He turned to Daisy, "I haven't been able to see Andy since the separation. I am shocked at how little his eyes have become. It's as though his eyes have sunken into his head. I can see how much he misses me. I was his main caretaker, and then I disappeared. He kept pinching my cheeks to make sure I was real."

There it was in a nutshell of one day; the many problems Ken and Daisy were facing had surfaced. The making of the problems had built over many years and it would take time to solve all of them. There were damaged children hurting, some with preconceived notions and chips on their shoulders. One toddler wanted to feed his mother and in that was a baby who strived to be the caretaker of a grown woman. There were friends trying to escape the line of fire. Money was a root problem for the children who believed they were being cheated. There were ex-wives who seemed to have no notion of how to care for their children without causing emotional baggage for the children to carry. It would not be a matter of working out how to live together as a family but the problem was more about how to care for children needing so much healing. And there was the resentment against Ken that he was dealing with personally. Clearly, Ken needed time to help Jane. Nobody, except Ken foresaw the seriousness of the problems. By including his parents and siblings, there were four families on the wheel of life with Ken at the hub, and it was his love for all that held him to the wheel.

Daisy took Ken's hand as the rippling seawater put on a moving colourful light show with reflecting city lights. Only Daisy could see it. Ken's sorrow was too deep and she was helpless to fix it. Not only that, she felt responsible for it. Not in her wildest dreams, did she want to ruin Ken's life. Who said, 'Love will conquer all'? Only time would tell. Dreams of relying on love had in one day become elusive.

EACH EVENING Carolyn telephoned just when the family was having their evening meal together – always with the same message until Daisy no longer answered the telephone and just let the boys get it. She was tired of being told that no one should tell the boys the truth. She had complained to Ken about the interruptions to the evening meal and his answer was to tell Carolyn to call at a different time. Not wanting to interrupt communication between a mother and her sons, Daisy let the calls continue, but was resenting the constant interruption of supper that for years had been respected as family time.

On one of their walks along the seawall, she asked Ken again why he chose not to tell the boys the truth about the divorce. He repeated that he did not feel the need to tell them something they already knew because they were not so young that they would not notice another man around. He also did not think it productive to inform them about adultery or lay blame of any kind. He said again that it would take time for the boys to be re-educated after all the years of alienation and expectations of him to be a doctor making lots of money. "A simple talk will not undo the years of brainwashing."

DAISY WAS STANDING in the open doorway of the boys' bedroom, trying to have a friendly conversation with them when the telephone rang. Out of habit, Daisy reached for the nearest phone on a desk in their room. Big mistake! It was Lana phoning from Winnipeg. Aware of obvious discomfort in the room, she kept the call brief but the call triggered something in the boys. They were making critical remarks about their father again.

Daisy decided enough was enough. If Ken would not defend himself, then she would do it for him. She paused with a flicker of conflict in wanting to say what needed to be said and what she may not like herself for saying after she said it.

"And you believe your mother's story about why your father left you? Enough!" She sounded determined and got their attention. "I won't have you criticizing your father. Your father is too much of a gentleman to tell you his story. You are old enough to hear the truth. Your mother had another man in her life. Your father was forced to leave. It's time you stop blaming your father. Anything to say?"

Having come up against Daisy's fury, the boys were silenced for the first time with the realization they were not in charge.

She continued, "One more thing, your father paid maintenance to your mother for you guys and he had a right to start a new life for himself when he was divorced from your mother. Now he has taken the responsibility for your college or university education if you choose to go. Don't ever insult your father again!"

That evening while walking on the seawall, telling Ken what she did was difficult. He quietly accepted the news.

BETWEEN PETER'S CONSTANT complaining at dinner that the food was not like his mother's cooking and his mother phoning every evening as though she knew exactly when they were sitting down to eat, the peaceful family time of dining together had become a time of disenchantment, with the main focus going to one person.

Peter grunted again, "My mother makes a better roast beef."

Daisy looked sympathetically across the two candle flames to where he was seated. She knew her roast beef was always cooked so that no blood ran. She never was able to stomach blood on her plate and would never feed blood to her children. In actual fact, the beef was quite grey with a brown garlic and mustard flavored crust but she made terrific gravy and Yorkshire pudding to go with it. Having been a vegetarian in the past, she thought meat well done was a stretch. She responded to Peter, "You obviously miss her, maybe you should be living with your mother."

"She doesn't want us there." Peter's head sunk low toward his plate of food.

"Maybe you could be doing something you have always wanted to do. What would that be?" Daisy asked.

Peter's face brightened. "Ballet! Like your daughters." He chuckled, "That way I will meet lots of girls." He continued to giggle.

"Okay. Tomorrow we shall buy you proper gear and get you into ballet classes at their ballet school. It's straight up the hill from here." At that the telephone rang. Stifling a sigh because she knew who was calling, Daisy left the table to answer again because she had something to say.

As usual, it was Carolyn, just in time for another interruption of a meal. Carolyn spoke especially loud this time. "How's everything?"

"Peter misses you," Daisy said, bracing for an argument about Peter.

"Never mind that. I just want to be sure no one tells them anything."

"You mean other than your version of why your marriage ended in divorce."

Rather than responding, Carolyn had another agenda. Her voice was loud and bossy, "Daisy, I think you should be ashamed of yourself for taking a man away from his small child and the child's mother!"

Daisy answered quietly, "Oh? I don't think you understand the situation. Bye." She hung up to stop an impulse to say more.

Stunned again, Daisy's head rushed with anger at what that woman did to Ken by cheating him out of years of fatherhood and now Carolyn was brazen enough to criticize her. With the family eating their dinner within earshot, she had managed to hold her tongue and not retaliate, as she wanted to do. She sat at the table pretending all was well. Her face burned. Ken was having pleasant but light conversation with the family. It was extremely clear to Daisy that the boys were not to blame for their beliefs and desires.

PETER ENJOYED THE ADVENTURE into a previously unknown world of dance. Shopping with Daisy, he chose black ballet slippers and tights. He would wear a white T-shirt with them. Then they wandered down the street to sign him up for classes. There were dozens of girls in the school but only a couple of guys. This suited Peter just fine.

SUDDENLY THE HOUSE BULGED with unexpected guests. Ken's brother and sister-in-law had come from Vermont for a visit only a few days after Ken's sons arrived.

The day after arriving, the couple had been out for the afternoon without saying where they were going. Meanwhile, Ken and Daisy cooked dinner for their return.

"It's nice that your brother Dick has come to see you."

Ken responded happily, "What a surprise! Just to let you know, he prefers to be called Richard."

The door opened and Richard, a handsome middle aged man who seemed to have a permanent sun shining on his curly locks, and his wife Nancy, a pleasant heavy-set woman with dark hair enter the room. The energy that came through the door with them was intense.

Before the door closed behind them, Richard announced, "Nancy and I have just visited with Jane and Andy. She tells us that she is starving and having to sell her furniture for food, Ken!" His statement was accusatory.

Ken looked confused, "How can that be?"

Daisy stated, "She must have stocked a pantry for a year and bought a lifetime of bras on the credit cards that Ken is paying. She has her nanny paid for, mortgage paid. She receives the equivalent of several thousand dollars a month. That's a lot of money. What more does she want?"

Embarrassed, Richard looked at the floor, "That's what she told us."

Daisy felt her dander rising. With eyes flashing, she faced Richard, "That makes me angry! Obviously it is to make Ken look bad; a show for you and who knows who else she is telling that to."

Richard looked at Ken, "Remember? I told you years ago she would outsmart you. I told you to be careful."

Ken responded quietly, "I remember."

Richard went on, "I told you to watch out for her, not to trust her. She's smarter than you."

Daisy interrupted again, "Her intelligence obviously goes in a different direction than Ken's. I feel the need to protect Ken from conniving ex-wives. Ken has offered to give all the assets to Jane and he will take all the debts. The assets are substantial and include the house and car, even though he is continuing to pay the mortgage for her until she is ready to sell, and who knows how long that will take. He and I agreed this is the best way to make sure Andy has all he needs. We've got his first wife telling lies to his sons and his second wife telling lies to you and who."

Richard clapped his hands together and an embarrassed smile crossed his face as he tried to get out of this mess by proclaiming, "The food looks *great!*"

With the door finally closed behind them, his wife looked confused as she stood near the door. Daisy observed that Nancy was a strong woman managing to keep quiet.

But Daisy could not let it go. "You're getting to know me at my worst. I'm sorry about that. I can't stand these women causing Ken problems with his family. Ken is entitled by law to keep half of all the assets. He is giving them all to Jane instead. He will get nothing from the house and he will carry all the marriage debts." Daisy was feeling awful about her outburst but in the face of what people were doing to Ken, she felt an overwhelming need to defend him. "Let's have dinner."

Ken looked as though he was going to be sick. He helped to carry food from the kitchen to the dining room table. Daisy had been raging loudly but true to his character, Ken was quieter in his hurt and bewilderment. Quietly, he ran though his mind that he believed he had done everything to give Jane and Andy security; he had paid for her schooling right through and was continuing to help financially and physically in support of her becoming a lawyer; he had given her all the money and assets of the marriage right down to the last penny and was continuing to pay monthly on a mortgage he will get nothing out of. The only things he took from the home were books and clothes. Most of all, he had gotten out of her way, believing that to be what she wanted.

DAISY'S CHILDREN had always participated in kitchen clean up, each having a particular job. Ken, Daisy, Richard and his wife had followed dinner with a stroll on the seawall, coming home to thousands of glass shards of wine glasses covering the dining room floor. When Daisy asked what happened, she was told that Peter broke wine glasses in retaliation to being asked to participate in the cleanup instead of giving the job entirely to Faith, the only one of Daisy's children at home that evening for dinner. Faith had a broken shoulder in a full cast. With only one working hand, Faith needed help. All that was required was to help clearing the table and put dishes in the dishwasher. That was too much for Peter.

Daisy called up the stairs to Peter. He responded by racing thunderously from his room, down the stairs, past the stunned guests and out the open patio door into the darkness of the park.

Daisy was shocked at her own unraveling. As she cleaned up broken glass, she apologized to Richard, "I'm sorry. You are certainly seeing me at my worst."

AFTER A FEW more mishaps during and following the visit of their uncle, who had gone, the boys called a family meeting. In the wisdom of a sixteen-year old spokesperson, Peter explained what had been going on from his point of view. He felt that no household duties should fall upon him because they were used to having a housekeeper do chores, and sharing a bedroom was not his or his brother's style. He explained that they expected a Vancouver townhouse on the waterfront to be a mansion on a beach and this co-op townhouse did not measure up. He said their mother had told them that since Saul had taught at the university, he must have left lots of money behind and they were planning to cash in on it. Then Peter explained that their mischief was supposed to get rid of Daisy and her family, so that the boys could take over the house. He explained that it had always worked in the past to get rid of housekeepers, so the only question was, "Why are Daisy and her kids not leaving?"

Peter's reasoning put a new perspective on what had been a trying time. Out of respect, no one laughed but the absurd wisdom of a couple of rebellious boys in their teens was comical to Daisy.

Out on the seawall, Daisy told Ken how amused she was. Ken was less amused. He had known the depth of the problem and was not surprised.

In the meantime, unknown to Daisy and Ken, while they were talking by the water, the boys packed their bags and took off, making their escape to the house of the supposedly rich psychiatrist to bunk with his son. This was their solution to better their situation and stick their noses up at their own father.

DAYS AND WEEKS went by with no change. Ballet outfit and prepaid dance classes went to waste.

Ken told Daisy, "I don't want it to be a competition between my family and yours. I have a responsibility to my sons. I promised."

"Peter just hates the food I cook."

"I can't imagine why. Their mother has had housekeepers look after them while she traveled and did her own thing. Over the years, they complained to me that they were mostly hungry."

"Are they talking to you now?"

"They are unavailable to me. They were complaining about your daughters and now they are hiding out. They have no idea of how to live with girls. I need to rent an apartment for when they emerge."

The suddenness of the boys' arrival and leaving had caused a serious upheaval. Daisy considered it her own failure and wondered what she could have done differently but not be run over. Most of all, Ken was being bullied from all sides and she hated that, so how could she have stayed silent? Her own family had retreated. Her boys barely came around. Lana had been relieved to get back to Winnipeg summer school and get away from the antagonism directed toward her by Ken's sons. Loraine busied herself with her friends and work, and ignored them. Faith wondered what happened and escaped into the park with her friends.

Ken was determined not to abandon his sons and hopefully to re-educate them with some of his own values in life and work, but not at the expense of another family.

IN STANLEY PARK on Sunday afternoon, Ken and Daisy sat on the base of a large memorial to Canadian soldiers of Japanese descent who lost their lives serving in World War I. Andy was climbing around the stone base. The day was sunny and comfortably warm enough not to need coats. Many people of all ages milled about, enjoying the park. A soldier, dressed in a heavy World War I winter coat, cap, pants, black leather boots, and carrying a big, old-fashioned brown suitcase in his right hand, walked with large firm strides across the field from left to right, looking straight ahead. Ken and Daisy watched in surprise as the soldier walked into a wall of dense bush that had no opening or pathway and disappeared.

Ken looked at Daisy, "Did you see him?"

"Yes, I saw a soldier walk across the field right into that bush."

"Carrying a large suitcase? And wearing World War 1 clothes?"

"Yes, dressed for winter."

"No one else seems to have seen him," Ken said.

This was an obvious encounter with another reality. Ken and Daisy were able to share the same experience without any convincing or need for explanation. Life just got simpler on one level. They could be together in time and no time.

17

A Question of Reconciliation

"I'M WORRIED about my son."

"You must go back to Jane."

"Don't push me back to Jane."

"I don't want you to go."

"I have to go."

"You may as well go back to Jane, you are always on the phone with her."

"I have to go."

"I don't want you to go, but you have to go."

"I don't want to go, but I have to go."

"Don't go."

"I have to go. I have never before been away from my son. I was his caretaker. He needs me. Maybe her anger is because she wants me back."

"Have her friends moved in with her?"

"No, not yet anyway."

"Do you want to go back?"

"I'm frightened of what she will do to herself or to my son. I have to put that concern before my own safety."

"You must go back but I'm afraid you will die because of emotional abuse."

"She is managing that whether I live with her or not. I have a prior responsibility to my son and to her. He has never known life without me before I left them. I regret the way I left. I never meant to cause her pain. I believed she wanted me gone."

"Does she want you back?"

"She won't talk to me about what happened. I still don't know the name of the truck that hit me!"

"I'm afraid for you."

"I should never have moved in with you right away. I should have had my own apartment. Then it would have been clearer between Jane and myself. She is so angry about you that a clear picture is difficult."

"What about your other sons? She didn't want them living with her."

"They won't talk to me anyway. I had hopes you could help me with them."

EVERY EVENING on the seawall under the turquoise sky that became a starry blue-black canopy that summer, the arguments continued far from everyone who might overhear except when their voices rose and carried across the water that mirrored city lights in a duality that reflected the turmoil of Daisy and Ken. Back and forth, Ken and Daisy fought about who was breaking up their relationship and whether or not Ken should go back to live with Jane and Andy.

The miraculous magnetic attraction that caused their paths to cross for twelve years over a continent from seashore to seashore, then to cause a union, was giving way to responsibilities and promises made to others during those twelve years.

To resolve the problem, Ken arranged to attend therapy sessions with Jane in another attempt to honour his marriage vows and reconcile with his wife. The blonde hotshot therapist, recently making a name for herself on an anchored houseboat, was supposed to have the newest and greatest techniques.

AS THEY WALKED along the seawall, Ken told Daisy, "In the sessions, we do a lot of hitting each other with pillows. There is a lot of anger directed at me but no sign of her wanting me back. The only thing I get out of this therapy is that she wants to see what more she can make me do for her. I clean her house. I wash her car. I spend as much time as I can caring for Andy in her home and out. I take her out to dinner but there is nothing coming back other than that she can't stand having me around when the jobs are done."

"Has it ever dawned on you that maybe you were right to leave the marriage?

"I regret leaving my son."

"Yes, but maybe you had no choice in leaving. You only thought you did. Maybe she just wants the world to know that you left her and what a bad man you are. You know... playing the victim!"

With Ken trying to reinstate his marriage, Daisy found it easy to ignore her own divorce and to forget again that she was ever legally married. It seemed like another lifetime anyway. Divorce? What divorce? What marriage? Uppermost in Daisy's mind was her own conflict between supporting Ken's struggle to reconcile with his wife and child – the fear for his life in doing so – the dread of losing Ken once again – feeling responsible for his losses because of her own seduction of him – and the determination to remain lifelong friends through it all and not lose him entirely again... and wishing both ex's would go away so that she and Ken could settle down together.

Turning to divination with the I Ching, Daisy unwrapped the yarrow sticks collected so long ago from the grounds of the meditation centre in Ontario. The special orange scarf used to wrap them for safekeeping was spread out on the table. A burning candle and incense were centered at the top of the scarf. The I Ching book used as a reference lay on her left side. She centered herself with a prayer.

In answer to Daisy's question about any future with Ken, the I Ching was clear that Ken and Daisy would grow old together and be together until death.

The question then became: What is destiny? If this divination is true, and at the time it was hard to believe, then all the people jumping up and down trying to destroy a relationship could only make trouble but nothing more with destiny at work. The future will tell.

The outcome of several weeks of the hotshot therapy was an agreement to have a divorce with Ken taking the blame for adultery with Daisy.

18

A Lawyer's Agenda

EACH YEAR IN AUGUST, Daisy's family traveled from the three western provinces of Canada to meet at her brother Bill's apiary farm in Alberta. It was an ideal place for a two week family reunion; a place where each person in the large gathering had acres of space on which to visit, rest, take in nature, ride horses, stay up late or rise early, and to play or work. Most of all, it was a time for the children to know their extended family.

Harvest time, 1981. At the same time as Daisy's family was planning their reunion, Ken's family was planning a family reunion in Vermont. Ken and Daisy discussed the situation and decided to visit Alberta because going to Vermont without Andy and the separation of thousands of miles by air travel seemed unbearable and Ken's sons had not yet returned. He wanted to be close at hand for all three.

Daisy had been in the habit of piling kids, animals, friends, anything or anyone into the car for the trip. This time, with a dog and her two youngest daughters, she took Ken on the twelve hundred kilometer trip across the mountains. She also took a lot for granted, like traveling with a dog without consultation and expecting Ken to drive all the way without a second driver. Even though they spent a pleasant night in a cabin on a lake halfway there, Ken was tired. She had thought she was low maintenance but now the kind of pressure she put on a man was plain.

While driving, Ken grew quieter, mulling over disloyalty to his own family. Ken missed Andy. Daisy was aware.

As day gave way to evening and the farm was near, with their dog nestled between them, the girls sang as they always had. They had made up a song years ago about the bumpy, gravel road. As they neared Edmonton area, Northern Lights danced brilliantly across the sky. Waves and swirls of changing colour wove in and out of darkening blue. As the girls sang, Ken stepped into Daisy's past.

On a rough gravel road, they approached the farm. White boxes for beehives, not presently in use because the honey had already been extracted, were piled high between a grove of Poplar trees and the giant prairie barn. The driveway was on the other side. "There's my brother's barn. Turn in at the mailbox," Daisy instructed.

The extended family of all ages had been expecting them. Finally Ken could be introduced. Children, glad to meet with each other again, took up as though they had never been apart.

Ken had already met Daisy's mother and he had spoken fondly of her as a reminder of his own gentle grandmother. Her mother seemed somehow to be too good for this world, living innocently making friends in the garden with all the insects and birds; she would enjoy communicating with the smallest of this world. She sang lullabies to her babies as she rocked them and as they grew she would sing happy, lilting songs to her children and grandchildren. Her precious flower garden each summer provided hours of colour and peace – and a fond memory was of her amidst the glorious blooms handing Daisy a flower to draw. In the evenings, while her husband was working the night shift, Daisy's mother would read, and read, and read far into the night. Daisy got curious and was introduced to reading about the esoteric. Here at the farm, family looked forward to the grandmother cooking family favorites like Ukrainian cabbage rolls, homemade perogies, and German noodles.

Daisy's mother was the daughter of a Ukrainian man with a Norwegian name who had owned his own vineyard and hotel but was also a casual soldier on horseback in the army. He had defied government orders by refusing to carry out cruel acts against people. He helped the people instead. A close relative was nabbed and sent to hard labor in Siberia, never to be heard from again and only remembered through Grandfather's stories. With a bounty placed on his head, Grandfather left everything behind and escaped to Canada. Daisy grew up admiring the handsomely quiet and sad, real live hero. He spent the rest of his life and his money earned hard, by working for the Canadian Pacific Railway in Regina, to bring people, one by one, out of the Ukraine to Canada. Because of him, dozens of people live free in Canada.

One winter when Daisy was around twelve years old, her grandfather gave his wool coat to his daughter to make into a coat for Daisy. With five children to clothe, it was a blessing to have the coat. Daisy's mother took it apart, turned the material inside out and sewed a new coat for Daisy. The coat felt as though her grandfather's arms were keeping her safe and warm in the prairie blizzards – and she thought a lot about what he did, resisting war on people and bringing them to safety. She felt his feelings and his bravery in the coat.

Daisy grew up believing that often people are too stupid to question anything when carrying out orders on behalf of governing bodies. Having worked for the Saskatchewan government, she saw certain cruelties by salaried men who did not give a damn about human suffering. Daisy had grown strong in the knowledge that people must think for themselves and not succumb to simply taking orders from people who, under the umbrella and protection of a large organization, gave orders that might be harmful. That would become her refrain in bringing up her own children. She would demand of her children, "Think for your self! Don't be a follower! Question authority if it seems wrong to you." Nothing angered her more than followers with no thought of right or wrong. Her mother had taught her by example; she had terrific strength to parent quietly. In very few words and to the point she would tell Daisy what was being disapproved of, even after Daisy was an adult. The example was carried through in Daisy's way of parenting, which was to the point and privately. There was no yelling or embarrassing kids in front of others. The problem with that method was that sometimes the kids thought they were the only ones being disciplined and the others not. They were also headstrong after being told over and over to think for themselves and not follow.

Daisy's father, a rough and tumble kind of guy with keen insight into people, was looking forward to meeting Ken. Her father took over much of Daisy's care when the twins were born two years after her. Because of him, she never felt displaced. They would lie on their stomachs on the floor in the evening and he would read the daily newspaper comics to her, teaching her to read at the same time. He had taught her how to dance to the gramophone and his favorite records with her standing on his shoes. He taught Daisy how to behave with horses, how to ride a bike, to draw, to do math so that when she started school, she already knew how to read and do arithmetic. He was the man who came to her home the afternoon she was preparing a big dinner for some Saskatchewan artists. The professional artists never noticed the green tree with clumps of red berries in the fresh snow outside her window, but her father exclaimed, "What a beautiful tree!" and with that she saw her father as the truest artist of them all with no fanfare, just an ordinary man... originally a farm boy, who loved music and really enjoyed his surroundings. He was full of zest and comedy. When showing off his high diving skills to a neighbor, he did the largest belly flop off the high board that Daisy had ever seen or hoped to see again; his body was beet red on the walk home from the public pool, but he laughed about it. When showing off his skating skills to the young hockey players while teaching Daisy how to skate on the outdoor communal rink, he leaped over snow banks piled as tall as a man from cleaning the rinks. He loved to show off and sometimes he was successful and sometimes he flopped only to get up and laugh about it. From her father, Daisy learned to have fun, even with flops. He would come home from work at 4 a.m. and water the skating rink he had built in the back yard for his small children and he built a snow slide as high as the roof of the house and then stoked the furnace so that the house was always warm. He worked hard campaigning; dressed in his brown suit and fedora hat and a portfolio under his arm, he went door to door to speak with families on behalf of Tommy Douglas and the CCF political party that brought in Canada's medical insurance to cover all people equally.

Daisy's father was a diviner. Many farmers have water wells found by him. He was so good at it that he could tell how much water, how deep to dig or drill, which direction the water flowed, and whether it was clear or black while he stood over it. He took all his children walking with willow branches and taught those who wanted to learn how to be a diviner. He marveled that Daisy was good at it. But the lesson he also instilled was that gifts like that are to be used and given free; one should never take money for a healing or a foresight, or for the gift of divining.

His children were brought up on storytelling. When they were small, long before television, on Sunday the family would gather in the living room after dinner. If at home, Daisy's parents would cuddle together on the sofa looking very much in love with the children around in a circle and it was story-telling time; or if they were at the farm, it was with grandparent and aunts sitting in chairs, and uncles sitting on the floor with their backs to the walls, sharing stories by the light of a coal-oil lamp. There were stories about everything from the mundane to stories that spoke of another dimension – about experiences of magic and life beyond this life. Daisy never, ever, tired of the stories. She grew up accepting that life is larger than what is in front of a nose and that living with a sixth sense is more normal than living without it, and she developed a deeply ingrained strength to question rules and orders that made no sense.

It was Daisy's father's mother who taught her an important lesson: that is to never judge a person by how they look. Daisy was a small child when she accompanied her grandparents to buy a new vehicle. She could not remember if it was a car or a tractor and or whether the guy was a bank manager or a salesman. What she understood and remembered was that the guy thought that because he was dealing with immigrant farmers and the woman could not read and write the English language and especially not the papers he had drawn up, he skewed the dollars in his favor. What he had not counted on was that Daisy's grandmother was a wiz at mathematics – all done in her head and she spoke up. Daisy had been a silent witness to how some people will take advantage of others. Daisy watched and wondered about her grandmother over the years. She was a woman who looked like a simple peasant in a long white apron, running around barefooted in the snow to feed her flocks, and would stand in her doorway without fear to hand out fresh baked bread to the Indian people who came knocking; she gave birth to and raised ten children on the flat prairies and was a look-alike to her famous musician cousin, Lawrence Welk. Daisy would wonder about the inner life of the astute woman who was not afraid to share food and would challenge a businessman, while at the same time she had a quietness about her and Mona Lisa smile.

Daisy believed her parents to be the most honest people in the universe until she met their match in Ken. She remembers clearly standing beside her parents' bed, telling a fib to her parents who were relaxing in bed listening to music on the radio. She remembers just turning two because the twins had not been born yet and she had just started talking; she had not spoken until she was turning two because she waited until she could speak complete sentences, expressing whole thoughts. Her parents explained the difference between telling a story and telling a lie. She remembers clearly that she understood the concept her parents were explaining to her.

Through childhood, Daisy had aspired to become a saint as soon as she learned about them, but the career choice had eluded her as foibles piled up. She identified mostly with her father – robust, having fun, swear words, belly flops and all, because she knew she could not be as sweet, beautiful and patient as her mother who seemed never to have sworn in her lifetime.

Daisy's family had prepared her to understand Ken so well. He possessed the quiet strength of purpose that she knew in her own grandparents and parents—people who stood their ground to uphold their moral values and where they could, they looked after people and quietly worked toward significant change.

EVENING MEALS ON THE FARM were buffet style so that people could mingle and be comfortable in their choices of food, place to sit, and who to talk with. Seating positions changed like musical chairs as the meal progressed until some people wandered away while some cleaned up.

Daisy's parents, each in turn, quietly told her that they experienced Ken as a nice, gentle man – a gentleman. They let her know they were now very pleased about her choice of partner. Daisy confided, "He is genuinely a gentle man. He is honestly spiritual from the inside out with no pretenses. He has no superiority complex." Her parents understood the full meaning of that.

While walking the field in the daylight and looking the horses over, Daisy told her father that Ken was the first man in her life who treated her with honest respect. Her father listened carefully as she explained that Ken is completely honest and unselfish, and that she can talk with him about anything, emphasizing that she can just be herself.

The days passed with riding horses, children playing in the giant haystack, running around, and sometimes sitting quietly, talking in low voices to share their own stories. Every evening, children bathed – little ones in a row in the tub, older ones alone, and they laughed a lot as they washed the hay out of their hair, and horse or other smells off their bodies.

Ken and Daisy took on simple chores that seemed more like fun than work for a few days. They dug potatoes for dinner with the children. They watched horses in the pasture as Daisy told stories about her horse-riding passions of the past.

"My sister Terisa and I used to ride giant work horses bareback on our grandparents' farm. One day out in the pasture, one horse became determined to dismount my sister, so he ran in one direction and quickly sidestep at full gallop to the other. My sister fell off and laid on her back on the ground saying over and over, "I'm dead!" I looked way down at her from my tall horse and saw that she wasn't dead. I laughed so hard that she got up and walked home. Her horse and me on mine followed her. We were so resilient. It never dawned on me that she might have broken something. I just saw the comedy. Then when we were putting the horses back into the barn, mine stepped back onto my foot. I was pinned so hard to the ground and it hurt so much that I couldn't even yell and I couldn't budge him. He was so big and heavy that his rear end towered over my head. I guess I got paid back for laughing at my sister. Ironically, neither one of us was really hurt."

Ken laughed.

They ate peas in the pea patch, while sharing more childhood stories. Daisy said, "Some of the best times of my childhood were sitting in the pea patch in the morning sunlight, eating peas for breakfast, watching the caterpillars and butterflies, and wondering about the transformation of life. Just the warmth of sun, smell of earth, the taste of green peas bursting in my mouth, and watching nature at work."

"I wish I had been with you in the pea patch. I have wanted to be with someone like you all my life."

Ken's answer was like the most important words she had ever heard. She had truly come home in knowing that he wanted to be with someone like her all his life. The feeling was mutual. Very mutual!

BROTHER BILL took a step back to examine Ken from head to toe and laughed, "There, that ought to do it. Now you're ready for the bees."

Through the netting covering his face, Ken looked across the farmyard to Daisy watching with amusement. He was unsure of this challenge. Outfitted in white beekeeper's protective clothing from head to toe, Ken climbed into the truck to go out into the fields with Bill and to face millions of bees in the extreme heat of the prairies. He waved to Daisy as they took off down the gravel country road, leaving a plume of dust behind them.

IN THE DUSK of evening, Ken and Daisy walked across the pasture to watch the display of Northern Lights. Children frolicked up and down the rolls of hay stacked high near the small, red hay barn with just enough light to have fun in. Their laughter filled the cooling air. Sounds always seemed clearer in evening air on the farm – a strange phenomenon.

"I've been thoroughly baptized into this family with all the bee stings today. I think I have a dozen stings."

"You must be in a lot of pain. There must have been an opening in your outfit. Why did you go out with my brother?"

"I needed to prove I could be a member of this family."

"But you don't need to get hurt to do that."

"I needed to do it. It's a guy thing."

Ken stood still, looking at the sky for a long time. They could hear the electricity of the Northern Lights. "I miss Andy. I wonder how he is doing. I was his caretaker and now he is so far away."

Ken's words moved through the air, spreading into the universe on the wings of moving coloured lights in the sky. Comforting Ken by holding his hand seemed impossible given the immensity of his sorrow but Daisy tried.

THE AIR OF the next afternoon felt soft. The screen-door slammed behind Daisy as she entered the house. Ken was on the telephone near the door. She was startled to see his face had lost colour and turned white as he listened.

In distress he answered whatever he had heard, "I'm going to fire my lawyer. Jane, you can draw up the papers and I'll sign them. As we discussed, you will take all the assets. I will take all the debts. I will pay the mortgage until the house is sold and you can keep the profit. I will pay for the nanny. I just want one thing; that is to share in the raising of our son. I want joint guardianship and joint custody in writing. ...Yes. Okay. We agree. ...Yes, go ahead and do that. We don't need two lawyers to get through this."

He slowly hung up the telephone and looked at Daisy with a distraught face, drained with shock.

"Right!" Daisy tried to assure Ken that she was on the same page with him. "With that kind of legal settlement, she should be very happy. You're being extremely generous. What's the problem?"

"The problem is that my lawyer has gone amuck. He's doing things I haven't asked him to do."

"Like what?"

"While I've been out of town, he filed for sole custody of Andy. I have to fire him. In the meantime, he's caused a lot of trouble between Jane and myself. She's angry that I would do that. All I want is to see my son grow up healthy with two parents."

AFTER A HASTY, anguished trip back to Vancouver, Ken and Daisy sat in front of a large wooden desk. A man with flaming red hair was behind the desk that seems too big for him and made him look small. The desk seemed like a protective barrier between him and clients.

He had a bold voice. "I remember her. We both have red hair. In law school, she was known as..." his voice deepens in a mimicking tone, "'the rich doctor's wife who drove the new BMW car'. That car alone is worth forty thousand dollars. Considering that your wife is a lawyer and at least ten years younger than yourself, we should make an example of your case. I can put the child in your sole custody, get maintenance for him, and divide the assets and debts right down the middle. You get half of everything and because of your age, we can get you maintenance for yourself."

Ken was visibly distressed. "That's not what I asked you to do. All I want is shared guardianship and shared custody of our two-year-old son. My goal is to help her parent our son. I told you I want her to have all the assets with no debts." Ken's voice rose, "I have a medical practice, I don't want or need maintenance for myself!"

The lawyer argued, "We can make a precedent case. She is a lawyer and much younger than you. You should consider..."

The argument continued for several minutes as the lawyer tried to convince Ken of what he wanted to do. Ken defended his position to never take anything from Jane and he defended Jane in every respect.

Daisy listened to Ken defending his ex-wife. During the argument, she became convinced that Ken was still in love with his ex-wife.

Ken angrily rose from his chair and standing tall and strong, was louder than the lawyer, "You went ahead about sole custody contrary to my instructions. I am *not* interested in you making a precedent case. I don't want to hurt Jane. You're fired!" With that, Ken turned on his heels to walk out of the office, leaving a stunned lawyer behind his desk.

Daisy was also stunned and glued to her chair. After a second to digest what just happened, she managed to find her legs to follow him. She had never seen Ken so angry.

OUT ON THE STREET Ken walked fast as though walking fast could erase the error. Daisy tried to keep up with difficulty.

As she caught up, she breathlessly said, "You're in love with her."

Angrily, Ken answered, "I will not go along with that guy making a precedent case for himself on my back. My son is only two. I intend to help her be the best mother she can be to him, even in divorce. That's all."

"But... you love her!"

Ken stopped to face Daisy in the street. "As the mother of my child, I love her."

"You have to hire a nanny to keep your child safe."

"I intend to help her be the best mother she can be of a two year old. That is my way."

They both fell silent, deep in their own thoughts as they walked to the bus stop. Ken was concerned about repairing the damage this lawyer caused between himself and Jane. The fallout on his child concerned him more than what Daisy believed.

Daisy pieced this latest upheaval together by thinking... I still think he loves her... he's always protecting her... but he's right in more ways than one... I remember how I cared for Karl, father of my children even though I could not live with him... the caring was different than how I love this man. Oh, well, I love you anyway, Ken... maybe even more because of how you are... who you are...

19

New Beginnings

"We can grow our gardens, build our homes and play with our children and grandchildren in a happier more peaceful world, that begins right here with the free exercise of our intelligence in John Dewey's sense of that word..."
Kehnroth Schramm

HAVING A COUNTRY PLACE where people could come and heal was a shared dream between Ken and Daisy. Both had lived in something close to this idea, Ken in his commune and Daisy on the meditation centre. Both had farming background. They drove around the ribbons of lower mainland country roads looking for such a place to rent and maybe buy someday, to build a healing centre. They wanted gardens for patients to garden while slowing down and healing or preserving good health, and an art centre for the same reasons. It should have a large kitchen where meals would be created and eaten together. Most of all, it would be a place of safety where healing could happen and where loneliness would be forgotten.

Animals, well known for their healing abilities, would be helpers as therapists. Daisy imagined horses, dogs and cats. Stopping to stand in knee high gold and green grasses at the side of a dirt road by a farmer's fence to talk and to admire the herd of Jersey cows, Ken expressed a wish for a Jersey cow. He told Daisy the story about a happier time when his friend taught him how to milk Jersey cows, and about singing quartets with friends while farming.

Visiting a physician's home was both encouraging and discouraging. She had made the transition from Vancouver to a Fraser Valley acreage and, being a woman, had brought her children with her even though she had left a marriage behind.

They were reminded that the pollution from the lower mainland travels up the Fraser Valley by wind and natural airflow, causing health problems to some residents.

On an exploration trip across the water to Vancouver Island and during an evening social gathering at the island home of Ken's former office partner, one female psychiatrist made it clear to Ken that it may be war because more psychiatrists coming into her territory were not wanted. She qualified it by saying, "Nothing personal."

The last thing Ken needed was another unnecessary war. Anyway, the realistic barrier in the form of expensive ferries between Ken and his children made island living formidable. Later, arriving at the ferry terminal, they discovered that they missed the last ferry of the evening and needed to rent a motel. It pointed to another barrier if Andy and Jane would have an emergency, as they often did, there would be no easy transportation.

IT HAD BEEN a fun time to share a dream, but they had came face to face with the barrier of how to make it work with children they probably could not bring along, except for visits. Ken's promise to care for his children must come first. The distance between Ken and Andy was the biggest problem and he was still hopeful his sons would return to live with him for their university education.

Vancouver by the sea became the only viable choice; though pleasant with beaches, sea and mountains, it offered city living in confined spaces. A country place was put on hold but not forgotten; it became a dream for sometime in the future.

Meanwhile, word had gotten out that Ken was living in the housing co-op with Daisy. People were coming out of the woodwork to knock on the door. The friend from Regina, now a practicing psychologist and neighbor in the co-op, proposed sharing an office with Ken. A midwife, also living in the co-op, asked that Ken give the local lay-midwives free use of his office. So many people wanted something from Ken that Daisy was taken aback.

His own office partner had made a sudden move to the Island months ago and Ken had found himself on his own to make and pay for a new office space. In a political climate where it was well known that physicians were supposed to share offices with physicians and no others, and because of his problems with his family, he decided on time alone to sort out his own life.

WITH SO MUCH going on all the time between work and three separate families, Ken and Daisy relished rare quiet time with each other to indulge in sharing knowledge and bounce ideas around. They were spending a quiet evening together in the living room when Loraine and Lana arrived home. Standing in front of Ken, Loraine announced, "Ken, I want you to walk me down the aisle at my wedding." It was part question, part statement. This was the announcement of an engagement.

Surprised, Ken answered, "I would be honored."

This would be the first wedding of the children. Loraine and Ron were the true-life story of East meets West. Ron was a guy from East Vancouver with the black leather jacket and black Dayton boots, played hockey and was a man's man growing up with only brothers. Loraine was a slender West Side ballet dancer who wore pink toe-shoes and figure skated with white skates.

KEN GOT LOST IN THE BACKGROUND as the whirlwind of preparing for a wedding took over. There was shopping for material to sew a formal wedding gown and Lana's Maid-of-Honor gown. Ron, who had never baked before, helped Daisy make the three-tiered wedding fruitcake laced with brandy that is traditional to the prairies. He did not let on that he did not even like fruitcake.

Having already chosen their church, and searched for a reception hall, they decided to have a chapel wedding and a reception at home in the co-op.

Through all this, Ken spent as much time as possible with his sons. They were slowly achieving an easier relationship with him even though a severed relationship from Daisy's family continued.

It was Christmas time and during the preparations for the wedding, a group of carolers made up of a few co-op residents, stopped outside the townhouse. Opening the door to them, Ken and Daisy stood together to welcome the friends. In the middle of the front row stood Mary Murray with her guitar. She became memorable because a dark shadow crossed over her eyes. Considering that Saul had done his best to leave the impression with friends that he was leaving because Daisy was having an affair, Daisy wondered if Mary blamed her. Under the caroling circumstances, Daisy had no opportunity to talk to Mary.

Over time, something about Mary would continue to niggle in the back of Daisy's mind, but not important enough to follow up as other events took precedent. But feeling protective of Ken, Daisy wished they had not opened the door that night.

Sewing and fitting satin and lace was most important while an old sewing machine and old iron both act up. Ken and Daisy went on a food expedition for the wedding reception and then, finally, the icing of the cake and decorating it with live red roses meant... It was Time!

LORAINE HAD BEEN BORN IN REGINA on a day when there was fresh, fluffy snow like powder puffs covering everything. January 2, 1982, her wedding day had dawned fresh and clean, reminiscent of her birth. Unusual for Vancouver, fluffy snow had fallen over night. Soft, white, powder pillows covered everything. Traveling to the church, the sun shone on the snow so that it seemed every snowflake sparkled like diamonds, making everything seem especially new and fortuitous.

Halfway to the church they saw Ron and his Best Man brother in a car headed away from the church as fast as they could go.

Wide-eyed Loraine watched them, "Oh, my god! Do you think he is running away?"

Inside the church, as they waited for some news, Daisy fussed with the veil and dresses as Ken watched. Word came that the guys arrived back. They had abandoned their car in the street and ran through the snow with the ring they had forgotten at home. They were calmly taking their place at the altar as though nothing had happened.

The prelude to the Wedding March filled the air. Daisy fussed for no real reason, making a few more tiny adjustments to Loraine's veil. Ken, wearing a three-piece suit kept only for special events and conferences, was on the other side of Loraine. He suddenly looked uneasy.

"I am having a problem," he said to Daisy. "I abandoned my marriage vows. I don't know if I can go through with this."

Daisy flashed him a look, meaning Oh, No! Not Now!

He got it and recovered his composure quickly. He took Loraine on his arm.

Looking dashing in tuxedos, Marcel and Antony opened the heavy wooden doors leading into the chapel. The wood interior had a golden sheen from sunlight coming through stained glass windows, splashing hues of many colours around the chapel, punctuated by large lit candles on stately pillars on either side of the altar.

Daisy quickly took her place in a pew near the altar and looked back to see Lana, the maid of honour, in a long, rose-coloured satin dress, looking glorious with a band of ribbon in her long brown hair that matched her dress and a smile that lit up the room. With the Wedding March, Lana led the way down the aisle and took her place at the altar opposite the men.

Loraine and Ken, arm in arm, stood together for a moment in the doorway facing the people filling the chapel. Ken turned to Loraine and smiled, giving her a personal moment of comfort as he accompanied her through the threshold to the next phase of her life.

Loraine, dressed in a long white satin and lace gown with a sheen that softly reflected the light of the room, and a white lace veil framing her smiling face, looked very ready to meet Ron, her husband-in-waiting.

The minister in his flowing white garment stood at the altar, ready to unite the couple. As Ken and Loraine approached, Daisy stepped out to join them.

The minister asked, "Who gives this bride in marriage?"

"We do," Ken and Daisy said in unison.

OUTSIDE THE CHURCH, Christmas lights were all around on the trees and houses, adding magic and colour to the white and green winter scene. Family and friends had come out of the church. With Andy in his arms, Ken stood with Daisy, watching the bride and groom receive the good wishes of everyone.

The irony of this was that Ken and Daisy had wanted to be married this Christmas. It was supposed to be their own wedding but for family responsibilities, both his and hers, they had put their own wishes aside for now.

All three of Ken's sons were surprisingly present. Among the guests, seated in the pews, two older sons cared for the young son while Ken was busy.

Ken whispered to Daisy, "This is a reminder of my own promises that I couldn't keep... my marriages... my hope to marry you by Christmas."

They were now entering a new phase of their lives; children were growing, changing, multiplying. As they stood in the snow, watching the family at the first wedding of their children, Daisy could not help thinking about their life so far – life with Ken. They shared the strong belief that family is of utmost importance. She was in awe of this man standing beside her, holding his smallest son close to his heart... a man who had worked so tirelessly for others, and who was heartbroken over his own broken family. Had she really been prepared for the transition of working in medicine with him?

Ken's two older sons had come back into his life. Now outside the church, having come to the wedding, they took their places to stand together with their father and their young brother. For the first time, Daisy could see the four united as family. Their work could begin. Daisy stepped aside.

Three new beginnings were happening that day – a young couple newly bonded in matrimony... a father and his three sons newly bonded... and a father living separate from all women for the sake of his children.

[A glimpse into the future: Ron's walk down the aisle with Loraine was his step into figure skates. The first time his toe picks hit the ice, he will nose-dive and slide across the ice on his belly into many years of ice dancing with Loraine. From Dayton boots and hockey skates blending toe shoes and figure skates – along with having children, the couple will find a shared artistry on the ice and in dance.]

20

The Written Word

SON PETER had followed his wish to go back to the Kootenays to complete high school. Instead of being able to live with his mother, he had been placed to live with her previous boyfriend. It turned out to be the secret Ken heard about at the wedding.

Stephen had entered university, choosing to live in student housing where fraternity life happened.

Ken followed through with renting an apartment as a catching mitt for himself and his sons.

Even though the older sons had been avoiding Daisy's family, their attendance at the wedding had been a breakthrough for Ken. The bottom line for Ken was that he continued to hope for a change in the dynamic influences of the ex-wives on his sons. In the meantime, he was available for every small and large opportunity to be with and talk with his boys. Sunday brunches, usually Chinese food, became regular for any son available to meet with him.

GETTING TO KNOW each other over the many months, Ken and Daisy had found the other even more fascinating. Ken was a morning person, waking early in the routine of years working in hospitals. His preferred hours suited caring for his small son by going to sleep early and waking early. Daisy's creative juices ran in the evening until the tiny hours of the morning while the world was quiet and children slept. He was audio – she was visual. He was an intellect and scholar – she, an artist. They fit like pieces of a puzzle – opposite but filling each other where there were spaces to make a whole. Though they were different, their hopes and dreams were in unison. They had reverence for all that lives and deep devotion for a higher power. Each had a lack of interest in money and little need for material things other than books, art supplies and music; both had given everything they owned away more than once. His wealth was in family and in knowledge; hers was the same. They both loved books and the wisdom and history contained in them. They were mutual admirers of each other's minds. They both had indelible memories. Each day brought new surprises from old memories to new ideas. They kept each other hopping with ideas and beliefs and sharing of knowledge. He excited her. She excited him. Each wanted to know intimate details about the other and the past; they could never get enough.

"I want to know you fully," was Ken's refrain.

To that, there was always the quest to know each other so intimately and truthfully that there was complete unification. Daisy wondered if that kind of knowing was ever possible in the physical plane and she constantly wondered if Ken carried a yearning for the kind of knowing that may only be obtainable in the spiritual realm.

The other refrain was about transformation – meaning it in a spiritual way. He read and wrote about transformations. It became Daisy's quest to understand what he was searching for.

Though at times he was absent in order to be available to his sons, Daisy admired his determination and struggle to keep his promise about caring for his sons.

While Ken needed space to focus on his sons, working together became the focus between Ken and Daisy. As she worked alongside him, she was constantly amazed at his knowledge of medicine and was thoroughly impressed at the medical details he remembered. Names of things and understanding of symptoms that he learned somewhere would surface at the right moment. In turn, he was amazed at her keen interest in learning medicine.

Ken's knowledge reached into other areas and astounded Daisy. His claims that he knew nothing about music and art were unfounded as Daisy, who has studied both music and art, found out. He constantly surprised her by knowing names of composers and recognizing their music. His interest in art had obviously been an undercurrent and he taught Daisy as much as she taught him.

Enthusiastically, he searched out and brought home to her, books and pictures of paintings he had known but she had not. Of special interest were those on the Dartmouth Campus, and those of the Spanish painters around the world who painted political statements.

Daisy experienced Ken as an open vessel of wisdom that had taken in knowledge of everything he had ever encountered. She felt a unique comfort and excitement at being chosen to be in his aura and to gain knowledge from him.

She marvelled at the depth of his understanding of people. A finer teacher she could not imagine.

He had asked her in the beginning of their relationship if she would mind him spending time in the library. Daisy thought that was an odd question since books had always been her fountain of wealth and comfort.

"Of course I don't mind."

By his reaction she knew instinctively there had been a problem in his past around time spent in libraries. What she discovered was that he spent every chance he could get to research many subjects in all the libraries. Ken researched in the university and the College of Physicians & Surgeons medical libraries. He spent time researching religion and philosophy in the Theology school libraries and bookstores. The university main library stacks and the city-run libraries were also home to Ken. He spent hours reading in the stacks of all the libraries and always left by carrying bags of books along with his backpack full of books. He researched and brought books to people he knew who were working on or questioning something. He was always looking for ways to guide family and clients into higher learning. To Daisy's astonishment, he read with lightening speed. She watched as he read all the books he had not handed out to other people, and then went back for more. And of course, there were the bookstores that he dove into on a regular basis.

His own library was extensive in subjects of history, philosophies old and new and of many cultures, anthropology, Greek mythology, Greek and Mandarin and Lakota languages, books written by aboriginal writers from around the world, allopathic medicine – including surgery and science based research along with psychiatry, alternative and complimentary and integrative medicine, other culture medicine from around the world, orthomolecular medicine, self-help, and much more – like self-sustainable farming, milking cows and building environmentally correct houses, just to name a few. Ken was interested in and read everything he could lay his hands on about man and ancient wisdoms that continued to be integral to many indigenous cultures.

As Daisy browsed his library, she was most surprised by the many volumes and sets of books on advanced mathematics.

Ken was eager to discuss any of the subjects with anyone willing, but he was mostly alone with the books and his knowledge. There was a lack of people willing or able to sit and talk with him. He often expressed appreciation for the farmers he had met because they had been the most willing to take the time to talk and stretch their ideas with another person. Those farmers had been more open minded than most physicians he met. He found that too many physicians had their comfort zone where they worked but did not have time or inclination to spend time discussing life unless they came up with a shtick to make money and needed to draw in people, then they were available on a limited basis.

Inviting a physician to dinner, or to lunch in hopes of communication, usually ended in disappointment. After Ken spent hours cooking or traveling to the restaurant, the physician would arrive, eat and leave in a hurry instead of staying to talk. But most disturbing were the closed-minded physicians who believed they had cornered wisdom in a few years of studying allopathic medicine that was fairly new in the years marking life on earth. Ken's brother Richard and one other non-physician colleague turned friend had been the most reliable over the years to have intellectual discussions with, but now both lived on the other side of the continent. That pretty much left Daisy as a talking companion, while Ken hoped his sons would one day be able to have these discussions.

Ken's library was a dream come true for Daisy. She had a lot of learning to do because she never before delved into some areas, like higher mathematics, or the volumes on medicine, but his library complimented her large library. As a child she dreamed not of money but of a treasure house with walls lined with books and she had achieved that. Her parents had a bookcase filled with the *Books of Knowledge* for which they had paid a whole month's income for the benefit their children. Her home was the only house she knew of that had its own *Books of Knowledge*. Her mother had mail-ordered a set of books for ten-year old Daisy about famous scientists of medicine but when she took them to school, her teacher stole them. Daisy could only stare at her books sitting on the shelf behind the teacher's desk and wonder about the lost information. Daisy's mother's early efforts to educate her child about medicine and having the information stolen haunted Daisy and just the memory would bring up a thud in her stomach for years.

With that in mind, books were important in trying to give her children a better education. The neighbourhood kids would arrive from school in a rush to play school or whatever with Daisy's creative kids who became the play-teachers. As one neighbour girl who lived in an expensive looking house explained, "I have a drawer full of socks, but I don't have a piano or books at home."

THOUGH DAISY ATTENDED school in the evenings and weekends to formally make the transition to medicine, she found the courses lacking in many areas. While gathering some credentials, she mainly relied on Ken, whose superior understanding of people, medicine, therapy, and mediation made far more sense to her than what others taught in credited courses.

To compliment all that she was learning, she found a treasure in the medical journals that arrived like clockwork with articles of newest research and quizzes of cases. Every spare moment was spent with these magazines that usually made their way to the stack in her bathroom because she did not want to miss a minute of reading time.

Books from Ken's library, filled with poems and storied cases written by physicians Robert Coles, Walker Percy, William Carlos Williams, and Milton H. Erickson were handed to Daisy with the advice, "These are physician authors who wrote about their work in differing styles and maintained patient confidentiality." Groundwork was being laid for the writing to come.

Ken handed Daisy a royal blue, hardcover binder embossed with gold ornate print. It was the Hippocratic Oath written in beautiful script. He explained, "You need to know and honour the Hippocratic Oath so long as you work with me. The oath of doing no harm and keeping patients' secrets is important."

It was as though the Hippocratic Oath, even in this written form, held age-old power that was now in her hands.

21

Magician of Healing

"PATIENTS IN PSYCHIATRY may be called clients." Ken said.

This newest revelation caused Daisy to research the current rights of the patient. The name 'clients' somehow liberated a person to make choices in his or her own power.

She told Ken, "What a revelation to realize I did not have to feel like I was in prison when I had babies in a hospital. I had rights! But, more than that, my children were not prisoners. **We** had rights! I just didn't know."

"MONEY IS NOT the reason I work in medicine," Ken explained. "Never do I put money ahead of the well-being of a person needing care or guidance. I would prefer to do what I do for no money." This statement was said in many ways over time.

Daisy watched Ken spending time with people for extended hours that could not be billed for. He never billed a person for missed appointments, which was time a psychiatrist could bill a client outside of the medical plan – a sort of punishment for bad behavior. Ken was adamant that the collection of money from his clients for specialized letters and forms was never permitted even though other physicians did bill for this service. As Daisy learned, Ken did not bill for nearly half the time he put in and if he had a choice and no family responsibilities, he would work for free.

"I would rather work on a salary than to bill for time spent, or for procedures. I believe in universal medical coverage, equal to all, but I don't want to be doling out my time for money, and making money on someone's grief or illness. Medicine should be a right and I should not have to worry about money to be a physician. If I could share the money paid to me with the clients, many would no longer be ill, but that is also against the rules of Medicare. Too many people suffer illnesses caused by poverty."

Daisy agreed with every word he said but mused that he clearly needed a keeper.

"The problem is that I get fired from salaried jobs when they find out that I work for the people and not for the financial bottom line of an institution, government or the courts. I have gotten fired at Christmas time. Sometimes it was over a lack of funding and I'm the guy they cut. I have been fired for trying to change things when I saw how the staff or the institution didn't work for the people they were suppose to serve."

"You mean, people protect their jobs or their castle and get rid of you." Daisy managed to get a smile from Ken. He felt understood but made no comment.

FOR HIS CLIENTS, Ken was on call twenty-four hours a day, every day of the year with no holidays. Daisy discovered that people and crisis go together during religious holidays and Ken insisted on being available. He said, "Illness and troubles don't take holidays." Consequently Daisy found herself working along with him, taking long troubled telephone calls during Christmas dinner and other holidays. It was not unusual for Ken to spend hours of a holiday with a seriously distressed client.

If Ken was away for a couple of days at a conference or for a rare visit to his own family in Vermont, that was when some clients had a case of jitters and need reassurance. It could be a busy un-billable telephone time for Daisy.

When the physicians in British Columbia quit working by going on strike, Ken continued working. He told Daisy, "I took the Hippocratic Oath. I will not quit seeing patients because of greed for more money."

As a result of working through a strike in the early 1980's, Ken received a letter written on stationery with the British Columbia Medical Association letterhead, threatening that he will suffer the consequences later.

Ken was unmoved by the threat and determinedly continued to see his clients. In reaction to Daisy's shock at reading the letter, Ken said, "I am not afraid of threats. My clients are not on strike."

That was the first but not the last time Daisy experienced Ken's determination to take care of his patients regardless of threats from people who could hurt him.

Psychiatrists around the lower mainland of British Columbia usually had waiting lists as long as several weeks and running into months; six months waiting was not unheard of. By booking appointments several months in advance, those psychiatrists had a secure income base.

Ken booked client appointments one week at a time, allowing for flexible treatment and changes as necessary with current clients because they were not locked in. He did not believe that any person needing help should be put on a waiting list but instead, he responded to crisis immediately, often working long hours to do so. Refusing to have a waiting list and by booking this way, Ken never knew where the income would come from for the month ahead.

Ken told Daisy, "Most psychiatrists work with individuals and because there are so few psychiatrists who see families – families and aboriginal people are always given preference in my practice. They are the under-served population. Individuals who refuse to include family members or close friends that are involved in their problems can more easily find help elsewhere."

All referring physicians were sent a written explanation of Ken's practice, outlining that treatment would include family and friends, and possible lifestyle changes that might include diet and orthomolecular treatment. The letter explained that no psychotropic drugs would be prescribed.

"Confidentiality must be kept. Never give out client information and never discuss a client in public. If there must be a discussion with me or another physician where someone might overhear, never use a name or any identifying information. This rule is never to be broken under any circumstances."

Ken had a few rules for clients who wanted to work with him. At the first meeting, he explained to each client that confidentiality would be honoured no matter who asks for information; for that reason, other than history taking and a treatment plan, he would not be writing down conversations between them. "In other words," he explained, "your secrets will never escape my office, even under threat, theft, subpoenas, or any other means because secrets won't exist in writing. If I am subpoenaed to court, I will have a bad memory." With that promise, clients expressed relief in found trust. They opened up, expressing themselves in ways that would otherwise remain locked in fear of being betrayed.

On the first appointment with all clients, Ken adamantly promised never to label anyone with Diagnostic Mental Disorders [DSM] codes for psychotic illnesses that are used by psychiatrists in record keeping and for billing medical insurances. He explained that he does not believe in black and white labels when there are grays and many colours in all people. Ken told clients he only uses code 309 Adjustment Reaction for billing the B.C. Medical Services. Ken explained that 'Adjustment Reaction' could explain all phases of life, allowing people room to grow, change, and not be stuck with a label, especially in government files.

Ken explained to the clients that he must have an open line to the referring doctor where prescribed pharmaceutical drugs and treatment plans were concerned, simply to allow direct telephone conversation between physicians to correctly understand the client's needs and to enable the physicians to work out an immediate care-plan. When necessary, Ken got right on the telephone while the client listened, to discuss with the referring physician a possible change in prescribed medications because of suspected interaction of too many or too much medication, or a diagnostic test that might be helpful. That way of working was immediate and could avoid misunderstandings in written material that might also end up in the wrong hands, or waste valuable time by way of snail-mail. [This was the 1980's, a time before computers in medical offices.]

On occasion, Ken would accompany a client to visit a referring physician or to the hospital for immediate clarification.

Ken instinctively picked up on questionable information on the fist visit. If the client objected to the idea of Ken talking with the referring doctor, that would sometimes be a clue to misinformation. Clients would sometimes give misleading information intentionally and unintentionally regarding medications. Clients were often unaware they were suffering side effects of medications or the 'domino effect' of more and more drugs to treat side effects. Ken helped physicians unlock these effects.

Ken took clients into his practice that were dependent on psychotropic drugs or other substance abuse. His reputation was that, if the person desired to stop the use of drugs, alcohol, or smoking, Ken would be the physician to help them do so. He would never insist that a person quit all psychotropic drugs in order to work with him; instead he allowed the person to work with him and continue a predetermined treatment plan with another physician.

Ken always explained to new clients that he would not give prescriptions for psychotropic drugs of any sort. That information got tested frequently. He refused to be coerced into writing a prescription for drugs at any time and if someone claimed to just need a renewal, the person was referred back to the doctor's office that wrote the prescription in the first place; the same went for pharmacies that had been given Ken's name to renew another physician's prescription.

Many patients sought Ken after having heard from others about his method of work. As he told Daisy, "I am deliberately not listed in the yellow pages. Clients come simply by word of mouth."

Inquiring people were always told that they must have a physician's referral to see Ken because he was a specialist. Daisy learned right from the start to follow-up on referrals by telephoning the referring office to ensure that the referrals were actually made. However, if the referring office slipped up, British Columbia Medical Services Plan [MSP] rejected the billing anyway and stated why on a twice-monthly statement, and did not pay for any session until the referral or correction on any other mistake came through. A time limit of six months was given to re-submit a corrected billing.

During the first session with a client, a discussion took place to explain that the first six weeks of the six-month referral period would be used for evaluation of whether or not the relationship with Ken was beneficial to the client and family. If necessary, the client would be referred elsewhere or additional resources would be explored. In most cases, the sessions continued for the remainder of the six months and could be renewed beyond that.

Ken told Daisy, "Treating a person and sending that person back into a sick environment can result in the person becoming sick again."

Ken worked by assessing the whole person and the whole family, health and history of the client, home, school, working conditions, and anything else that was going on in the life of the individual and family. Then a plan of treatment was discussed and written regarding lifestyle changes that might include diet, orthomolecular treatment and complimentary medicine. Any involved person might be invited to the next meeting; most often it was family but the invitation may be extended to a social worker, a teacher, or a group of people who could all work together to make a workable health care plan. If outside help was needed, a referral was made for additional therapy, advice, or back to the referring physician for further medical tests regarding a suspected physical problem.

OCCASIONALLY there were clients who needed to be referred on to the legal system during the first or subsequent visit. Usually, these people came with an agenda involving battles over children and assets in divorce. The scenario would often start with a demand for an appointment with Ken for her alone so that she could blatantly accuse the father of something and have it written up for the courts by a psychiatrist. She would expect that Ken should jump to it and automatically comply to make a defaming report on her say-so – and she would go on to say, "No, no appointment with the child or the father would be necessary either". Curiously, no man ever tried that story with Ken or Daisy.

If one of these potential clients got in the door on pretence, Ken would explain that he would not go to court in child custody battles. He always explained clearly that to enable him to be helpful to the family – especially to the children, *all* members of the family needed to trust him and neither parent could coerce him. He made it absolutely clear that the wellbeing of the children came first and parental alienation would never wash; a peaceful, supportive outcome was desirable and must be worked toward by *all* parties – even in divorce. With that information, the client either disappeared or made adjustments in thinking. With Ken's help, often there was a calming of parents as they gave up a selfish fight in favour of parenting their children regardless of whether they stayed married or divorced.

Where children lived in a single parent family, Ken was supportive by helping the family to cope and grow together.

IN A SESSION with Ken, he wrote essential health histories, and then laid down his pen. From then on he interacted with patients face to face and only lifted his pen again to record any health plan or referral.

Ken explained to Daisy, "Clients need undivided attention. A doctor continually writing and not really hearing is likely to miss visual clues. When a psychiatrist continually writes, then there is also distraction by the unconscious or conscious mind of the client; they worry and wonder about what is being written. Any accident can result in a subpoena of medical files to court. In the written file, the client is compromised by an external person's opinion. The physician's interpretation of a person may be incorrect to begin with. Then lawyers and judges follow with their own interpretation of the file, twisting written statements about a person to best suit their own desired outcome of a case. That's one reason I gave up working in family court. It was frustrating to have people who knew nothing about medicine make interpretations and not listen to me."

THE LESSON OF SILENCE was simple. "Every moment does not have to be filled with noise. Listen." Ken explained to Daisy, "Let clients come to their own revelations and decisions without coercion. You can give information when necessary. They are provided with a safe place to think and feel things through."

The slowing down often disarmed clients who came with pre-conceived labels and Daisy observed that sessions took on a relaxed feeling. The clients easily slipped into stories with free-flowing emotion and stopped acting out a label.

In the movies, Daisy had often seen a psychiatrist ask too many questions, and in so doing, lead the conversation with the patient responding. To watch Ken work was a revelation as he did the opposite of the movies. Non-coercion was Ken's way.

WHERE CONTROVERSIAL medical questions were concerned, clients were pointed in a direction to find information necessary to weigh pros and cons.

During Daisy's first years of medical study and observation, psychiatric labels such as Borderline Personality, and many others, fascinated her. The intriguing names seemed to be shortcuts in discussions. She wanted to impress Ken with her growing knowledge.

Ken was definitely not impressed. He encouraged her to get beyond using limiting concepts of the simplified labels other physicians liked to use and to learn more – to gain a deeper understanding of the people instead of labels.

EVEN THOUGH Ken's bookshelves held many books on all the various ways psychiatry had been used and the books were written by various expert authors about their views on how to work with patients, Ken had studied long and hard enough, clocking more than a quarter of a century experience in many settings to be confident in his way of gently working with his patients of all ages and in all settings.

In a private conversation, a Vancouver psychiatrist challenged Ken about working with children. The pompous older man told Ken that unless he took the course in the States that he had taken one summer to become a child psychiatrist, that Ken was not qualified. Daisy did not interrupt but she was insulted for Ken and surprised that he took the criticism quietly without flinching.

Out on the street after the meeting, she asked, "Ken, why did you not defend yourself? You have years of working in Pediatrics."

"The guy needed to feel good about himself and I let him do that. He can't harm me. He is about to retire. He's a guy who puts all of himself into writing what the client says instead of paying attention to the person."

"Oh! Good riddance to him!" Daisy was always taken back at Ken's insight and willingness to let things go but she struggled with her own emotions about wanting to defend him all the time.

KEN HAD ALWAYS been interested in universal energy and how it is feels between people, within the body, and connections with external forces. He could only wear a wind-up watch with no battery. His body reacted to battery currents. Daisy understood that because all watches stopped on her own mother's arms.

Among other things that included meditation, Ken had studied Wilhelm Reich's writings on orgone energy. He practiced a technique of eye movement with some clients to unblock body energy and when he taught the technique to Daisy, she was amazed at the flow of energy through her body. He commented that she was unusually unblocked.

He also studied acupuncture and energy flow through the body. In experimenting for the fun of it with his electronic box on body points, Daisy placed the point between her thumb and forefinger and sure enough, the tip of her tongue tingled. He told her that in childbirth, it helps if a woman can open her mouth and let out noise because the energy flow helps the uterus do its work. She was reminded of the nurses she had encountered who told women in labour to stop making noise because that was not lady-like.

It was the Chinese massage technique and the use of moxa that was the way a client could feel energy running through the body from one area to another around the body and from head to toe. If there were blockages, the energy would not go through and not reach the ends of the limbs.

Hypnosis had also been part of Ken's studies. The teaching of self-hypnosis was sometimes used to help clients explore the unconscious and bring to the surface what they needed. Ken taught self-hypnosis with built in safeguards to absolutely keep the clients in their own power, leaving no residual loss of power behind or with him. No questions were asked of clients. They were allowed internal work. If the client wished to speak about the experience, they could do so when ready. Those sessions often resulted in stories that would be unforgettable.

The only kind of hypnosis Daisy had encountered before Ken was in her teen years when a middle-aged showman had hypnotized a friend, and later at a house party proved the girl was still under his control. This exhibition struck fear in all present and horrified the teenaged girl's parents. Now Daisy learned that hypnosis could be entirely different, safe and beneficial with control staying with the client and not the guide.

Then there was Ken's germ theory. When Daisy questioned why he seemed so unafraid of catching anything from sick people who came to see him, she was amused at his explanation. As a physician, he believed himself to be immune to all germs and that if he were to be afraid of germs, he could not do a physician's job. With his example, she was determined her immune system would also guard her.

THOUGH TRAINED IN and supportive of science based allopathic medicine, Ken was also trained in medical anthropology and continually studied alternative, integrative, complimentary, and other cultural medicines from around the globe. He openly practiced orthomolecular psychiatry. He believed all medical practitioners from all cultures should work together and allopathic practitioners should stop excluding what they have not studied and do not understand.

Ken adamantly told Daisy to disallow pharmaceutical representatives appointments with him because he was not interested, would not stock their samples, and would never accept their gifts. She was also warned not to believe the studies funded by pharmaceutical companies, and that included university trials and studies funded by the pharmaceutical companies because they may be skewed; instead, to look toward independent studies.

Matter-of-factly, Ken informed Daisy that one-day they might take his license away if they find out his true interests – *"they"* meaning the British Columbia College of Physicians and Surgeons.

At first, Daisy thought he was just being paranoid. Then she discovered that he was not paranoid but simply vigilant of his surroundings. The fact that he did not use psychotropic drugs put him in constant danger about keeping his medical license in the province of British Columbia where the BC College of Physicians and Surgeons and the provincial government had been reluctant to embrace any other medicine than allopathic medicine.

Ken advised her to be careful to abide by the code of conduct to not criticize another physician to the clients. That advice made life easier. Where she might have gotten on her high horse in private, in the practice she was quietly accepting choices people made. Although, she occasionally thought, "If they choose to make a hero of a donkey's ass, then so be it."

Daisy's life had become an intense study of medicine. Ken facilitated her keen interest and concerns by having ongoing discussions with her about anything that she wanted to clarify or to discuss about the latest research. Daisy knew she would never be a physician or catch up to Ken's years of training and practice no matter how much she read, but working with him was easy because his gentle training was always with respect. He always included her in discussions with other physicians, making her his teammate.

After the first days of learning medical office administration, Ken had started inviting Daisy to sit in on sessions with clients. To her astonishment, seldom did a client question her presence. That way, the real training had begun while at the same time Daisy was providing physical protection for Ken.

She was getting lessons fast and clear about the climate that Ken worked in and the extreme dangers he faced. It was an unrelenting, daily danger to survive. There were the dangers that all physicians face of making a medical mistake. A complaint could be lodged with the College of Physicians and Surgeons about anything manufactured or real if a patient became disgruntled in any way. There was the stream of women claiming to be victims of sexual abuse. Separating experience from imagination was important because some of these women had already seen another therapist who may have – and sometimes did plant the suggestion of sexual abuse. As a result, the person would faintly 'remember' something – not really remembering – but it had built up in her brain until it became a real problem, often with the result of ruining family relationships long before Ken came into the picture.

Then there were real cases of sexual abuse and the work to help the client get on with his or her life instead of staying stuck.

There was a constant danger because a doctor could be accused of sexual misconduct by a patient in a climate of the time when it was widely known in British Columbia that any sexual abuse case could result in an easy settlement of Fifty-Thousand Dollars fast cash and more in some court cases. It was profitable to be a victim. It was almost impossible for any accused person to prove innocence. The supposed victim was usually believed just on the basis of a complaint even though nothing could be proven. And the doctor could be jailed. A detective of the time was known to have said, "It has to be true because she made a complaint."

Daisy learned to be extremely vigilant about the women coming to see Ken. Her antennas grew long and large. She felt it was Ken's right as a doctor to trust everyone, and her right to watch out for him. She learned that physicians are targets not only for marriage but much more – it could be sex, money, or both; or it might be simply for bragging rights with other women about having a relationship with a doctor. She came to understand the term 'Dragon Lady' that had been used to describe the medical office assistant. Daisy's intention was to be a terrific Dragon Lady.

NON-INTERFERENCE. Ken advised Daisy to listen and encourage clients in exploring and coming to their own conclusions in the questions around life and death, religion and abortion.

Immunization was often a subject questioning parents brought to the sessions. Ken advised clients to educate themselves regarding the pros and cons of immunization, and then make a decision. What he did tell clients was that when he did work as a paediatrician in baby clinics, each baby's health was assessed and no baby was immunized while ill or previously exposed to an illness; then each disease had a vaccine given separately so that if there was a serious reaction, there was knowledge about what caused it and perhaps that particular shot would not be repeated in order to avoid long-term effects. He explained that in his baby clinics, no cocktail immunization was given, expecting a small body's immunization system to deal with it.

For Daisy, vaccinations turned out to be one of the most mind-boggling questions of medicine. She read everything she could find about the subject. It was easy to read the print that said only one child in 100,000 might be affected. It was another story to deal directly with grieving parents whose child turned out to be the one. She confided in Ken, "I really have a hard time with the subject of immunizations. That one child... we see those families first hand... too many of them to be one in 100,000."

She could think of nothing that matched the impact of a substance or procedure that could be so profoundly beneficial, or so severely damaging to millions of young and innocent children worldwide.

She complained, "Ken, the war rages on between the companies who make the vaccines, the health care workers who believe that a pandemic might occur if immunizations are not given, and people who live in fear of an outbreak of disease, and parents who only want to protect their irreplaceable children. Even we know of children who suffered side effects and even death. So often these people come to us seeking help in making intelligent decisions or to help them with the damage already done. And I question ingredients used in those concoctions."

Ken's advice was consistent. "You can point people in the direction of information about the pros and cons. They can make their own informed decisions."

KEN'S CLIENTS came from all walks of life. There were physicians, nurses, lawyers, teachers, politicians, social workers, counselors, an undertaker, writers, journalists, artists, students, laborers, white collar, blue collar, rich people, poor people, Judge's kids, young children, old people, people living in mansions, street people, and every other walk of life experiencing anything and everything from birth to death – people who have difficult moments in their lives. It was a lesson that no walk of life is protected from stresses, family troubles, work overload or under-load, physical and emotional injuries, and especially the cycle of giving birth and dying. Regardless of who the people were or whatever age, Ken talked to the real person inside – the child within – the ageless person – the person without clothes.

Daisy soon discovered that some clients working in high profile jobs or in medicine did sneak under cover into the office, hoping no one saw them enter.

"What about the touchy, feely people... the ones who want to end sessions with hugs and kisses?" she asked.

"This is a medical practice. Physical encounters may be misunderstood by a client or by the old guard. Be careful."

"Well, that's a relief," Daisy responded, "I'm not the huggy type anyway."

He advised, "Also, it is against the rules to accept anything that can be misconstrued as an extravagant gift or payment for something. We cannot make a profit on anything in the practice other than to bill the government Medical Services Plan."

Immediately after starting to work with Ken, Daisy had seen people who came to Ken because they could no longer function after being given a psychotropic drug by another physician. The first person was a high profile professional woman suffering a complete physical collapse. She arrived for a first appointment not able to walk by herself. Alerted by a phone call, Daisy had to go out into the street to help her out of a cab and into the office. To Daisy's astonishment, within a few minutes, Ken figured out that the woman was suffering side effects of a commonly prescribed sedative that was given to her by her family physician for post-partum recovery. Without hesitation, Ken got on the telephone while the client sat next to him. He had a conversation with the referring physician to correct the medication. Within a few days, with the addition of Ken's care of the woman and her family in her own home by way of home visits, she was again her usual high functioning self.

What was interesting to Daisy was her own experience of consulting that woman's physician only once after Saul had left her. That physician was eager for Daisy to be on Valium, the same drug that had debilitated this woman. Daisy had taken it only once as prescribed and found herself unable to get out of bed. When she tried to get up, she could not walk. She never took the drug again but did not go back to the physician to explain what happened. Daisy realized that by merely avoiding that doctor and not educating her about the side effects, she probably contributed to this client's situation.

In Daisy's lifetime, her first introduction to knowing any person on a sedative was when living in an Inuit village and Valium was the popular drug for teachers trying to cope with unfamiliar surroundings. From September to December, the grade five teacher on Valium had become increasingly disoriented. By Christmas she was flown out of the north permanently.

It did not take long for Daisy to see what Ken told her about the severe dangers of psychotropic drugs. A man who was having hallucinations had been hospitalized after his general physician prescribed a drug known for hallucinogenic side effects. Ken received a call from the frightened family to come and intervene. Meanwhile, Daisy wondered why, when all the side effects were published, would anyone be given a drug that would hospitalize a patient and on top of that, the patient suffering the side effect was then given a DSM label to live with.

Another woman came seeking help because she was afraid of killing her children. She was suffering post-partum depression and could not cope. Immediate changes were made to her diet and included nutritional supplements. Also another habit was eliminated. Inability to cope with her children disappeared within days. Using Orthomolecular medicine, her cure was rapid and complete.

Ken always told his suicidal clients that they could count on him to be there for them so long as they worked with him, instead of committing suicide. Ken always kept his promise and no one broke his or her promise to him. There was never a suicide in Ken's practice of medicine.

EVEN THOUGH Ken could not solve the ongoing problems with his ex-wife and the fall-out on his own children, he worked magic with clients and their children. In awe, Daisy witnessed miraculous changes in people. She had never in her lifetime seen a physician so efficient with what seemed like pulling the correct fixes right out of the air. She was convinced Ken was a magician of healing.

Ken was Daisy's hero. She had been in love with the man. She now loved the teacher.

22

Storytelling and More

"WILL YOU TELL us the story about the well, Daisy?" Ken asked.

"Sure."

The room became quiet as clients waited in anticipation. Daisy centered herself in preparation to once again tell her story.

"This is a true story. ...A small group of people, including myself, founded the Dharma Centre, a Buddhist meditation centre in Kinmount, Ontario. It is still there today. We bought four hundred acres of beautiful rolling land with forest and a small lake. The land had two log cabins needing a lot of repair and a dry, stone well. Dead porcupines were at the bottom of the well. It was cleaned and the log houses were restored to a livable rustic fashion without modern conveniences. I was chosen to live in the main house with my four children, one just a tiny baby in cloth diapers that I had to wash by hand in a tub of water. Besides looking after my own family, my duties were to look after hundreds of people coming and going, including Buddhist monks from near and far. I had to make sure they all were fed and looked after.

"The well remained dry. Our only water source for drinking, cooking, and washing was a sparkling, pretty little stream that came out of the ground like a tiny fountain between some rocks on our land. To get water from the fountain meant a long walk hauling water in jugs or pails far up and down the dirt road with a large hill that ran alongside our land.

"After a member watched me working in the kitchen, he suggested a solution to water storage. He was able to get oak whisky barrels from the brewery he worked in. So the barrels arrived and were filled with water from the stream. Life seemed easier with two large oak barrels of water with taps sitting in my kitchen.

"Then came the weekend a few weeks later; a lot of people arrived and I cooked the meals as usual. Then they left. I thought it had been a successful weekend until during the next week a message reached me that many people had become ill. I was being blamed because they thought that I had probably cooked their meals with an improper frame of mind, causing illness. I knew this was not true. Water tests did reveal mold in the barrels. Then I did become desperate.

"That afternoon, I stood by the dry well and talked to it. I asked for water.

"My family slept in the top floor rooms of the main cabin and I was in the habit of looking out the window to view the countryside first thing in the morning.

"The very next morning I went to the window as usual, looked out to a beautiful sunshiny morning and saw the well filled with water even though it had not rained during the night.

"I ran out to the well filled with so much water that it overflowed, covering the ground for several feet around. I could not get close.

"Standing there in the morning sunshine, I thanked the well for the water. I talked to the well about too much water. I told the well I wanted the water to be about a foot below the top of the stone wall and not all over the ground.

"The very next morning I looked out the window again and saw that the ground was dry around the well.

"I ran out to the well and sure enough, the ground was dry around the well and the water level was exactly as I had requested. But I looked at the water and it looked a little dirty with dry leaves and bits of dirt floating on top.

"I thanked the well for giving me water to the measurement that I had requested and for the dry ground around the well. Then I asked the well for clean water.

"The very next morning I looked out the window at the well and it looked good. I ran out to the well and it was sparkling clean, to the level I had requested and the ground around was dry.

"I thanked the well and started to use the water that day. It tasted really good and clean. The level of water maintained itself as I had requested.

"We did send a bottle of water for testing and the test came back clean.

"Then I found that I could get water but not everyone could get water. Some people were not allowed to take water from the well. Their pail would not turn over and fill with water no matter how they tried. Only certain people could get the water.

"The well provided clean water as long as I lived there. I heard that when I left the meditation centre, the well went dry.

"So, that is the true story exactly as it happened."

KEN LIKED DAISY to tell this story to clients in need of a new spring of hope and a little stir of magic.

Ken and Daisy told stories that were meant to give clients permission to be comfortable remembering, realizing and telling their own stories from within and beyond their own lines drawn in the sand. The practice was an endless stream of stories, all meaningful and many far outside the constriction of accepted societal thinking, allowing clients freedom to explore and grow in a safe place where they knew the safety net was Ken, who had promised verbally to each client to do no harm and to keep confidentiality.

To engage clients into play and laughter, Ken and his clients occasionally would don silly noses or big eyeglass frames and talk with their disguises on – opening new vistas of communication that clients had not dared to delve into before; at the least, people would have much needed laughter, often followed by floodgates opening to stories and emotions that lay in wait. Playing seemed to be beneficial often.

To help married couples understand each other, Ken sometimes asked them to trade places by sitting in each other's chairs.

"Take the time to feel the energy left behind in the chair."

After a few minutes, someone might start speaking. Most often those sessions had the effect of revelations about the partner's point of view and feelings.

THOUGH THE EXPLORATIONS between married couples often resulted in a saved marriage, not all marriages could be saved regardless of the responsibility to children.

"I am asking each of you to carry an egg in your pocket for one week. The egg is your marriage. You will treasure it. You will nurture it. You will realize it is fragile and can break and cause a mess if not protected. You will help each other to protect the eggs in your awareness that your partner is also protecting the egg. Come back in a week."

A week had gone by and a husband arrived alone for the appointed time. "She smashed my egg! I was trying really hard to save my egg and one night she just turned on me. She slugged my shirt pocket deliberately and smashed it. It ran down my clothes and into my shoe."

Even though the man's situation was no laughing matter, later Daisy joked with Ken about record keeping. "It would be funny for medical records to read about smashed eggs, big noses, and clients saving their marriage because they traded chairs to feel their partner's energy."

Smiling, Ken responded, "They would never understand. It's much easier for administrators to believe in labels and medication, than healing by other means." Then he became serious. "It is exactly this that I expect one day will cost me my medical license in this province."

KEN PASSIONATELY WORKED non-stop attending working committee meetings on health, housing, and environmental committees, supporting and giving talks about healthy change for all. As he did years ago when he was a much younger man starting out, he continued to work humbly as a volunteer, never expecting a return for himself.

Ken spoke about the earth that supports life and how we need to take care of the earth, just as we need to take care of all life. Often speaking to deaf ears, Ken tried to convince groups of people to take care of an ailing environment that many did not see. He wanted people to turn lawns into vegetable gardens to feed the hungry in our society. He wanted all children to be cared for respectfully, housed, and fed healthy food. He wanted the aboriginal people to have proper health care. He worked toward steering aboriginal people to train as physicians and teachers so that they would be able to care for their own communities rather than rely on people with lesser understanding of their culture.

Daisy had always been concerned about the same issues but by being with Ken, everything was revved up as she watched him go from seeing patients to attend hours of meetings and conferences, working every waking moment to convince people to wake up and take care of their children and the earth that supports them.

As Ken told her, "I was a kid like 'chicken little' telling everyone the sky is falling. They paid no attention."

THE FIRST TIME Daisy attended a conference with him and listened to him speak to a crowd, she was struck with surprise at his eloquence of speech. While standing at the podium, he seems to shine with an unworldly light, exuding assurance and light out into the room full of people.

Ken told his audience:

> "...Making things better for our children and grandchildren is an essential human need often disregarded in the name of progress. We are fortunate to have the aboriginal presence to remind us of the need to care for our human and natural resources in the name of our grandparents and our grandchildren. Without this continuity, human beings lose our abilities to make things better at home and in our communities. ..."

Daisy was in awe when Ken walked toward her, smiling. All she could think to say was, "I wish I would have recorded you so I can hear you speak again. I am so impressed."

"You will remember," he assured her.

She was not sure she could remember. She felt the immediate loss of a missed opportunity.

She heard him again, and again – always with another way of explaining to people that they should wake up. He told them how to make good change.

At another podium, giving another speech, Ken told this audience:

"...Over the span of less than fifty years, we have been losing the rights and the skills to build our own homes in which to give birth and education to our children, as well as to care for our sick and dying loved ones. Now we are told that public money for housing, hospitals, and education is short, and providing for these needs becomes a private responsibility while international corporations avoid their tax, environmental, and human responsibilities. In my career, I have found that 'better living through chemistry' makes more people sick faster than I could ever hope to heal them as a physician. ..."

23

Letters

A LETTER ARRIVED from Jane's lawyer, stating that Daisy told Jane not to phone the house regarding Andy. The letter also stated that Jane has never asked for money from Ken.

Ken answered the lawyer by letter, explaining that Daisy only told Jane to stop harassing him and it had nothing to do with her calling about Andy or about arranging care of their son, and that he had gotten on the phone to Jane right at the time to explain and appease her about any misunderstanding.

Immediately, another letter from Jane's lawyer arrived to complain that while in Ken's care, he had allowed their two year old to go on an 'excursion' with a six or eight year old child. This second letter was a clear indication that two separate tracks were being laid. One track was the assembly of information for public record and the other was a hidden track about what was going on in Jane's private relationship with Ken.

There was no child in existence as described in the lawyer's letter. Daisy's children were teenagers or adults and Andy was never allowed to go with strangers. The only person other than Ken who had taken Andy out into the park fronting the townhouse was a daughter, sixteen years of age. The same daughter answered the door when Jane came to pick up Andy that evening. The daughter was visibly shaken for hours. Later she told Daisy she never, ever wanted to encounter Jane's nastiness again.

It had been hard to be helpful to Ken and Andy when any help or attention paid to Andy caused further problems.

Even after Jane's lawyer wrote those letters, the child was withheld, alternating with cries for physical or financial help. The never-ending yoyo behaviour led Ken to try for more joint counselling with Jane.

Nothing helped.

Ken had protected his ex-wife by firing his lawyer and had not hired another lawyer in favour of trusting Jane. Now he was paying the price. There was no one to defend him except Daisy.

Having had enough, Daisy blurted out, "Ken, how could you have married a person like that and had a child with her?"

He paused, then responded, "Look at the guys you were with."

They stopped and listened to themselves. Months of stress had reduced them to an argument going to go nowhere fast. Daisy knew Ken would never tolerate her calling the mother of his child down and Ken was right, she could not defend her past relationships any better than he could.

The feedback from brother Richard on his visit and the explosion that took place when Ken picked Andy up that first day in July were only preliminaries to never ending torture, as Daisy saw it. But more than that, the fallout on Ken was that his health was suffering under the constant emotional abuse, accompanied by his heartache for having moved out on his son. He had been running in the park each morning. That stopped. He was either looking after the child or he was trying to negotiate the latest problems with his ex-wife early in the mornings instead of running. He had been on call constantly to her needs. He was unable to resolve the problem of having had a child with Jane. He was damned if he got close and damned if he was separated.

There was nothing he could do to fix it. Ken cried a lot in those days.

The good news was that with Ken's unwavering physical and financial support regardless of the ups and downs, his ex-wife completed her Articling stint and got on with being a lawyer.

ANOTHER LETTER ARRIVED, this time from the False Creek Housing Co-op Board of Directors. As Daisy read it, she replayed in her head what Ken had said just days before, "Jane told me that you are going to receive a letter from the co-op Board of Directors, giving you notice to vacate because of your dog."

Stunned, Daisy had asked, "How would Jane know of any letter coming to me from the Board before I receive it? And how can my dog be a problem? Other co-op dogs run loose and mine never does and he is not a barker."

"I don't know. I'm telling you what Jane told me."

"Under no circumstances should Jane know of a letter being mailed to me unless she is involved behind the scenes. After all, she used to live here, too, and knows people here."

Ken had also said, "She also told me that False Creek is not up to the standard she wants for her son. She doesn't want her son visiting here."

Holding the letter that just arrived, Daisy was stunned to read that as foretold, the letter was an eviction notice because of the dog; no warning about how to fix a problem, just eviction with no explanation of why the dog was a problem.

Renting a home in the at-large market meant giving up the security of a 90-year lease on lower rent in the co-op housing and a four-bedroom waterfront home that can never be replaced. Daisy had always paid the highest possible rent rate in the co-op even when her income was low as a single parent so that the Board could not find reason to bother her, but for some reason they were bothering her.

Instead of fighting, Daisy willingly gave up her secure housing for the benefit of Ken and Andy, in the hope that Jane would have one less reason to complain and Ken's access to his son would be less strained.

Daisy forgot the message from the psychic, "Don't give up the security of your present home. Stay put regardless of outside forces."

Giving up the co-op home proved to be an enormous sacrifice. It would be a giant mistake. It began several house moves in fast succession with huge financial loss after renting from several unscrupulous landlords.

Soon after moving out of the co-op, at a downtown bus stop, a former co-op neighbour approached Daisy; she was also one of the Directors on the Board of the False Creek Housing Co-op. She was also a red-haired woman but much older. She said, "I want to apologize for what we did to you. My husband and I miss your family."

Daisy smiled and simply said, "Thanks."

On the bus ride home Daisy wondered why she had not asked for an explanation of what happened. Missed opportunity! Instead of labouring over it, she told herself... oh well, let it go... let it all go... I've got better things to do than to dwell on what's lost.

APARTMENT LIVING proved difficult for Ken. His youngest son had been named in rental agreements but regardless, every time Andy made a sound there were complaints. Moving to a new apartment followed by another was always the same. The older sons had not yet come to live with Ken. Preferring a family atmosphere, Ken and Andy spent most weekends and some weekdays and nights in Daisy's home where they always had their own private room out of respect for Jane and Andy.

Waking Ken up from a night's sleep, there were constant weekend late night phone calls from whatever social gathering Jane was attending. It was Daisy's theory that Ken was supposed to get jealous. Ken's separate apartment provided Daisy some welcome respite from what felt like a constant intrusion by a woman who rejected Ken but would not let him go. The apartment also provided Ken with choice as to when he should include his youngest son with Daisy's family.

Ken and Daisy needed the comfort of each other through the continual difficulties that Ken was dealing with.

Sympathetic to Jane, Daisy continued to stay in the background. It was a balancing act to be available to Andy but not take over a mothering role out of respect for Jane. When the tiny boy voiced that he must take food to his mother after he had eaten a full meal, Daisy packed a plate brimming full of the latest dinner for the boy to give to his mother. Jane's never ending complaints and constant need of extra help financially kept Ken occupied. He was determined to grant Jane's every wish and be available around the clock. And Daisy lost dinner plates. When Daisy questioned that Ken was continually trying to please an ex-wife who seemed never to be satisfied, Ken explained, "Jane is just young... really a child."

"Are you kidding? She is only about five years younger than me!" But it was futile to argue when relevance of age was in the eye of the beholder.

24

A Trip to Vermont

JUNE 1982. Ken's mother had a stroke while driving her car. Luckily no one was hurt. Ken wanted to visit her. He was hopeful that because his mother and Daisy had so much in common, his mother would like her. He wanted to show Daisy the small farm where his brother Don, who he was environmentally conscious, harvested maple syrup with the help of horses rather than using a gas tractor. Ken also wanted to introduce Daisy's family into his own roots.

Ron and Loraine and Daisy's youngest daughter Faith came along on the trip to Vermont.

Meeting at the Montreal airport with Ken's mother and youngest brother, Ken was taken aback. He had walked into another problem. Daisy and her family were not so welcome as he had hoped and he had not been forewarned.

Ken's family was made up of strong achievers and this white-haired woman with a soft voice had been a strong achiever herself, and had been the driving force to keep her family together. Daisy had not yet figured out why she and her family were intruders.

The car ride through the green of Vermont was immediately relaxing with promise of a temporary escape from commerciality. There were no billboards. The white buildings sprinkled among green hills gave a feeling of cleanliness and space to breath. And with the green miles, hope did spring that the greeting was a mistake.

SHOWING DAISY the Vermont Medical School Campus was important because Ken wanted to bring her into his life experience. Alone together in the dusk of evening, lights and shadows played dramatically on the impressive old buildings that held so much knowledge and many secrets – and Ken's past. The campus looked as though someone had swept the ground, and it looked mature compared to the young, wilder feeling of western Canada. Daisy was in awe to actually stand with Ken in front of the stately old house where he had lived across the street from the university and where he had walked the ground beneath their feet while studying medicine. He was infused with memories and she did her best to know and feel him in those years by osmosis as they stood together with his arm around her waist under an old tree that was here all those years ago and saw everything. The years melded together from a time past into timelessness.

KEN'S MOTHER introduced the family to the doll museum and toyshop that she built up and had owned in Manchester. She was quick to pick up on Faith's artistic interest and gave her an exciting new material for sculpting. Up to now, Faith had mastered the use of plasticine to make intricate small sculptures. The new material allowed her to make permanent figurines and kept her busy for the rest of the visit.

Ken took Daisy to see an acreage that his family had owned for a while. As they stood on the hill overlooking the home, he explained this was where he tried to convince his parents to turn it into a small farm. He explained that at the time, his sisters had horses but to his disappointment, his parents were not interested in farming.

Green Vermont – rolling hills, white houses dotting the green, lake on one side and mountains in the distance on the other, Morgan horses with luscious tails long enough to touch the ground, the medical school, and family. All put together, Daisy now understood why Ken was so very homesick.

ON A DAY TRIP to the Morgan horse farm, the family watched the beauties frolicking in the green grass. This was an education for

Daisy because she had never known Morgans before; now she fell in love with them.

In making their way as tourists around the farm, they were unexpectedly led into an area to witness breeding. When the female horse was brought into a confined, off the ground stall like a stage, and the already stimulated 'ready' male horse was led up the ramp to mount her, Ken and Daisy simultaneously had emotional reactions like being kicked in the gut. What bothered each of them was the enforcers – the captors – the rape of both the male and female. The staged rape reminded them of the confinements of certain relationships and laws that bind. They reacted physically by leaving. They could not watch. Besides, they had a young girl with them and this type of mating was not family entertainment. Ken's words of former days rung in Daisy's head, "I can't mate in captivity." He meant that he could not *live* in captivity. Neither could she. Somehow the event brought even more understanding of what Ken was objecting to in his former marriage. But it also brought up why she had been on the run from a first marriage. As they walked away, each in their own way shuddered and wanted to shake off memories of being in captivity.

IN KEN'S MOTHER'S house with some time alone together, Ken took the opportunity to take Daisy on a tour of pictures on the walls. "This is my wedding picture. Who do you think Carolyn is marrying if you look at the picture?"

The picture did show a bewildered Ken almost standing alone while his new wife leaned closer to the minister.

What a surprise! Daisy reminded herself that even this story was true.

Another framed photo of an aunt caused Daisy to wonder if Ken had been attracted to Jane because of a resemblance to this aunt. She decided not to mention it.

In the midst of stories about the family, they became aware of two cloth dolls of several feet in height, representing a woman and man, sitting on a chair by the fireplace. They had been given as a gift to Ken's parents. The male doll was disturbingly crooked, somehow characterizing the illness that had kept Ken's father in hospital.

Together, they straightened the doll's face and body to look healthier and set him back beside the other doll. Once again, they were on the same wavelength and worked together to fix something.

THE STROKE HAD obviously affected Ken's mother but she could still enjoy planting flowers. Daisy took the opportunity to sit beside her in the garden and try to be friends. Ken's mother was eager to relive the past by telling Daisy all about her son. Stories tumbled out of her, including truly intimate details about Ken's earlier life. They were fresh in his mother's memory.

NEAR THE END of the visit, the anticipation that Ken was leaving again had his mother wearing her heart on her sleeve. She missed their talks of so long ago just as much as he missed them. She would be losing her first born to the far Northwest all over again. She was upset with him for going off with this new family.

In the conversations that got testy, Ken reminded her that he originally left the United States because of the Vietnam War – not because he wanted to go away.

Her response was, "What war?"

Though his mother had keen memory of family and past business affairs, she had lost some memory of worldly affairs and had forgotten the war that took her son away.

It had become apparent to Ken that there were various opinions floating around family members about his leaving the brothers to look after family affairs because of their father's ongoing hospitalization and now their mother's stroke that caused a certain amount of impairment. With three sons on the opposite side of the continent in another country entirely, Ken had to live apart from family in order to take care of family.

His mother's pain became palatable. Ken was distressed because he could not fix it – and he would love to return to Vermont, so much so that Daisy and her family started looking briefly at how to do it.

The newspaper ads regarding housing in Vermont were extremely attractive. Being able to work and be self-supporting as Canadians in a foreign country was the problem. It was a nice dream for a few hours, but then reality set in. Ken knew he could not leave his sons so far away because his first responsibility was to his children. Daisy understood because of her own children. It was agreed that a move without all their children could not happen – at least not now.

Ken's mother had been a kind and generous hostess to the new family, but in an emotional breakdown, she made it clear that this new family was no replacement. "I want grandchildren of my own blood to come home!"

And there it was. It was not personal that Daisy and her family were outsiders. It was family by blood ties that Ken's mother wanted around her.

AT HOME A FEW DAY LATER, Daisy answered the telephone in the office and then handed the telephone to Ken. "You need to take this."

He listened, and then asked, "What is the pain like?" Ken was standing and straightened to his usual alertness pose, looking toward the ceiling as he often did so that he could hear and 'see' better.

Ken asked the obvious question, "Have you called your doctor?"

"Stay calm. Is your husband with you? ...Good! Have him take you to the new hospital immediately. Immediately! We'll meet you there."

Ken turned to Daisy as he hung up the telephone. "Please cancel all the afternoon clients quickly. We need to go to the hospital. I think the placenta is tearing away. She is caught in the middle while the hospital makes its move. She can't get anyone on the phone so we have to make sure she is taken care of right away."

KEN WAS RIGHT in his diagnosis. The mother and her baby were in grave danger. Ken had chosen the best obstetrician he knew of to care for her throughout her pregnancy. Because she was family, Ken had hired a nurse-midwife, one of the two that were new to working in the new hospital under new rules. Ken's own sister was working as a nurse-midwife in Vermont; he was familiar with how they worked.

The obstetrician chose not to rush into a caesarian as another doctor might. Instead, he monitored mom and baby closely, hoping for a natural outcome.

Then the obstetrician insisted Ken and family get away from the hallway close to the room. With Ken out of the way, and without a consultation with the birthing mother, the obstetrician invited a crowd of hospital staff and medical students to fill the birthing room. There was standing room only to watch as he heroically managed this difficult birth.

Through extremely painful labor because of the shots of Pitosin, an artificial hormone that simulates the body's natural hormone Oxytocin to facilitate labor, and though long, in the end the birthing was successful.

ON BEING BORN, the baby was immediately transferred to the Newborn Intensive Care Unit, a protocol and a precaution for a baby born a bit early, adding to that the condition of Placenta Abruptio.

During the night, a person stood over the mother to give her the news that the baby breathed so hard she blew a hole in her lung and was on life support. It was a harsh awakening. Then, rather than offering to take the mother to her baby, the person walked out, leaving the now sleepless mother alone for hours to worry in the dark.

The morning after the birth, Ken and Daisy looked through the nursery window at an incubator holding the newborn laced with tubes and breathing apparatus. The baby was battling for her life.

"Placenta Abruptio. Ken, if it hadn't been for you, the mother and baby might have bled to death. I'm always amazed at your knowledge and how you know things, even through a phone. ...But

I believe someone carelessly blew a hole in the baby's lung. I think they covered it up by telling the mother that the baby blew a hole in her own lung. In other words, blaming the baby for her own possible demise. How could they be so careless, then lie about it?"

"I can't give them medicine while they are in hospital but you can give a Homeopathic remedy to your family." Ken suggested a remedy for the trauma. "Mom and baby are still attached by an invisible connection – energy. If we treat the mom, the baby may benefit."

"Right. Who on earth but you and I would understand that?"

[IN FUTURE, this baby will tell her own birth story. No one will ever describe this birth to her, but at the age of three, the information will come from her memory. The child will say that a spot on top of her head hurt. (The spot was where the monitor hook was in her head during labor.) She will describe moving through a tunnel and coming out into a room filled with people all dressed in green and how they frightened her. She will give testimony that newborn babies do feel, do see, do hear, do have a range of emotions that they can describe – meaning that they have knowledge of a range of emotions, and they do remember and can retain memory of details like colour.

This child gives testimony that these senses do not just start at birth but they develop and function in the womb long before birth – putting to rest the beliefs as late as the 1970s when new babies, and even babies several weeks old, were thought to see only shadows and could not feel pain.

Moreover, as a newborn, this child reacted with extreme sensitivity to emotions of people around her and to words of people around her; it became obvious when she reacted with strong embarrassment and even cried when talked about.

The baby born before full term already had a range of understanding and emotion that was more than just feeling – she had advanced understanding that at age three she could articulate.]

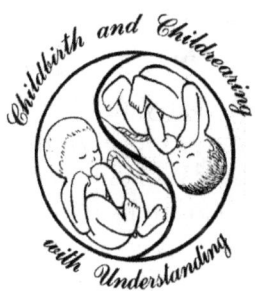

Childbirth and Childrearing with Understanding

part two

25

Pioneer Health Centre

KEN WROTE in his notebook:
The Story of Pioneer Health Centre
"In the Spring of 1981, Daisy and Ken got together and decided to develop a place for people in love. At that time, we were utilizing the theories and methods of Wilhelm Reich, M.D. in our work with couples and families. By November '81, we rented and renovated an office at [address] for this work. In the Spring of 1982, we joined the Task Force on Midwifery and Ken wrote... paper on the relevance of personal therapy for natural childbirth. At about the same time we met [naturopathic doctor] and began discussing the interrelations between Chinese medicine, acupuncture and Reichian bodywork. These discussions led in October to the foundation of the Pioneer Health Centre..."

IN HIS RESEARCH, Ken had discovered and read all the books and papers he could find on the Peckham Experiment that had been originally established in 1926, closed in 1929 and re-established in 1935, continuing until 1950 at the Peckham Pioneer Health Centre in Peckham, a suburb of London, England. Founders, Dr. Scott Williamson and Dr. Innes Pearce proved that the centre could provide hundreds of families, who lived within walking distance, with a place to take care of their emotional, physical and social needs and potentials.

It was an experiment of health. It was believed that health, rather than illness, would thrive and be contagious to people if they had a place in which to be healthy. Organic food was provided to the premises by way of their own small farm with gardens.

All family members of all ages were able to participate in physical activity in the large swimming pool, gym and other activities within the building. Children could play among themselves and parents could participate or socialize while watching over their children in the wisely designed building. Social activities for all members allowed freedom to move about and not be tied to schedules. There were regular health check-ups, and continuing prenatal and postnatal care all in one place.

The founders believed that prevention of illness could be obtained for a whole community by looking after the whole person; this was the key to good health and healthy family living.

TO REPLACE the idea of a country-healing centre, Ken got excited about building a place like the Peckham Pioneer Health Centre right in the city of Vancouver.

In eagerness to share his research and build on the work of the Peckham Experiment, he had spoken with a physician who was partially retired with a continuing hand in at the University of British Columbia Medical School, and in the past he had establish a health centre in East Vancouver. This elderly physician invited Ken to give a talk about the English model to medical students at UBC.

Ken asked Daisy to come with him. She expected a theatre in which Ken could address at least one class of students with the use of an overhead screen but they were ushered into a lunchroom with a long white table and a few wooden kitchen chairs.

A few students in their white coats sat around the table while others meandered casually in and out, or lolled in the doorway rather than commit one way or another. With such inattention, it was an awkward situation for Ken to explain what the Peckham Experiment was about. As people shuffled noisily, Ken's soft voice did not carry well. He passed around books with pictures for show-and-tell but it was obvious that no one had the least bit of interest.

Ken was still speaking as one student, who had not committed beyond the door-jam, took aside the older physician who also had not committed himself beyond the doorway. Daisy was appalled to overhear the young man complain about wasted time, to which the older physician was heard to deny his involvement and meandered away down the hall with the student, thereby wiping out any connection to Ken and left Ken dangling.

Shocked, Daisy yearned to protect Ken, who only meant well and was, as usual, giving of his time and research for free and at least deserved respect.

Listening to a few following remarks, it was made clear that for this particular group of students, the notion of keeping people healthy rather than just looking for symptoms and cures was lost on them; their time was too valuable to consider health.

Walking away from the campus, Daisy burned with outrage at what she considered stupidity of some medical students. She was even more outraged at the old doctor who invited Ken and then turned his back under the influence of a young student, who was not much older than a boy and was supposedly at school to learn something.

Her opinion spilled out. "This, in a nutshell, is what our medical system is suffering from – doctors graduating who are only taught to cure and not taught how to help people avoid illness; a system that only wants to support paying doctors for illness, rather than support doctors to help people to stay well; doctors who will protect their own rear ends when challenged even by a kid pretending to be a doctor."

She really wanted to lash out at the people left behind in the medical building, to wake them up and quit their holier than thou idea of medicine. Being new at this, Daisy felt righteous that she had not been brainwashed and could see through the sham of a system and why it was so lacking.

She continued, not able to shut up in her disgust, "Science based medicine, my eye! They don't know their asses from their elbows!"

Through it all, Ken listened quietly. He was dealing with feelings of having been humiliated.

Daisy's respect for Ken grew by leaps and bounds even as he faced adversities and disappointments. She had a growing enchantment with Ken's ideas and his constant battle to make a better world. Her battle was to keep him safe.

She told Ken that the problem was that these kids, meaning the medical students, do not understand the difference between the Peckham Pioneer Health Centre and the present day community centres that have scheduled activities with no larger health plan for families.

"You know Ken, today reminds me of wanting to protect my mother when I was just a baby. My memory is clear at a very young age. I was really tiny and could not even walk yet. I was told I walked at nine months, so I had to be younger than that. My mother allowed her two girl friends to take me out for an afternoon. I remember them clearly... one was my mother's long time best friend from childhood, my Godmother. I even remember them asking my mom to take me out and then I remember my mother dressing me up nice for the occasion. They took me to a third friend's house and we were in a basement kitchen. At that age I was even aware of where I was. I remember my Godmother sitting me on the kitchen counter and I was looking up at all the water pipes just a short distance over my head. They started talking about my mother, criticizing her, and I was listening. Even though I was a baby, I remember the angry emotions I felt and I did not want to be there with them because I knew these women were doing wrong by talking about my mother behind her back. I was horribly helpless because I could not talk to defend and protect my mother but I understood everything they were saying. Every word! I feel the same now. I have insight into people but I cannot speak to defend you in situations like this... but I want to."

She wanted so much to make him feel better with her story.

ENTHUSIASM FOR BUILDING a Pioneer Health Centre kept Ken studying and talking about it. The experience at UBC was behind him.

Word got around. Coming out of a sabbatical spent being an artist, a general physician needed to start a new practice in medicine. A naturopathic doctor and the artist approached Ken about wanting to share a clinic with him. Meeting for lunch in a restaurant, Daisy quietly sized the two up. Normally another artist would be of interest but her reaction to this guy was aversion for no obvious reason and Mr. Handsome Charming Naturopath did not charm her either. She would not put her body in front of either one even if her life depended on it.

Ken listened to their needs. Then he explained his. "I am interested in a health centre based on the principles of the Peckham Experiment that was done in England. You can read about it in this book, *Quality of Life*, by Dr. Innes Pearce. The principles are that whole families are looked after in a holistic way. Between the three of us, we should be able to do it. I would want a business plan with a mandate in writing."

Mr. Physician and Mr. Naturopath agreed verbally to the terms and that Daisy would set up and manage the office.

GOING FORWARD, the four met again around Daisy's dining room table. They agreed to lease and renovate an empty space in a local medical building. The guys played broke so Ken agreed to pay the rent for all in a smaller space in the same building until the new health centre was built. Daisy offered to do reception and administration as an unpaid volunteer for the guys so that they could start working together immediately. The two new partners would get a free ride for months, but it was a new beginning of the Pioneer Health Centre and a dream.

"We will need another person to manage a three doctor office when we open the new office. I suggest Daisy's daughter Lana be in training with Daisy as our part-time medical office assistant. This will be the beginning of her medical training. I expect she will be a physician one day." Ken made this suggestion because Lana had come home from Winnipeg. Though she loved dancing, she had become disenchanted about the lifestyle of leading ballerinas she had met and watched. Unknown to Ken, when Lana was age one and a half, Daisy's son had an accident and it was a question about whether or not to have the ankle x-rayed. Lana got up from across the room, walked toward the ankle, pointing at it and said in a clear, strong voice, "It will heal." That was the first hint that Lana would one day be a doctor. Ken was right.

In the background Daisy's sons were replacing a glass pane in the door of the newly rented house. Daisy watched the men leave the house with an air of superiority as they walked past her boys.

Ken saw this, too. "Watch out for those two guys," he warned Daisy as the door closed behind them.

CONSTRUCTION OF THE new Pioneer Health Centre on the first floor of the medical building had been underway for weeks. The walls were up, marking spaces. There was the sound of a hammer banging nails and a saw sawing wood in the background. Some lumber lay in stacks. Ken and Daisy observed the progress.

"It's a far cry from the Pioneer Health Centre in England but it's a start." Ken sounded hopeful.

He told the man in charge of construction, "I don't want any glue under the rug because of fumes, and no paints that give off fumes. This is a medical centre."

The contractor/builder was a friend of Mr. Naturopath and was at the same time remodeling Mr. Naturopath's home. "Oh, sure," he smiled assuringly.

IT HAD BEEN months coming. A party marking the opening of the new Pioneer Health Centre was underway. A large crowd of clients and friends who knew the doctors had gathered. Daisy had arranged the reception area with trays of food and drinks that had been paid for by Ken with no contribution for the other guys. Even this part was a free ride for them. Ken's new therapy room, large enough to see whole families in, was turned into a ballroom for the night. A buxom, attractive, young blond lady with thick red lipstick was Mr. Naturopath's date. They danced up a happy storm. Mr. Physician watched by himself at the sidelines.

In the reception area, Ken was busy setting up large air filters, one that he bought and a couple rented.

Daisy said to him. "Here we are, opening the Pioneer Health Centre at last. I love your room. Your cork flooring is great."

Ken was not happy as he fiddled with machine settings. "We have gone ahead on good faith but those guys have resisted putting an agreement in writing so far."

"Yeah," Daisy agreed, "and renovations have taken a long time."

"I asked them to avoid gluing rugs down but they did it anyway. The fumes are too heavy. It's not a healthy place. I hope this will filter out particles in the air."

OPEN WITH PATIENTS coming and going, Lana was working at the reception desk while Daisy moved Ken's medical files from boxes into his filing cabinets. She was also working out a method of colour coding the charts so that at a glance it would be known which doctor or doctors in the clinic the patient had seen.

She opened another box and while lifting out files, two small pieces of paper with handwritten notes on them fell to the floor. At first glance they seemed insignificant but noticing each was titled 'Wish List', she read them. The information hit her solar plexus with a thud. After a pause to digest the telling tale, Daisy glanced through the thick manual they had fallen from; it was an elaborate financial plan clearly put together by a financial planner.

THAT EVENING, Daisy and Ken walked along the seawall. City lights were mirrored in calm indigo water of the bay.

Daisy was disturbed. "Ken, there is a file in the office probably by mistake. I read it anyway because two small notes fell out. They are wish lists... one written by you wishing for *love* and *family, and home, peace, health*. The other paper is in Jane's handwriting. I saw with my own eyes the difference between you and her. She wished for Power! Money! Prestige! Her list is very scary."

"We wrote those wish lists in therapy. I was trying to save our marriage so I took her and our baby to Ben and Jock on Cortes Island for couple therapy. I know what she wrote. Those are our differences."

"You mean she was there with her baby and that's what she wrote? How sad! Most women would have been feeling nurturing hormones and reflected that... In the same box, I found a financial plan. The way I read it, the planner had your wife playing with money and assets while you worked for them."

"That's right. Jane and I had agreed to a different plan, one where I would pay for her to go to school and when she got her degree, I would have an opportunity to change careers in return. Then I got presented with another plan. I told her she was killing me with her need for material things. "

"You always protect her but you know, some of the things you have told me seemed extremely farfetched, but as I have met the people in your life and see things, I realize you are always telling the truth. The way I see it, unscrupulous people take advantage of you."

"People don't realize I mean it when I say I don't do things conventionally and I never expect to make lots of money. The way I see it, my ex-wife thought she could change me into a man who wants the prestige of a three-piece suit when I prefer to dress casually. On that note, I expect to be in trouble one day because I practice differently than other Psychiatrists."

"But all the billings are correct. You never do anything wrong with your clients. You have *outstanding* success in helping people."

"That may be true but in this province there is an expectation that a psychiatrist gives drugs as treatment. I don't prescribe drugs."

"I know. You change things around for people where other doctors are stumped. That's often why you get referrals."

"The big problem is that everything I do as a Psychiatrist is under one umbrella of the Medical Services Plan. I believe in universal insurance for all but they have made it illegal for me to do any alternative or complimentary medicine. I've probably told you this before, but a physician high in the ranks of the BC College of Physicians and Surgeons has already told me that if he catches any physician doing Homeopathy, he would take away the license to practice medicine. I can't practice medicine without a license but my license prohibits me from doing anything except allopathic medicine. And it's illegal for a physician to barter or work outside the system of the Medical Services Plan."

"You mean trading medical care for bread and chickens instead of money like in the old days."

"That's right. That's illegal. And it's illegal for me to share my earnings with the patients who may not be sick if they had more money with which to feed healthy food to their families. One day, they could come down on me just for being different. Before that happens, I need to change my career. Preferably to teach again."

"The problem with breaking into teaching here on the West coast is that everyone is protecting their own ass and won't let people like you in easily because you may have more experience than they have and upset their apple cart."

"I gave up tenure in Regina because I needed to move my family."

"It may have been a mistake to give up tenure."

"I was trying to save my marriage."

"Ken, I prefer your casual dress! I prefer your high-class intellect. I like that you are a gentle human being with morals. I feel safe around you."

Holding hands, they walked along the stone walkway by the water in silence, deep in their own thoughts.

Ken turned inward, thinking about his moves and why he made them.

Daisy feasted her eyes on the deepening surrounding colours and how the scene should be captured for posterity.

OUTSIDE KEN'S THERAPY ROOM near the reception desk but out of the way of people traffic, Ken had furnished a children's play area with toys and small table and chairs for doing artwork. A four-year old boy was talking to the toys while his mother was with Ken behind closed doors. Daisy and Lana kept an eye on the child from their desk.

Suddenly, Mr. Naturopath's door flung open. He angrily marched a few feet to confront Daisy at her desk. "Keep that child quiet!" he barked and marched back into his room, slamming his door. His commotion was noisier than the child.

At that, Daisy knew this project was a fail. While Mr. Naturopath wanted quiet for whatever reason, he seemed insensitive to his own patients. Many times Daisy had stopped patients that he had just treated from leaving the office because they were unsteady on their feet. She would give his patients a cup of tea and ask them to wait until they could leave safely.

The stubborn streak running up Daisy's back was enough to keep her in her seat just watching the bad behavior of Mr. Naturopath and to ignore his demand.

Meanwhile, Mr. Physician had been doing another vaginal exam on the same woman who came in regularly and she could be heard making a familiar sound. Daisy could never figure out if she. was in pleasure or pain or why the child's noise bothered Mr. Naturopath when this woman was noisier and apparently did not bother him. Daisy only knew she would again have to scrub and sterilize the metal non-disposable instrument being used for the vaginal exam. Daisy was not looking forward to it.

It had been a few months since the Pioneer Health Centre opened. It had become clear that the centre was not functioning anything like the Peckham Pioneer Health Centre. There was no interest by Mr. Naturopath or Mr. Physician as to what Ken was trying to do. They simply appeared to be happy for all the patient referrals they could get out of Ken.

IT WAS EARLY MORNING. Daisy slipped into Ken's therapy room as a couple left with their child. The sunlight streamed into the large room tastefully and comfortably furnished with casual chairs, a lounge with bright cushions, area rug, lamp, plants, and shelves of books. It was too nice a space to spoil with her information, but she had to.

"Ken, I need to talk with you. The accounting ledger for renovations doesn't look right to me. I think someone has siphoned off a lot of lumber and supplies from the renovations."

"Are you sure?" Disappointment had been building but he had not expected this.

"I'll take the ledger to your accountant today," she offered.

THE LARGE, THICK LEDGER lay across the accountant's desk. His brow furrowed as he flipped pages.

"It has been kept by the contractor," Daisy explained.

"I can't make head or tail of this. It's tax time. I don't have the time to audit this now. Bring it back in a couple of weeks."

BACK AT THE health centre, Daisy placed the ledger into the bottom drawer of a filing cabinet and locked it, believing this to be a safe place.

SUNSHINE POURED THROUGH the window from down the hallway onto the filing cabinets, starting the next day. Daisy unlocked the filing cabinets to find a blank space – the ledger was gone. She turned on her heels and went to Ken's open door.

"Ken, I locked the renovation ledger in the filing cabinet last night. Now it's gone! Over night someone with a key has taken it."

"We'll just ask the guys where it is." As he said that, the two men arrived together through the main door.

Daisy approached them, "Have either of you seen the renovation ledger?"

Mr. Naturopath said, "No!" and slipped into his room without missing a beat.

Mr. Physician said, "Nope," and rushed to his room while looking straight ahead as though dismissing Daisy.

Their doors closed simultaneously, leaving Daisy feeling the air that moved as they had rushed past her. She was suspicious that one of them had overheard her speaking to Ken about what she was up to the day before.

On Ken's advice, Daisy arranged a picnic lunch paid for by Ken, as usual, and called for a noon meeting out on the lawn behind the building. They sat in an informal circle. Neither man showed interest in eating.

It seemed to Daisy that the two guys were grinning like Cheshire cats with a pact to not participate, so she started the meeting by laying out the agenda. "We need to discuss the mandate of the health centre and we need to discuss the missing renovation ledger."

Mr. Physician answered, "I don't keep the ledger."

Mr. Naturopath said, "I have nothing to say about it."

Daisy continued, "The ledger went missing overnight. What about the contractor? Does he have a key to the filing cabinets that contain confidential medical records? Someone removed the ledger after the office was closed."

There was no answer.

Ken changed the subject to the other outstanding problem. "We have yet to sign the business plan and health centre mandate,"

Silence continued.

The meeting bombed. There was a solid wall. The two men appeared resolved to be silent, not to participate, and not keep promises made to Ken while expecting that Ken would continue in this sham.

IT WAS A SAD DAY. Ken cancelled clients in order to pack up his room.

Since all the furniture belonged to Ken except for what the two guys had in their own rooms and the autoclave, there was the necessity for all filing cabinets to be cleared. Daisy was busy separating his files from any the other doctors had in the filing system. The two men had been told they must find their own furniture because after the workday, the reception area would be empty.

Daisy approached Mr. Physician to retrieve the several examination instruments that Ken loaned to him because Mr. Physician came with nothing, not even the basic tools of a physician, like a stethoscope. To Daisy's surprise, he denied having any of Ken's instruments. Angry at this outrageous denial since she knew the equipment well and had been witness to Ken's generosity, Daisy marched into the examining room and opened cupboards. With basic instruments in her hands, Mr. Physician approached from behind and tried to grab them back while slamming the cupboard door closed on her hand as she was reaching for missing parts. He ordered her to leave his room.

She left with instruments missing a few attachments. He had been unsuccessful at taking back what she had already retrieved.

Daisy told Ken, "Mr. Physician has kept some pieces of your medical instruments, insisting they are his. I think he thought he has kept more than he has. The attachments are no good without the main instruments."

Daisy expected Ken to go in and insist on the return of his equipment but typical of him, he did not. "I won't argue over things." He continued packing.

She was thinking about the soft yellow flannel sheet that also belonged to Ken and used to be on his day bed. It was beyond retrieval in Mr. Naturopath's guarded room. It was her fault that it was now lost. She had been doing the laundry for that room and when Mr. Naturopath asked to use Ken's sunshine sheet, she had allowed him to borrow it, expecting it to be temporary.

She could not help but think what a ride these guys had with her even taking the laundry home to do for them.

Ken brought her out of her thoughts. "I have already spoken to my lawyer about my legal position. I have no interest in pursuing them legally. They can rent my room to someone else and keep the assets of the building. I don't think they want to end up in court under the circumstances. It's an experiment that didn't work. They have resisted putting anything in writing. Now this! I'm walking... starting over again."

Daisy had additional news a few minutes later. "They have just given me a letter to formally fire me and they also fired Lana. They are covering their asses, just in case we thought we would stay on. I hope I never see them again. They had better not ask me for the time of day! I have used up all my rolls of rice paper that I used for Chinese painting; I covered their windows with it and they did not even thank me. Ken, I have looked for the beautifully embossed Hippocratic Oath that is yours. It also was stolen from the filing cabinets."

26

War of the Women

THE ENDING OF the Pioneer Health Centre was supposed to be a new start for Ken. The new office was a large, airy space with surround windows that opened on the sunny side of the street, on the second floor of a building that already had another medical office with three doctors on the same floor. It already had a reception area separate from the spacious main room. Other than a coat of fresh paint, this time Ken did not have to renovate. It seemed perfect.

Things sped up. Ken was inundated with the women in his life and his three sons were larger than life.

Andy had been enrolled in a privately run pre-school and was taken care of all day long, five days a week. Andy's nanny was out of work because Ken could take care of his son evenings, weekends, and even weekdays when necessary. Ken had been grateful to the nanny for keeping his son safe over the years. Even though he had personally paid all of her salary all those years, he felt he owed her more. To solve the obligation, he hired her to do the reception work in the office.

Daisy liked gentle Janet as a person and was also grateful to her for helping Ken with Andy all those years. On the other hand, Daisy had gone to school for ten months, giving up several evenings a week to train as a medical office assistant, so she was quietly miffed that the nanny was not expected to do that.

THE REALESTATE AGENT, who had sold the house to Ken and Jane, was the agent for selling it again to give the proceeds to Jane. He had been anxious to talk to Ken about what he said he had been told. Ken and Daisy met with him at his place of work.

Derrik said, "She told me the crack in the basement window was caused by you. She said you broke it in a fit of rage."

Ken was visibly shocked. "I wonder why she would tell anyone such a false story."

"To make you look bad?" the agent questioned. "Considering she is reaping all the proceeds, it seems strange that on top of that she wants you to look bad. I just thought you should know."

The revelation of that story sat unattended but for Ken and Daisy, it was worrisome, sitting in the background. What else was being said or what was to come?

WAITING FOR KEN to come out of the bank, Daisy dawdled, looking at book covers in the window of a second-hand bookstore. As Ken came out of the bank, his face showed extreme concern.

"The bank has confiscated my total income for this month to close a loan. I took the loan to repay Jane's father for a down-payment on her house."

"Why would they do that?"

"That's what I asked. The manager told me they are calling in all small loans because they made bad investments in Africa."

"And you have to pay for that? But you never missed a payment. Every cent of your income arrives automatically twice a month to this bank. I think you should move your account before your next paycheck arrives."

"They won't do that twice."

TWO WEEKS LATER, Ken arrived at the office, having come from the bank. Daisy was sitting behind the front desk checking up on work done by the nanny.

Still in shock, Ken said, "They did it again! The bank took my total income a second time! I have no money!"

Daisy was always amazed at the innocence of this man who lived his life by trusting that there was goodness in all people but in turn got dumped on and stolen from.

FOR MANY YEARS Ken had been studying other cultural methods of understanding the human body. Together, he and Daisy studied Chinese Medicine and Tai Chi with a respected Traditional Chinese Medicine Acupuncturist of Chinese decent. Ken had been referring some clients with severe physical pain as a result of bodily injuries to this healer, with amazing results. With Janet at the front desk, Daisy was encouraged to do other things like accompanying willing clients to their treatments so that she could give support while learning techniques. One such client was a man with a frozen neck as a result of being tortured while a he was political prisoner in another county. She watched as a correctly placed needle in the opposite end of the body unlocked his neck that moved pain free within seconds.

DAISY'S MOTHER, sister and niece had come from Regina for their yearly visit. While walking on a Vancouver street, her mother tripped on uneven pavement, fell and chipped a bone in her elbow. The same acupuncturist treated her.

At the same time Ken's mother arrived from Vermont to visit with her grandchildren. Ken was surprised that his brothers forgot to buy traveling health insurance for the elderly woman who had health issues. This meant Ken would have to pay for of all her health needs. When she was told that Ken had given up his partnership in the Pioneer Health Centre she became upset and tried to convince him to reinstate himself.

Because of his work schedule, Ken asked Daisy to take his mother for necessary allopathic medical tests. Over a snack in a restaurant following the tests, Ken's mother used the opportunity to tell Daisy that she must convince her son to continue with the Pioneer Health Centre partnership. Daisy explained clearly that in her opinion Ken had been in partnership with a couple of guys who took advantage of him and they did not share his idea of a mandate for the health centre.

An hour later, Ken's mother and Daisy arrived back at the house where Ken was waiting. As they walked in, Ken's mother wasted no time in announcing, "Daisy and I have agreed that you should not quit the partnership and you should go back."

Ken was surprised and suddenly angry as he looked at Daisy, who was taken aback.

"Ken, I did not say that. Your mother must have misunderstood me."

Now all three were upset. Ken's mother was saying one thing, Daisy saying another, and he was caught in the middle, not wanting to accuse either woman of lying or to accuse Daisy of betraying him.

Ken's mother thought she had convinced Daisy to back her up and she felt betrayed by Daisy.

Daisy was in a bind because she did not want to argue with Ken's mother who, however mistaken, only had her son's best interest at heart. Misrepresented, Daisy did not know how deliberately mischievous this was or if it was truly a misunderstanding by a woman who had suffered a stroke, but she felt betrayed. Knowing indefensible damage had been done between herself and Ken, and between herself and his mother, she walked out, leaving mother and son to work things out.

She could hear their voices rise as she walked away. Ken was determined that his mother must understand he would not go back on his decision. His mother wanted him to understand that her keen business sense told her that a partnership in a medical clinic is desirable and he must not give it up.

KEN'S MOTHER had been a strong businesswoman. Following in her father's footsteps, she made a lot of money as he predicted she would, but most of her earnings were being spent taking care of her husband's medical costs. She was a woman who remained faithful to her hospitalized husband, carrying his framed picture everywhere she went. Expectations of her children to be successful and well educated were high. There also was her version of high moral standards expected of her family in their personal lives. Divorce was not condoned. To her, the first wives were the true wives; a second wife could be tolerated if she produced grandchildren; a third wife was forever just "the other woman" and Daisy had stepped into that role with her never-to-be-blood-relatives children. In private, the gossip in Ken's family was that

Daisy and her family must be in it for money – an accusation all too familiar to Daisy.

AMIDST ALL THE ongoing drama and in a convergence of women, the first ex-wife arrived to visit with Ken's mother. Carolyn and second ex-wife Jane took the opportunity of their ex-mother-in-law's visit in her weakened state to gang up on Daisy. Word got back to Daisy early in the day that the two ex-wives and Ken's mother were in a restaurant for lunch and the two ex-wives loudly made a joke of Daisy in public.

Later that day, Ken relayed the same description of the event to Daisy as his second ex-wife had told it to him.

What could Daisy say? The three women in Ken's life before her had happily ganged up on her; and now there was a fourth, the nanny, who was always nice and polite but had been added to the ranks of privilege and power.

THE HOUSE KEN had rented for his sons was also comfortable for his mother's visit. It had two suites so he lived upstairs with his sons and his mother. Daisy's oldest son and his partner rented the bottom suite.

Daisy lived in a rented house a couple of blocks away. She and Ken had fallen in love with her house on their first visit because of the smell of oil painting that the previous owner was doing in the large upstairs bathroom beside the hot tub under a skylight. Even though Ken and Daisy lived in separate residences, they managed to get together in her place under a skylight over the bed to enjoy reading Chagall's book together. They spent time in the hot tub and dreamt about painting pictures if they could only find the time between working and the turmoil of caring for three families – his and his and hers.

In private stolen moments before Ken's mother's arrival they would dance in his home, in the living room to music he loved – just the music and being together. He told her he loved the natural heartbeat of the music. Little did they know that even those times together would become fragile memories in days to come.

Their mothers met and had a cordial conversation, promising to keep in touch. Daisy watched as her mother seemed so innocent, trusting that she had just met a friend in Ken's mother. Her mother did not realize that Ken's mother, as a result of her stroke and continuous efforts with her own grandchildren and the problem in making Ken listen to her, would simply forget the meeting.

IN PREPARATION FOR a planned day to honor the two grandmothers in a combined family gathering, Daisy had gone shopping for a smorgasbord of food and filled the refrigerator in Ken's part of the house. Because of the expected sharing, it was an innocent assumption that there would be no need to put the food in her son's refrigerator in the lower suite.

Uninvited to the gathering, Carolyn unexpectedly arrived to usurp the afternoon by loudly holding court with Ken's mother inside the upper suite of the house. No one dared to enter the house or to start serving any food.

As Carolyn could be heard loud and clear through open windows, Daisy and Ken gardened in the back yard. Daisy's mother watched in quiet serenity from a chair under the shade of a tree with her first great-grandchild on her knee. Photos were taken of several generations. Daisy's family was so far unaware of major trouble brewing.

Tension was building in Ken. He was familiar with how his first wife bent his mother's ear. He had already explained to Daisy that Carolyn had always been determined to be a favored daughter to his mother even after divorce and had refused to give up the Schramm name even though she had remarried. In fact, he had admitted that one of the reasons he had not gone to his own family reunion was to avoid Carolyn, who he understood would be there.

As a result of Carolyn's presence, his anxiety level grew as he waited for trouble to hit him. He knew he would be the target at some point. Daisy knew what he was waiting for and was caught up in the tension. Like children squabbling over mud pies, they started to disagree over how deep to make mounds of dirt for planting as Daisy's mother watched.

Then the dreaded moment happened. Carolyn suddenly appeared, leaning over the white railing on the porch above them. In her loud, stern, sergeant-major voice, she sharply ordered Ken into the house.

Ken's back was to her. His back stiffened. He had been expecting her just like that. After a frozen pause, he stood the garden fork in the dirt, silently turned, and walked toward the house.

Daisy wanted to protect him from that woman but knew she had better stay put as she watched him make his way into the house to face whatever the women had in store for him.

Daisy's mother clued in and knowingly watched in silence.

The baby on her lap had jolted and sat straight as her back stiffened when Carolyn's voice had jabbed the air.

The rest of the family in the back yard fell silent.

In total self-absorption, Carolyn had shown absolutely no recognition or regard for Daisy's family in the garden, including Daisy's mother, and she had shown no respect for Ken in front of everyone.

In a continuation, Carolyn's crisp voice resonated through the air from open windows and doors for the neighborhood to hear her ranting at Ken about their life together, his education, insulting his work, and about herself. She clearly was determined to air all her complaints, real or imagined, for Ken's mother to hear and to make Ken her scapegoat once and for all. Even though she was a nurse who should know better, the ex-wife showed no regard for a repercussion on the health of a woman who had suffered a serious stroke not too long ago and was known to have a compromised heart.

Ken's voice was too soft for his words to carry to the outside.

After a couple of hours Ken emerged frazzled and unhappy.

When Daisy asked about the meeting, Ken simply responded, "That woman will never change. She is determined that my mother and everyone else should see things her way. She continues to drag up issues from years ago. She likes to complain about me."

Daisy wanted to console him, but knew she could not because Carolyn was the mother of his two sons and would forever have a line into him.

The family gathering was ruined. Ken's mother no longer felt up to socializing with anyone and closed herself in her room.

On one hand, Daisy understood Ken's loyalty to all these people but she remembered the "half married man" story and realized that he would forever be a half married man until his youngest son became an adult. She could hardly wait!

DAYS LATER, Ken was still hurting. He and Daisy were standing in his kitchen, when he commented that the women in his life should all put on boxing gloves and fight it out among themselves – without him. Then it slipped out, "My mother has wanted me to promise never to marry you because I have children with these other women".

Fed up with the women in his life and in no way wanting to duke it out with them, Daisy flung her ring at him in a fury. The gold ring hit the floor with a *ping* and *swoosh* as it slid into unknown dark regions down the hallway. It was as though time stopped. The flying ring was another blow. Daisy realized with shock what she has just done. His oldest son appeared like magic from the other side of a doorway and there was instant knowledge that he had been listening. That was enough for Ken. Turning on his heels, he walked out of his own house and was gone with his son trailing him.

Suddenly alone and confused, Daisy wondered if she meant it. She had expected Ken to pick up the ring and possibly give it back, or at least pick it up and put it in his pocket, but here she was searching for it. Finding it, she decided there was only one place for it. She hurriedly put the ring into his pillow. The pillow was made of oats with a zippered cover, one of those pillows that were supposed to be good for you, and Daisy knew that only the pillowcase could be washed but never the oats. She only hoped he would never discard the pillow with the gold ring buried in it. She felt he should dream on the ring and on his hopes to marry her. Then she took the expensive perfume he had given as a gift to replace the cheap perfume that he did not like the smell of and she sprayed his pillow and futon mattress until the container was empty. Determined to be finished and get a new life minus his family, she did not want him to forget her so easily.

The mountain of food that Daisy had put into the upstairs refrigerator was still sitting there, largely untouched. Carolyn had managed to cause such unhappy feelings all around that the two families never did get together over food. But in some strange way Daisy still believed that she could simply tell her son and his girlfriend to use some of the food since she had paid for it anyway, rather than removing the food and putting at least some in the downstairs fridge. This did not go over well with Ken's son. He made it clear no one was welcome in his space for peanut butter or anything else.

Ken's sons had the backup they needed in their mothers, to continue treating Daisy's family as outcasts. The idea of blending families was continuing to be a blatant mistake.

SINCE LEAVING the housing co-op, Ken and Daisy had been playing musical chairs – actually musical houses where their chairs took residence. Twice, landlords took advantage of Daisy by renting houses to her and when their divorces got settled, took back their houses. After one month, the same scenario was happening to the house with the hot tub and skylights. Ken decided that since his sons were not happy with the shared arrangement, he would rent another apartment for his three sons so that Daisy could have his rented house to share with her son who was living in the lower suite.

Ken spent time alone in his separate apartment, believing he had forever severed ties to Daisy. He made another attempt to restore his relationship with Jane by taking her and Andy on a weekend holiday to the Oregon coast, and falling into his old pattern of doing something special and expensive for Jane in order to have a relationship. His reasoning was that he believed she wanted him back or else she would not spend so much time and energy trying to get rid of Daisy.

IT WAS A CHANCE meeting on the same day of his return. After a miserable weekend of knowing Ken had been with Jane, Daisy saw him coming toward her on a busy street.

Glad to see her, he could not help smiling but he was also wary as they approached each other.

She thought he looked healthier than she had ever seen him look. His face looked rested. He was wearing a loose white cotton shirt that she had never seen before and his skin against the white looked beautifully tanned. She was convinced that whatever happened with Jane, it had finally come to a resolution, probably in Jane's favor.

Silent for a minute, they faced each other. His gentle smile and kindness in his eyes were inviting.

"Hi," Ken said softly.

"Hi... How was your holiday?" she almost whispered, trying to find her voice.

"We went to the Oregon coast and stayed in a cabin by the beach... and shopped for toys in Bellingham."

"Yes, and how was it?" She thought she knew the answer, did not want the answer but wanted him to say it, all at the same time. She also knew Ken would never lie about anything.

"We don't get along, even for a short time. It was disappointing, as usual."

Surprised, she asked, "Where does it go from here?"

"Nowhere. She doesn't want me."

Daisy wondered if finding a resolution was why he looked so healthy; he seemed relieved – or resigned but not unhappy. "Oh! ...Maybe she just wants to prove she can take you away from me any time she wants. Is it finished... finally?"

"There is nowhere to go with it from here. I believe I have done all I can do except to help her with our child. ...By the way, the perfume is a bit strong." He smiled.

TOGETHER ONCE MORE regardless of baggage, one day Daisy asked, "What are we going to do about your mother? She disapproves of me."

"Keep in mind that she has had a stroke. Her health is frail. Throughout my childhood, she was my best friend, the only person I could really talk with about everything. But she was also tough on me, pushing me into being the person I am. She was determined to protect me because of my birth defect but in so doing she constantly made me face my fears and forced me to work through them. It was probably her way of working through her own fears of having a child born with Spina Bifida. She tried to protect me but she often chose the wrong way to protect me. She is attempting to protect me now, and once again I am opposing her as I have often done. She dressed me in a sailor suit and told me I was to have my tonsils out, and then abandoned me while they circumcised me when I was nine."

"I am a mother and sometimes in hindsight, you know the advice has been wrong. I am sure your mother was only doing what the doctors advised her was the right thing to do."

What a turn around! Now Daisy found reason to defend the woman who could not accept her, and Ken made it all right to accept her – as is, and even feel compassion by understanding what it means to be a mother and make mistakes.

27

Midwifery

OUT OF THE DARK AGES! Into the light! Liberation! The midwifery movement was on the rise. Ken and Daisy had joined forces with the army of midwives who knew that the decades old way of birthing babies in Canadian hospitals had been wrong. Ken encouraged Daisy and Lana to train as lay-midwives. They followed through. In training with lay-midwives, Lana was generously brave, allowing her hands to be punctured with needles by women practicing those skills. Daisy preferred they practice on grapefruits, refusing to submit body parts to be touched or punctured even in the name of 'teaching'.

IT WAS IN THE 1970's that women began to take back their power and the fight was on between physicians and midwives. During the past sixty or so years, men in the western world had taken control of the field of Obstetrics. Women lost human rights and dignity. Women were not innocent; nurses and the few women physicians were complacent enforcers in the name of science. Men in government and College of Physicians administration positions laid down laws against midwives and promised punishment for physicians working with midwives.

Women had been kept in the dark about the whole pregnancy process and given no choice about the birth. Women felt lucky and safe just to be allowed into the hospital, so usually they headed for the hospital at the first sign of labor. There was no question of comfort as a woman was shaved, given an enema and swabbed in an attempt to sterilize her body inside and out. She was told to stay in bed until it was time for the birth and allowed only tiny sips of water or ice-cubes to suck on, subjecting her to ketone levels going out of whack in a long labor. For the birth, she was transferred to a narrow, hard stretcher where she must lay flat on her back and rushed to an operating room. Under bright lights, her legs were parted and her feet were tied to cold metal stirrups. Hands were tied down to the sides of the gurney, rending her totally imprisoned under the control of others. There was no family member allowed to be present but the room might fill with a dozen uninvited onlookers to observe the extraction of a baby, and to pass on the technique of how-to-do-it. Aware of suffering indignities, her objections were silenced by a heavy hand clamping a mask over her nose and mouth so that she had no choice but to breath in ether or chloroform that rendered her unconscious; it was called a sweet name like 'twilight sleep'. The woman would then be an unconscious vessel from which the baby could be extracted. An episiotomy, known among midwives as the 'unkind cut', was automatically performed on the unconscious woman whether she needed it or not. The cut was to ensure a larger opening for a baby to slide out or for large steel forceps to get in and drag the baby out of a woman who could no longer participate in pushing the baby out. Then the placenta would be extracted and if the physician was a novice, he might pull on it to hurry it up. The woman was then sewn up, sometimes crookedly leaving scars and large indents from the thick stitches as though rope had been used – and some doctors left a larger opening by not entirely closing the wound end to end.

All these procedures were considered progressive and non-negotiable because in about 1915 midwives and home births were publicly denounced in favor of more progressive hospital procedures, which only the middle and upper class could afford. In 1920, a male doctor announced that these procedures could save women from the evils of labor and the dangers of damage from a pathological process.

Rough handling of newborn babies as they left the warmth of amniotic fluid was consider okay because it was believed newborn babies could feel no pain, and were dumb and blind. The baby's first experience after birth was pain as he or she was held upside down in the cold air by ankles and slapped hard on the buttock, followed by the realization that the mother's comforting heartbeat had disappeared. The babies were rushed away to a nursery and placed under bright lights. Strange fingers poked the baby as rotating strange faces appeared above. The baby has left a protective fluid home where he swam with the sound of his mother's heartbeat and where he played with his fingers and toes, and sucked his thumb but has found himself bundled tightly, like a football, and cannot move a muscle. He had been fed continually through the umbilical cord. Baby's born to so-called progressive mothers of the Americas would now experience a strict schedule of feeding only every four hours. It was training for feast and famine – overeating alternating with hunger – and to be ignored and feeling alone.

Four-hour intervals seemed like an eternity to a newborn baby. The constant food source dried up while mothers with painfully engorged breasts were allowed nursing visits only every four hours with no relief in between the hours. If baby was tired after crying for a long while, and slept through a feeding, he just went hungry for another four hours. Mothers were strongly encouraged to keep this schedule at home because otherwise they may spoil their babies. There was no understanding of the nourishment that passed on certain immunities from mother to baby through breast milk. Breastfeeding was discouraged for scores of years while bottle-feeding formulas were pushed onto women as a better food source for their babies. In the name of progress, women nourished the pockets of big companies.

In some hospitals, women got the best care every morning by starched nurses washing stitches in rows of beds and setting up heating lamps under tented bottoms to dry out stitches.

This describes Daisy's and other women's experience with giving birth – and it was Ken's mother's experience. So when Ken's mother told him that his birth was the same as all the others, this is why.

THE MIDWIVES OF the eighties were teaching how to do things differently. They taught gentle birth. Women's rights were recognized and respected. Women were instructed about the stages of pregnancy and labor. They made birth plans that included the baby's father. They expected the physician to go along with the birth plan and only resort to more drastic measures in case of emergency.

Old ways were replaced with comfort and the use of gravity in labor and birth. Fully conscious women brought fully conscious, contented babies into the world. Umbilical cords were not cut until they ceased to pulse so there was less chance of damaging babies' brains by accidentally being without oxygen. There was less pulling on babies' heads and yanking of necks where damage often occurred in the past. All in all, there was less chance of injury in the gentle births.

Bonding was immediate as babies were placed on mothers for warmth and nursing. Fathers were able to hold and touch newborn babies. Siblings could be present. Newborn babies know familiar gentle touch and the voices they heard while growing in the womb stayed with them. Entry into the world was not so scary because there was continuity.

IN THE 1980'S the army of midwives began to have an impact. Birthing centers started to dot Canada, so that women could bypass old-school hospital maternity wards. Some hospitals started their own version of more comfortable birthing rooms where women could labor with family in the room and then birth their babies in the same room with a bed instead of on stretchers. The rooms may have patterned wallpaper, a reminder of home and bathrooms with showers because laboring women feel better in water.

The war was still on between many physicians and lay midwives but when Ontario legalized midwifery, it was hopeful that the rest of the country would follow.

Daisy thought often about the '70s when she was kicked out of a physician's office simply because she dared to just ask about a possible home birth. Even though that same doctor wanted nothing to do with her, he then gave her name and telephone number to another physician who wanted to run her blood through a machine to take the proteins from her blood for kidney patients. The physician making the request for her protein did not want to take "no" for an answer even though Daisy explained she was nearly six months pregnant. He tried to convince her that taking her protein would not harm her baby and because she had many pregnancies before, she had lots of protein that he was determined to have. She refused.

Three days after the doctor's physical examination, she developed a stubborn infection, causing a miscarriage of the perfectly formed baby boy. A week later, the on-call doctor at Lion's Gate Hospital, yelled, "Get the bottle!" He did not care about the fact that Daisy was in grief as her perfectly formed fetus was bottled and whisked away – stolen.

WHEN ANOTHER REQUEST came for the use of Ken's office to start a new midwifery school, Ken generously gave time and space free of charge to the nurses and lay-midwives involved. The idea was to get a head start on gaining credentials for when midwifery became legal but still at a time when it was illegal for physicians in British Columbia to be involved with lay-midwives. Hanging over Ken's head was the threat from the BC College of Physicians and Surgeons regarding physicians' participation with lay-midwives.

Ken was undeterred by the threat to him and, in fact, requested to take the training along with Daisy; he had worked as a physician delivering babies in Vermont and did so in his own progressive gentle way but he wanted the midwifery training that was happening in his office. The women did not mind taking advantage of his free office but suddenly there was grumbling and murmuring, "He is a *male*!"

They told him, "No!" in no uncertain terms.

Never the less, typical of Ken, he kept his disappointment to himself and continued giving with no hard feelings.

WITH NANNY JANET and son Stephen carrying the office work for Ken, Daisy was free to do midwifery. She had been invited to work temporarily with a couple of midwives. Though they had more experience and taught her a lot, they clearly lacked the quality of knowing about good emotional patient care. Daisy learned that they had little respect for patient confidentiality and were showing videos of births without consent of the birthing mother.

Very soon, Daisy was asked to do labor support to replace another midwife who was quitting at the last minute. The woman's physician told Daisy that the woman had a septum that caused the cervix to have two openings but not to worry about it. His instructions were to keep his patient at home as long as possible and only bring her to the hospital when she was almost fully dilated.

Daisy had immediate problems and wished she had not taken the job. The first problem was the discovery on examination that the septum was a scary thick, wide muscle across the opening of the cervix, causing Daisy to wonder how dilation could happen without cutting it first. She worried and while her patient rested, she scanned medical books brought with her to search for a clue about dealing with this condition but found nothing helpful. The second problem was the woman's female friend who kept vigil and was determined to be between the laboring woman and her husband, and now between the woman and Daisy.

A long afternoon and night passed. Dilation was not progressing, as it should. Several times by telephone Daisy expressed concern to the woman's doctor, but he remained adamant that the woman should labor at home as though this was a normal situation.

Concerned, Ken insisted on keeping in touch with Daisy even though he was not the woman's doctor. By the second evening, Ken advised Daisy to transport the woman to the hospital while the baby's heart was still healthy, regardless of the other doctor's demands. She did so.

An angry doctor arrived at the hospital. A short dark-haired man, with chest puffed to make his size seem larger, immediately loudly reamed Daisy out in front of the birthing parents and several hospital staff for bringing the woman to the hospital when dilation was so small.

After filling the room with angry noise, he did an examination. Without further comment he cut the septum to make one large opening of the cervix. Regardless of his rage, Daisy stayed close beside him to watch and learn. She could see the septum was as thick and wide as she thought – kind of like a swollen tongue, and common sense was that it had to be cut for dilation to progress. A healthy baby boy was born within a couple of hours.

Daisy stayed for the birth, watching from the far wall. Somehow she had become the enemy in the room. No one bothered to acknowledge her for anything. In fact, the doctor continued to treat her with silent hostility.

The lesson she took away with her on the bus ride home late that night was the determination never to take on another birth where a girlfriend came between her and the laboring woman – and never again to go along with bad instructions, even from a doctor. Reflecting on whether this doctor had been lazy or just stupid, she also wondered why of all the midwives available, had she been chosen for this difficult labor support job and why the doctor would insist that this could be a normal labor. The doctor would not have taken any heat if things had gone wrong at home because he was not present. There was so much danger of the baby being held back too long and being a stillbirth or being born brain damaged, resulting in Cerebral Palsy because of lack of oxygen. Daisy could have ended up in jail, like another midwife had done, if something had gone wrong because the witch-hunt by the British Columbia College of Physicians and Surgeons was hot and heavy about practicing lay-midwives.

As was usual after a long labor with no sleep, when Daisy finally did lie down to sleep, the bed hit her hard in the back.

The almost catastrophe bothered Daisy for a long time afterward. She was grateful for Ken's watchful guidance. Extreme harm to the mother and her baby, and to Daisy was averted but the mother would never know of Ken who was the physician behind the scene who really saved her baby from harm.

[In future, after never seeing each other again, this little boy, at two years old, will cry in a bookstore. Daisy will hear him from behind another bookstall and immediately feel recognition just from his cry that she only heard once at his birth.]

THE BABY ABOUT TO BE BORN had been active, turning and kicking throughout the pregnancy. The day Mom was in labor, the baby changed position again and turned feet down. Daisy decided to try gravity to encourage the baby to turn again in time for birthing. She had mom lay on her side in the direction Daisy thought the baby would move easily and hoped the invisible cord was not going to become constricted. It was necessary to keep monitoring. The baby turned like magic, and wonder of wonders she birthed with no problems, head first.

[In future, this baby grows up to be a gymnast.]

THERE WERE MANY successful birth outcomes in Daisy's work. Happy babies and parents were dreams come true most often and what all midwives strived for. But Daisy often secretly thought things could have gone smoother. She found it difficult to overlook anything that could be done better. While most caregivers were good and caring, some caregivers seemed oblivious so long as they got their job done.

She found it necessary to argue with hospital technicians and eventually administration about giving the PKU (Phenylketonuria) test to babies too soon. Due to changing attitudes and overcrowding, babies were leaving hospitals within hours of being born. But the PKU test depends on a baby's consumption of milk protein over at least forty-eight hours and doing the test earlier rendered the tests useless. It annoyed Daisy that a major hospital would play a game of Russian roulette with babies and their eventual mental capabilities. The reasoning given was to do the test before leaving the hospital in case the parents would not get it done after leaving the hospital. As a result of Daisy's pressure, permission was finally given to have community health nurses do the tests at home after the proper time lapse.

[At the time of writing this book in 2010, some major hospitals continue to do the PKU test too early without informing parents that the test is useless. When challenged, some offer a second PKU test.]

THE DOCTOR HAD left the room to call home. A nurse sat at a corner table, writing notes with her back to the room. Daisy had been walking in circles with the laboring mother when suddenly the mother felt the baby dropping fast. Daisy quickly squatted and caught the baby's head, and waited for the whole body to drop into her hands.

At the sound of the commotion, the nurse leapt from her perch in a panic and ran past the birthing woman. Out of the corner of her eye, Daisy could see the nurse's legs run right past to the door, open it and stand there screaming down the hall for the doctor.

The nurse was providing amusement for Daisy in the pause of waiting for a baby to slide out. Getting no response, the nurse returned and tried to shove Daisy out of the way. She was a heavy-set, middle-aged woman with strong arms giving Daisy a few good knocks. Instead of offering assistance in patient care, the nurse had turned it into a turf war. She resorted to pushing at Daisy's body with all her body weight and continued banging her hips against Daisy's right shoulder even as Daisy had the baby's head in her hands and it would be dangerous to let go. In the midst of this, Daisy reflected momentarily on her luck to have strong legs holding firmly to the ground as the baby was born into her hands while she was being punched hard.

Daisy was concerned if the woman did not stop punching, she could not manage the next stage of delivering the placenta. In a firm voice Daisy instructed the nurse to stop punching and to help instead in guiding the woman to the edge of the bed while Daisy continued holding the baby because the umbilical cord was still attached to mom.

The nurse gave up fighting and started to help.

With the baby resting comfortably on mother's body, and placenta released, the doctor arrived. He stood in the middle of the room looking lost and embarrassed.

The nurse was red faced with anger and in a flustered way told a story to the doctor.

Daisy was just relieved that the baby did not land head first on the cold, stone floor because of the stupidity of the nurse.

The parents with baby in their arms were sent out of the labor room to the maternity ward for rest and recovery. Daisy tagged along to keep a watchful eye.

With mom resting in bed and baby comfortably wrapped in her arms, the happy father took pictures. All seemed well. The worst was yet to come when a young nurse entered the room and snatched the obviously healthy baby with good colour and breathing normally out of Daisy's arms right after she had her picture taken with the baby.

The nurse had not taken the baby's temperature or even felt her body, but said she needed to take the baby due to low temperature. Daisy objected. But the baby was rushed out of the room. Daisy followed. The baby was placed in a bassinette in a corner of the nursing station behind a solid glass window – not taken to the newborn intensive care unit or even a nursery. The parents could not get to her behind the guard of solid glass and front desk personnel. Daisy could see through the window that nothing special was being done for the baby except that she was being separated from her mother. In fact, she was ignored and alone. It was a clear collusion by nurses with nurses.

Daisy argued that the best way to keep a baby warm is against the mother's warm body, preferably bare bodies cocooned together under blankets, and being breast fed instead of the bottles the nurses were now plugging her with against the parents' wishes. Nursing by the mother was not being allowed. Daisy pleaded with the nurses and tried to educate them about what is known as the kangaroo method of caring for babies.

For his own reasons, the doctor refused to answer Daisy's many telephone calls to his office. He did not visit. He actually abandoned his patients. Without the doctor telling the nurses to give back the baby, the punishment continued to the detriment of the mother and baby, interrupting bonding and nourishment. This continued all the next day.

Through the grapevine, word got out that the reason for punishment was that though Daisy could do labor support in the hospital, as a lay-midwife she was not supposed to catch a baby in hospital regardless of how or why. And because she did so, nurses ganged up and took it upon themselves to punish the family.

The parents packed up and demanded to take their baby home, at which time because the nurses had no medical reason to keep the baby, they relinquished the healthy baby.

THE SAME DOCTOR was a physician hired for another birth and Daisy was again the labor support. It turned out to be another case where a girlfriend was determined to be the centre of attention during home labor. Even though Daisy had been determined never to do that again, there she was. When it came time for the birth in hospital, the friend took over as labor support while Daisy watched over an older daughter outside. Eventually the friend gave up, not knowing what to do. She had come between the woman and her husband but now conceded to him. He asked Daisy to come in. The friend and Daisy traded places.

Daisy entered the room to find the mother suffering extreme fatigue and gave her a homeopathic remedy. The woman revived immediately with strong energy for the imminent birth and took a standing position with one foot raised and resting on a low rail of the bed. Her doctor came into the room and demanded that she lay down on her back for his convenience. Daisy gave him a stern look and insisted that the mother be allowed to stand. He was not happy. Daisy imagined another scene where she would catch the baby, but regardless of his disapproval, this time he stayed with it. The standing birth was successful.

THE MOST UNUSUAL birth support request came through a long distant call to Ken's cell phone from a midwife in a birthing centre thousands of miles away. A young woman who was a former child client had moved to another city. She had been in labor all night with her first baby.

Several people, including the young mother in labor, had seen an old man hanging around the birthing centre the previous day. Another woman laboring in a neighboring room claimed she recognized him as her deceased grandfather. Then during the night, the neighbor woman gave birth to a stillborn baby boy. Several people saw the old man again that night as he took the dead baby's spirit away.

The fear expressed in the phone call was that the baby had been stolen and that another baby might be taken. Out of terror, the former client asked the midwife to call Ken and Daisy for help. Over the telephone, they counseled on what to do for protection and how to calm the situation. They did labor support for both the mother and the midwife, who was sweet and knowledgeable but was shaken to the core. The birth was successful and the baby born was healthy.

WHY, OH WHY, Daisy wondered, do I get these difficult cases to deal with? This time it was a twin pregnancy. The woman was wheelchair bound. In the ultra-sound there were two absolutely beautiful and perfectly formed fetuses – a boy and a girl, at four months gestation. The problem was that the little girl was growing in a thin bubble projecting out of the upper right quadrant of the uterus. It was clear that the bubble would eventually burst as the fetus grew larger. The medical consensus was that all three might lose their lives. The specialist decided the answer was to save two lives by destroying the third.

The mother wanted Daisy to accompany her for the procedure. Daisy would rather not but needed to be supportive regardless of her own queasiness. At the appointed time she took her place at the patient's side in the tiny low light room along with two specialists.

The ultra-sound pictures showed the beautifully healthy female fetus was moving and contentedly sucking her thumb. The first physician held a long needle with the intent to stab the fetus in the heart. He tried several times. With needle poised in his hand, sweat poured off his face. He tried again. Pain gripped his face. He could not do it. He turned his back as the second physician took the needle to puncture right through mom's flesh and into the heart of the fetus. The heart stopped beating instantly. She was dead.

The intent was to leave her there until the birth of the twin boy.

Daisy did her job of watching over the woman during the remainder of the pregnancy and was again in attendance as support at the cesarean birth. This time she watched as the same doctor, who had difficulty before, was again having difficulty.

The second doctor looked at him in shock, exclaiming loudly, "You cut the placenta!"

The second doctor took over in a hurry and lifted a lovely baby out of the cavity. The boy was handed to Daisy to hold and share with his mother while the doctors continued working. The boy was beautiful but grunted a little as he breathed. He would have to go to the newborn intensive care unit but would be fine.

Then the little girl, perfectly beautiful as that fateful day but now grey, was laid on a terry cloth-covered table at the side of the room. Daisy walked over to spend a few reverent minutes with her and wondered – what if? She experienced profound sadness for the little girl.

A young, disapproving nurse offered painkiller drugs to the mother who accepted them until she could hardly function. The nurse used the woman's fog as an excuse to have the baby taken away from the wheelchair bound mother and placed in foster care. The doctor who had difficulty at the birth backed the nurse. Daisy called a meeting. Ken and people from supportive agencies showed up to help protect the mother and child. The astonished naysayers were fended off in the meeting in a hospital boardroom.

In the following days, Daisy picked up the ashes from the crematorium for the mom.

And then she went home to feel the comfort of Ken.

SOMETIMES DAISY WENT without sleep for two or three days and when finally she made her way home, the bed hit her body instead of the other way around. It was painful until her body got used to the bed. Daisy was disenchanted and often at odds fighting for change in a world that was changing but not fast enough. This was no dream job. It had risks. It was a hard life.

She worked hard to make birth plans with the pregnant parents and then to consult with each attending physician to have everyone in agreement. Mostly, the plans worked and everyone was happy. Occasionally, there was the one that seemed like the doctor only agreed to the birth plan in order to pacify the patient but had no real interest. Daisy had kept mom and dad at home until 8 cm dilated and labor was progressing fast. At the hospital, nursing staff called the physician to let him know. It seemed the staff knew this doctor and they relayed the message that he was probably at a dog race and not to expect him any time soon. And he did keep everyone waiting.

Meanwhile, because of over-crowded conditions even in this new hospital, there was no private delivery room available anyway. If the woman gave birth any time soon, it was going to be in the busy and noisy holding-room with four beds where she had been plunked. Women moaning and groaning in labor filled three other beds, with support people coming and going. In other words, she will give birth in public without her doctor. Daisy's patient's labor took a hiatus. There was no reason to panic during the waiting period because the mom and baby's vital signs were normal and she could not be sent home at eight or nine centimeters dilation. They waited.

They had arrived at the hospital around noon and labor only resumed when a private delivery room became available around the same time that the doctor arrived at 6 p.m., dressed like he had come from a party.

The birth was smooth as eagle-eyed Daisy reminded the doctor of the birth plan every time he tried to deviate to old practices.

The actual birth was amazing to watch as this baby boy came head first, his fully focusing eyes searched around for his parents even before he was fully born. He literally swam his way out of his mom's abdomen. The motion of his legs kicking behind him in a swimming pattern could clearly be seen through her abdomen. He was born completely alert. The room had grandparents present. Though several people wanted to look at the baby up close, he looked past everyone, searching the room for his mother and then past people to his father, visually latching on. Happy parents cuddled him and nursing began.

Just as suddenly as the doctor had appeared, he disappeared, bow tie and all. The attending nurse filled a basin of warm water and picked up a washcloth and towel. Daisy assumed she was going to help the patient get cleaned up but she thrust it all on a side table, saying, "Now you can wash yourself. I have to get to my next patient."

After a birth, Daisy continued to stay on duty at the hospital with parents around the clock in recovery, offering relief for a tired father who often needed a break for a meal or a little sleep; but the point was also to watch over postpartum care regardless of being in hospital. In this way Daisy uncovered problems that were ordinarily ignored and unchecked.

Up in the postnatal ward, the contented baby boy lay against mom's bare chest, nursing with mom's warm arms wrapped around him under a blanket. Just when everyone was relaxed, thinking all problems were over, a nurse entered the room. She was a tall, lean but big boned older nurse with a hardened face moving swiftly toward the mom as she barked, "Your baby must be swaddled!" She grabbed the baby away from mom's breast and laid the baby on the bed to show the mom how to wrap a newborn. In so doing, she wrapped tightly by pulling the blanket across the baby with adult strength. The baby became a hard, stiff bundle with a head sticking out. The swaddling was so tight that it shocked mom and Daisy. Knowing about hip dysplasia, Daisy suspected the condition might sometimes be caused by over-zealous swaddling, resulting in life-long disabilities. Babies were checked soon after birth for the deformity.

As soon as the nurse left the room, Daisy loosened the wrap and again laid baby against mom's breast while explaining that swaddling is one thing, but smothering or causing damage to limbs is another.

The same nurse came back into the room several more times throughout her shift and went through the same routine. It had turned into a fight about the handling of the baby until mom and dad were fed up. They packed up to go home with baby.

Before leaving the hospital, the flying pediatrician who moved air as he rushed through the hallway, made his way into the glassed-in nursery and to a row of ten bare bottomed babies laid out for him. He flicked legs one after the other in fast succession, looking and listening for hip dysplasia. Daisy watched through the window as 'her' baby's hips were checked. She sighed in relief when he was pronounced okay.

This successful but unusual birth had been a lesson in watching how the subconscious mind might be in control, even in labor. More than that, this baby knew his own parents – *both* parents, not only by sound, but also visually. And in the follow-up, this baby took to swimming easily with great joy.

DAISY HAD EXPLAINED to Ken that she found some midwives in serious breach of confidentiality. There had been troubling conversations in front of clients. Daisy was convinced the midwives she had been working with had valuable techniques but that they were in desperate need of understanding people, not just technique—the very thing that Ken was good at teaching. Ken offered free classes.

Daisy had been learning by hard knocks to understand Ken's calling to help and heal people but also his disenchantment with front-line medicine where there were so many blocks and hurdles put up by old guard not willing to budge from their own comfort zone or power position. Daisy had entered midwifery with a glorified idea of bouncing babies and being able to make a difference one baby at a time. Bouncing babies and happy births did happen and she had been present to many of them but it had been quite an education along the way. Through her work, it became obvious in a tangible way that though medicine had come a long way, more change must happen, not entirely from within where, yes, there were good people and lots of great outcomes, but change was also too slow and wore a person out. Change must happen from within and without. That is why, as Ken always said, "Good teachers are so important," and, "Learning and changing must be a constant." Daisy understood Ken's passion and determination to work with like-minded groups of people to push for change, and he did so with every ounce of strength he could muster. She now had even more in-depth respect for Ken and all he stood for.

Daisy was cut from the same cloth as Ken; helping someone was the only reason for working in medicine. Like Ken, she refused to overlook problems that could be fixed to provide safer patient care, and as a result the work was not easy during a transitional stage. She was rather proud of the experience of being likened to a most respected social order of old-fashioned barefoot doctors when, for payment, she was given a bag of second-hand clothes that she could not wear.

After all, no matter what the shortcomings may have been with some midwives Daisy had known, she was convinced that by legalizing them into the medical system, they would humanize the birthing process; they would normalize the process, lessening the need for medical interventions by people who think giving birth is abnormal. And this larger picture is what Ken was so adamant about in his support of the movement, regardless of what it may bring down on his own head.

"DOCTOR KEN, I was on the pill and I didn't want to be pregnant. I am five months pregnant. On mother's day it gave me a kick. On mother's day! That's the first time I felt it. That's the first time I thought I might be pregnant."

The large woman sat in the chair across from Ken and Daisy. Daisy could see that even at five months she might carry a baby hidden in her frame – but not to feel it?

The woman continued, "I want to sue my doctor!"

"Why?" Ken asked.

"Because he gave me the new birth control pill that has less strength than the one I was taking. I want to sue."

In conversation with Ken, her face lit up whenever she spoke of the baby. She finally admitted that a new baby would be nice. Within the hour she decided that suing a doctor because she would have a bundle of joy made no sense.

Four months following that first meeting, the woman gave birth to a baby boy by cesarean section because she believed strongly that her vagina was too small to give birth. Never the less, the outcome was a good one. The woman was in love with her baby.

At the same time there was an unusual number of clients coming to Ken in hopes of solving their problems of being pregnant because of changing over to a new pill. Commonly, couples came in fighting over whether or not to have an abortion. Rarely did they follow through, but there was sometime the one that did. Others fought over whether to live together or marry because of the coming child.

With advancement in medicine, new problems also came alongside. In Ken's non-biased way, he helped the clients work though their anxieties and make their own decisions.

At about the same time there was the pregnant little person. She was a woman no taller than four feet with well-proportioned tiny frame. She showed up at Daisy's door explaining that she thought she could not get pregnant while on the pill but here she was – pregnant. Even though she was single, she wanted to keep the child and have a natural birth. She went through a perfectly healthy pregnancy and gave birth without intervention to a healthy five-pound baby. She had been the one Daisy most worried about and the outcome was perfect.

ON A NIGHT of work, Daisy had been waiting for a bus. A man emerged from the shadows of a darkened street, walking quickly toward her. He paused a few feet away and asked, "Do you have the time?"

"Sure." Daisy lifted her sleeve to look closely at her watch without looking up. "It's 8:30." Then she looked up. To her astonishment, she had just given the time of day to Mr. Physician.

Neither one acknowledged knowing the other. He continued down the street.

AT HOME Daisy shared what seemed outrageous, "Ken, you won't believe what just happened. I swore I would never give the time of day to Mr. Physician and I just did! I just wonder how on earth this happens, that he should approach *me* in the dark to ask for the time when I've put out to the universe that I will never give him the time of day!"

28

Wishes Dreams and Illness

KEN WROTE in his journal:

APRIL 1983. ...What I want to accomplish... with Jane: I want to relieve the anguish of the past four years of failure while building a secure base for her growth and Andy's development into manhood. Concretely, this means developing a secure economic base, mutual understanding about shared and separate goals, clarity about what may be good for Andy...

AUGUST 18th 1983. These are the resources which I bring to my relationships as a lover, friend, parent and sometimes, husband: At times these resources may also be troubling!

I am strong, self directed and totally loyal to my feelings, beliefs and actions with regard to the emotions I share with those close to me. These emotions and the actions through which I embody them are all I have to share with anyone. I work hard to keep the promises I make to myself and those with whom I share love as knowing recognition of the needs and abilities of individual human beings, including my own needs and abilities. My allegiance is to my extended, voluntary family in which I freely choose to be a member. I hope to extend these bonds to include Chinese people with whom I can speak and write and discuss living issues. [Ken had been studying Mandarin, speaking and writing.]

I want to have people in my life who are energetic, self-regulated and willing to work with me on life projects freely, keeping for themselves and sharing whatever they choose. When I share love with someone, that bond is lifelong and individualized, specific to our relationship and none other. My troubles often arise from conflicting loyalties and promises made to different individuals and to myself at different times and in varied situations.

At fifty years of age now, I feel a strong urge to "own" a piece of land on which to nourish my family, friends and future grandchildren. I plan to integrate my life and my work even more closely than before so that I can become a wiser, more alive person, capable of sharing my life fully with loved ones. So help me Life!

SEPTEMBER 15th, 1983. *I have a family and I need help with their care, especially with Andy. He will be spending more overnights with me this fall and winter. Essentially, I need help with my life plan, which is:*

1) to pay off all my outstanding debts... by next summer so that I can begin to make a new life without credit cards and with a

2) good credit rating so that buying land and building a house becomes a real possibility.

3) I want to establish a new career for myself in community medicine, medical and ecological anthropology, specializing in Chinese medicine. Accomplishing 1 & 2 will make it possible for me to consider seriously staying in the Vancouver area as a consultant to developments in acupuncture.

4) Whether or not I stay here past next summer, my goal is to develop a home for my family and grandchildren where land, food, clean air and water are available. My preferred way to do this is to develop cottage industry on the land where my family members can join with other concerned families to explore freely alternative living styles and technologies.

5) I want out of the BC Medical Plan tyranny. I want to be able to make a living by growing food, people, books, projects, etc. I am uncertain about having more babies because I am having so much trouble with my present responsibilities that I do not have time and energy to help develop adequate midwifery services and places for family nurture at this time. I want to settle this issue by next fall.

WITH DAISY: *I want to know that I have her support in caring for my sons and living with them while remaining interested and concerned about her welfare, (i.e. well being) as* *well as her family. I would like her support for my life plan and I would be willing to negotiate with her on principle about any issues that she has with that plan or with me...*

SEPTEMBER '83. I want to be able to talk with Jane about her life and Andy free of financial manipulation... I want an end to the war!

Ken's notebook: Afternoon October 14th, 1983 *"My partner is surprising and is my closest friend. I am a person who wants to share his life and feelings with loved ones so that I can help build a better world with my family and friends."*

Daisy's notebook: October 1983 *"My partner is a very special person who deserves respect and care, certainly more than he has ever received."*

AS AN EXTENSION of their interest in healing methods from cultures around the world, Ken asked Daisy to join him in auditing an Asian Studies class at the university. While walking the UBC grounds, they had a chance meeting with a professor of Hindu philosophy and were welcomed to audit her classes also. Studying and working together filled a need for each other's companionship where no other person could come between them – no ex-wives, no children, nobody. Side by side, sharing thoughts while exploring information were happy times.

A morning in early November 1983, Ken could not get out of bed. He was ill.

Leaving Ken in bed, Daisy attended the Asian studies class for both of them. She wrote extensive notes intended to bring Ken up to date in preparation for the next class, not realizing that this illness was going to be life changing; recovery would take – not days, not months, but years.

At noon she arrived home to find Ken still in bed with Andy crawling over him and bouncing on him as if he were an exercise mat. Ken's face, hands and body were greatly swollen with large fluid bumps covering him. He looked grossly disfigured. He was feeling worse. His illness had progressed in the past three hours. His face expressed his concern.

Daisy stood at the foot of his bed in shock at the large bubble swellings that were somehow different than the extreme blistery allergies she had seen before. She remembered that her own tiny daughter had blown up like a balloon, her skin like sheer paper over bubbles after eating goose one New Year day; and her son always had hay fever allergies that caused his eyes and face to swell up horribly. Both children had been taken to emergency hospitals and released as 'non-life-threatening'. The illness in front of her eyes was a reminder but similarities ended there.

Andy had been dropped off and not delivered to school for some unknown reason and had been plastering Ken with his toys and books for hours. Daisy noted that the little boy was just happy to be with his father.

Ken was extremely weak. "Daisy, please help me. I'm too sick. I can't think."

"What is it?"

"Read about it in the Merck Manual. It may be a side effect of the blood pressure medicine taken for too long. Kidneys. It can be life threatening if there is internal swelling, especially around the heart."

Daisy was in the middle of reading the Merck Manual, getting more concerned about swelling in Ken's head along with other organs when his two older sons arrived. Walking in, they could see Ken through the open door to the bedroom near the front entrance and headed straight for him.

Standing at the foot of his bed, they announced, "We need money for food and rent." Both sons were living in the apartment that Ken had rented for them and where he normally spent time with them, but because he had not shown up, they came looking for him. Lost in their own concerns, they seemed oblivious to Ken's illness.

With difficulty, Ken wrote a cheque. The boys left as quickly as they came.

Daisy had been watching, saying nothing until the boys had gone. "Ken, I shouldn't be critical, but they didn't even acknowledge that you are sick... just asking for money. Jane sends Andy over even though you are sick."

"I know. I'm sure I scared the boys." Ken's voice was soft and kind. "They don't know what to say. I want Andy with me! I need to know he is okay. I just need your help, Daisy."

She had to agree that young people sometimes do not know what to say or do and then compensate by pretending not to see. She remembered doing that to her own parents.

More importantly, she heard Ken's plea for help.

THE ILLNESS that dragged on for weeks was acting as the illness by an old name of Brights disease that had taken the life of Ken's Great Grandfather and namesake, Dr. Charles Kehnroth, and also a long list of famous peoples' lives. Ken's maternal grandmother had died at age sixty-five of hypertensive heart disease and pulmonary edema. His maternal grandfather died of a heart attack. His mother had recently suffered several strokes, one while driving her car. Clearly family history was reason to be scared for Ken's survival.

Daisy entered the bedroom with a tray holding cups of tea. "Ken, you continue maintaining the boys and paying maintenance to Jane. You look after Andy like a full time parent and all the while you've been so sick. You're the one with no income when you can't work. Is that fair?"

Ken looked distressed, "Daisy, it's okay. I want Andy with me at any price so I know he is okay and I miss him when he's not with me. He's my son. It's okay."

Once again, Daisy realized that no matter what, in health and in sickness, Ken will always put his children and Jane, who he thinks of as another needy child, ahead of himself. It was no use arguing about it. Better to be understanding and supportive.

She rested her head lightly on his chest for a moment of closeness and a brief rest together. The sound from inside his chest startled her. Never before had she heard a heart swoosh and gurgle loudly instead of distinct beats. She told Ken what she was hearing. His reaction was fear. Now they were both frightened.

Daisy tried to help. She had learned from their teacher of Chinese Medicine, a massaging technique that might dispel the extra body fluids, hopefully from within toward the outside of the body and from the head down to the feet, rather than the reverse.

Ken rose from the bed. Still in a weakened condition, he went back to work.

29

Endings and Beginnings

JANUARY 1984. Ken collapsed a second time. Over and over he had been suffering the balloon effect cropping up over various parts of his body accompanied by overpowering weakness. It became necessary for Ken to acknowledge the difficulty in continuing to work front-line medicine. Clients became frightened when an eye swelled to distort his face, or an ankle swelled so that he could not walk. Ken realized that he must follow advice that he so often gave to his clients.

He discussed his problem with Daisy. "I have to maintain a complete change in lifestyle from here on. I need more time with my children and less stress. I need a complete change in diet. When I'm recovered enough to work again, I'll have to take it slowly and be in semi-retirement. I want to teach again instead of a private practice. I want to be alive for the children!"

That statement was a plea for Daisy to understand but more to the universe for healing for the sake of the children. His son Andy was constantly on his mind. Ken continued to suffer sorrow over the disastrous marriage that caused him to leave his child.

"But Ken, you are with your son more than some fathers who actually live with their children." Daisy had said this before and his answer was as before.

"It is not the same... because of a divorce. I was his caretaker. I cannot make up for leaving him. I can't be with him too much."

"I understand. Allopathic medicine has done nothing for you. In fact, I think the side effect of your blood pressure medicine has caused more problems than it was helpful."

"I need to approach this another way if I'm to live."

To Ken, always having been an ivy-league scholar for whom learning, researching in the libraries, always physically active and enjoying the outdoors, and believing that working was the honorable lifeline to life itself, the weakness and incapacity to do all those things brought about by ill health had been difficult.

"I was never housebroken," Ken had said long ago. Now he added, "Being ill and housebound is not easy. I need to walk in the forest as much as possible."

A medical doctor in a high administrative position in the office of the B.C. College of Physicians and Surgeons once told Ken, face to face, that if he discovered any doctor practicing Homeopathy in this province, he would take his license away.

Threats had not deterred Ken or another physician, who at this time arrived back from Greece after spending time with the world-renowned guru of Homeopathy, George Vithoulkas. With this doctor's Homeopathic remedies and a complete change in diet, supplements, and Chinese massage, Ken made progress. Between visits to their teacher, Joe Wong, Daisy was able to continue the massages and moxa treatments.

Now they dived into intense study of Homeopathy. Ken's medical background gave him a head start in understanding constitutional remedies.

Daisy was drawn to understand acute remedies for everyday accidents and minor illnesses that parents and grandparents deal with. She experimented on her own family of animals and babies because they could not speak in judgment and they were not Ken's patients. It was clear in an unspoken language whether or not a remedy worked. Her reasoning was that if the remedies are simply sugar pills containing nothing at all, then they could have no effect and were safe. In every case studied, the remedies had clear healing effects. Croup disappeared after one remedy; but when her child had croup years before, she had been hospitalised. A kitten in shock after falling out of a high tree onto hard ground was fine after one dose of a remedy. Cats who came out of surgery and refused food would suddenly eat. Strep throat and purple swollen tonsils would get better after one remedy.

The concept of Homeopathy was easy to understand in Ken and Daisy's continuing study of energy, auras, and how water retains memory of energy. It made sense.

At that time, Nanotechnology and Nanomedicine were in their infancy. Perhaps Homeopathy had been the forerunner to understanding the science of Nano. Or was understanding the Nano a way to understand Homeopathy? Ken and Daisy mulled over questions.

DAISY'S MOTHER ARRIVED at Easter time for her yearly visit. She looked especially pretty, glowing with happiness. She had lost a little weight, so prior to the trip she had purchased the new, sweetly feminine wardrobe. As they waited and searched the terminal, it becomes apparent that the airline had lost the suitcase.

All her life, Daisy's mother had been intuitive. Standing empty handed in Daisy's living room, she had a sudden ominous feeling that this was a prediction of her death and that she was never going to wear all of the new clothing.

Her suitcase arrived late in the night by courier, but the emotional damage had been done. After arriving full of life, she lost strength. The radiance she had emanated, faded. Over the following days she relied on a thread of strength just to get out of bed or to eat.

Determined to take care of her, Ken searched the community for help. During this time while Daisy's mother obviously had a compromised immune system, Ken asked Jane not to deliver Andy to the house with Chickenpox because they did not want Daisy's mother to be subjected to any form of varicella-zoster virus, like shingles or herpes zoster. As though it was a cue to do so, Andy was plunked into the house the very next morning with blistering Chickenpox on his body.

Peter, Ken's middle son, also came to stay, which was good. He and Daisy's mother, both night people, had conversations in the kitchen while others slept.

Things had changed. Peter was older, no longer challenging his father or Daisy. Instead, Peter was clearly on a path of service to people. Ken loved the boy and was having an enjoyable time in sharing ideas about what Peter was doing and could do.

In the midst of all this, the midwifery school moved to a new location. They gave no explanation for the sudden move out of a large, bright, clean and free space in a legitimate medical building to a place that looked to Daisy like a dark, less clean dump. It was left to the imagination that they probably took offense to Ken telling them to put their babies' poopy diapers in the bathroom down the hall and not leave such a stink in his office waste paper baskets for clients to smell; or did they take offense to the session discussing the need to respect confidentiality?

SEEING HER MOTHER off at the airport, accompanied by Ken and Andy on June 10th, was the first and only time Daisy silently resented Andy's presence. With only four seats in the car, there was no room for another member of her family to accompany their grandmother because Andy, who clearly did not care, had to come with Ken.

Daisy's mother mustered up strength to do the trip to the airport. Before heading into the boarding area where no one could follow, she turned toward Daisy. With a wan smile, she told Daisy, "I love you."

It was a brief intimate moment between them. This family had always put more stock in how people treated each other than in words. With those words, she let Daisy know that she believed they would not see each other in this life again. They exchanged 'knowing' without words. It was in the soft brown mother's eyes meeting her daughter's green eyes, and looking deep into each other's souls, they acknowledged a primal knowing that went far into lives lived together from before birth.

Then she turned toward the doors that would swallow her up.

In deep sadness, Daisy watched the back of her mother's legs walk slowly away toward security doors where she could not follow – knowing she would never see those legs walking again.

The cold grey metal doors closed. Daisy's mother was gone. Daisy panicked about whether her mother would fall on her way to the plane. But it was too late.

Memories of her mother's legs that she used to cling to as a small child flooded in, reminding her of finding safety while hiding under her mother's colourful cotton skirts.

IN JULY OF 1984, a month after her mother went home, cars traveled from the western provinces to meet in Regina. A car carrying Daisy and some of her children and grandchild sped over the jagged mountains to follow paths of grey ribbon roads laid out in the flat checkerboard of green and yellow grasses and tall grain fields of the prairies to be at her mother's side.

During her mother's last visit to Vancouver, Daisy's son Marcel had dreamt that his grandmother was in a large brick building and died. He had reported this to his grandmother and she had responded in a strong, determined voice, "I am not dying!"

A couple of weeks later, Daisy's father, innocent of knowing about the dream, had taken his sick wife to the hospital to seek help. In the parking lot, she looked up at the brick building and remembered the dream. She clung to the bumper of the car in one last desperate move to stay out of the brick building but he, in desperation to get help, had picked her up and carried her inside.

From three provinces, the family gathered in Regina. Though emaciated in her hospital bed, they found their mother and grandmother determined to recover, not willing to give up on life.

No sooner had everyone arrived and had a brief visit, their mother was whisked away for a test that required a dye to be administered through her body. Ken had always told Daisy about tests that can cause severe side effects and had described just the condition that she would now witness. His words and warnings rang through her head as her mother was delivered back to her bed completely paralyzed on her right side.

The room was tiny and cramped, two beds and two patients with only a thin white curtain hanging between the beds. There was cramped standing room only for visitors. Daisy and her sister stood at the bedside as their mother ate the noon meal from the hospital tray with her left hand, not wanting to be fed. She was managing quite well, seeming to enjoy the food, and, true to her nature, did not complain about the paralysis of her right arm. She was trusting that things would get better.

A doctor arrived. He was a tall, graying man who did not greet the patient. Instead, he asked the sisters to step outside.

As Daisy turned to follow the doctor, the last image she had of her mother was of her carefully lifting a fork of food into mid air toward her mouth.

Right outside the wide-open doorway, only a few feet away from the patient, with no preamble, the doctor's deep voice boomed loudly as he towered over the sisters. "Your mother is going to die!"

Those words echoed against the marble walls and floor, reverberating everywhere and much to Daisy's shock, she knew her mother had heard. How could she not hear?

As her sister asked questions, Daisy hurried back into the room. Clearly, the damage had been done. Her mother had not moved. Her hand held the fork with food on it, exactly where she had last seen it – in mid air, and her mother looked straight ahead as though frozen. Then slowly her hand lowered the fork to rest onto the plate, never to be raised again.

Daisy had just witnessed another mistake that Ken had told her about and she had been unable to stop it. The guy was too self-absorbed and insensitive to his surroundings that it did not occur to him that he was leaving no room for hope or for the mystery of a miracle, or at the very least allowing some peace for his patient by being sensitive to her. Instead he spoke about a patient loud enough and close enough for her to hear, announcing her certain death to everyone as though his self-perceived expertise held the only true and absolute knowledge.

From that moment Daisy's mother did not eat another bite of food and refused all fluids except for a tiny sip of water now and then from a straw, just enough to appease her daughters. She now was starving to death, hastening the process. No amount of coaxing could change her quiet determination.

In one last attempt to fade away by herself, she asked Daisy to go home. Refusing to leave her mother alone in such an inhospitable climate, Daisy stayed around the clock. While sleeping under her mother's hospital bed on the bare, cold marble floor, she was thankful for the summer's hot prairie heat. She only had her mother's new soft, pink housecoat as a pillow. Her mother wasted away quickly above her, turning yellow, then orange with jaundice.

A SURPRISE MOVE into a private room across the hall happened only days later in the late evening. The room had two chairs and a lot of hospital junk piled in one corner. This was where the two sisters would keep vigil in relative comfort now, not realizing another plan was in store.

In the new room an air mattress was on the bed but the pump was not working even though it ground away noisily. The deflated air mattress had hundreds of sharp edges of hard plastic cells that dug her mother's frail body, causing large dents in what thin flesh she had and caused pain in her bones.

Right away Daisy was at war. "This is worse than having no air mattress!" Daisy argued with two nurses who insisted nothing could be done to change it. Daisy was having no patience with their callousness; she angrily ordered that the air mattress be removed immediately. Without a word but only backward glances, the nurses disappeared. As Daisy and her sister were trying to move her mother off the hard plastic, low and behold, the two disgruntled nurses brought in a working air pump.

During the night, Daisy's sister slipped out to sleep in the lounge. She had worked all day and could not keep her eyes open.

There was a picture of a cottage with a luscious flower garden on the wall near the foot of the bed. A little more comfortable now, her mother's eyes drank it in. She signaled with her eyes that Daisy should look at it. It was a reminder of her mother's summer flower garden. But because her mother could no longer speak, Daisy was not sure of what her mother wanted her to know except that it was a reminder of her mother's flower garden and the security of her childhood home – a security she has never since known. She could imagine her mother standing in that garden handing her a flower to draw as she once did.

Daisy's mother had been refusing pain medication, wanting to be lucid of mind. Just before the morning shift change, one of the nurses came back into the room and leaned over Daisy's mother to ask if she would like a painkiller. Mother responded for the first time with a nod. She not only had her illness to deal with but the bed had bitten painfully into her body. A few minutes passed and the same nurse returned with the needle, quickly did the injection and disappeared on a run, not waiting even for a moment to see what affect it had or even to say a kind word to the patient.

Immediately, mother's breathing was suppressed. Daisy recognized that her mother has been given a lethal dose of Morphine. Her life would end in a few minutes.

There was a thunderous sound all around, like armies marching in big boots in the hallways and staircases. It was a shift change but should not sound so loud. Daisy was preoccupied with her mother and could not investigate. Then the sound stopped.

Her mother realized she was about to die and panicked briefly as she could feel her internal organs shutting down completely. Daisy was able to offer a small bit of guidance to crossing over. A look of peace came over her mother's face as her eyes lifted to look into the blue space of a clear early morning sky outside the window.

It had taken a week for her mother to starve to death. Now, in the morning, with her mother lying dead, Daisy stubbornly refused to allow hospital staff an immediate removal of the body, insisting on three hours in which she and her sister could sit with their mother to allow time for her spirit to leave peacefully. Nurses that had just come on duty, found themselves facing stubborn determination that rivaled their own. A morning doctor intervened, giving the sisters permission to have three hours.

Now came the realization that they had been put into this room with junk piled high, just before the lethal dose of morphine because it was the room to die in.

Daisy and her sister kept a vigil with their mother. With time to think, Daisy was amazed and saddened that death and birth are so close in nature. Fights with hospital staff were similar even though the events are a beginning and an end of life. She wondered why things like birth and death could not be simply peaceful with everyone doing a caring job with no mistakes and no battleaxes to deal with. Hospitalization had done nothing, absolutely nothing to help the patient this time. Daisy wished her mother had been kept at home to either live or die. At least she would have had some peace in a loving environment.

Daisy could not help but think about her mother losing her own mother at the age of six. Daisy's grandmother had given birth to four babies at home but when she was having her fifth, she was given the special gift of an expensive hospital birth. She never went home again because she contracted a hospital borne staph infection and died three days after giving birth. This had always been a part of Daisy's reasoning for going into midwifery regardless of the essay she wrote on entering midwifery school after being told that no midwife should have longstanding personal birthing issues. Daisy had quite a few.

With the death of Daisy's mother, there was a passing of a bit of the old world culture. It had been a world of creating everything from nothing by putting simple ingredients together – taking from the garden and making classy, hearty, healthy meals before the word organic came on packages. It was a time of weaving and sewing cloth into well fitting clothing and hand-embroidering colourful designs on household linens.

Having lost her mother as a child, and being the eldest child, Daisy's mother would run home from school to cook a hearty meal for her father and the younger children, not because she had to but because she loved her father so much, she wanted to. She taught herself to make all the cultural foods of the Ukraine and daily she would cook a whole meal from soup, main course, to the dessert.

As Daisy watched over her mother's body, she remembered the hours of standing with her mother over a large roasting pan half full of boiling water, rolling every noodle between their palms of floured hands and watching every noodle plop, being careful not to splash on any hands. Everything her mother made was from scratch. She was an expert at pulling dough paper-thin in a large circle across the kitchen tabletop to make apple and cinnamon strudel. Perogies meant rolling large sheets of dough and cutting them into hundreds of squares that were then filled with anything from mashed potatoes, cheeses, to berries.

This day not only meant the disappearance of a woman but all that she did and taught, and all the health she bestowed on people with her healthy foods and kind heart. She had been a healer without a medical degree.

No more would her voice be heard singing to her babies, "You are my sunshine, my only sunshine. You make me happy when skies are gray. You'll never know dear, how much I love you. Please don't take my sunshine away." And no more would her sweet lilting humming be heard. Daisy remembered brother Bill on her lap every afternoon of his young years and her mother singing lullabies and humming as she rocked him back and forth.

DAISY WORE a white dress embroidered across the top with an array of brightly coloured flowers in honor of her mother's love of flowers. She had never seen her mother wear black so she thought it inappropriate this day. In the receiving line at the funeral, as the eldest child, Daisy stood beside her father. To her surprise, her first husband took his place on the other side of her. Daisy had not seen him in twenty years but today he came because his Canadian mother had died and he also grieved.

Daisy noted that Karl was as handsome as ever and he still had an adorable accent when he spoke. She was unprepared for him to claim he was still in love with her. She had always cared for him but they would speak this day and go on with their lives separately. It was not possible to step back in time with him.

Daisy had lit a large candle on top of a metal angel candleholder on her sister's dining room table and insisted it continue burning during the funeral. Her brother-in-law had objected because he was working for the fire department and knew the dangers. But Daisy told him a higher power would watch over the candle.

Following the funeral, they came back to the house. The many relatives would follow a little later. Meanwhile, her father was drawn to sitting beside the candle. He suddenly burst into weeping that seemed to come from such a deep source, as though his body turned inside out and the crying penetrated eternity. The candle immediately began a fast drip in an unusual way so that large tears gathered in the angel's eyes and run down the angel's face as though crying real tears. It was so heart wrenching that Daisy left the room to give her father some privacy.

OVER THE NEXT days, out of curiosity, Daisy tried to repeat the dripping as an experiment, even providing a breeze, but there was no way she could repeat the experience of the crying angel. It appeared that the angel truly cried with her father, supernaturally.

ON THE DIRT road running past his farm, brother Bill walked alone in the country air to remember his mother. With no other person closer than a quarter of a mile, he heard a female voice singing to him in a high octave... a reminder of his mother singing to him. She was singing without words, much like lullabies his mother used to hum to him. The phenomenon caused him to wonder about the experience. He called Daisy.

HAVING STAYED IN Vancouver at this time by himself to continue caring for his son Andy and to work, Ken was devastated. He had fallen in love with this mother-in-law who reminded him so much of his own maternal grandmother. He had wanted to help her and in the vastness of Vancouver's health care professionals, he had failed to find appropriate help. He felt his aloneness acutely in the absence of Daisy and her whole family. Having wondered at times what life would have been like without this adopted family, he now had a chance to know. Surprised at how much he missed Daisy and had come to rely on her, he begged her to return, "I need you!"

On boarding the airplane for her return trip, as Daisy reached her seat, she felt an excited swoosh of air. Daisy felt her mother's presence as the plane lifted into the air. Her mother had always enjoyed the trips to Vancouver.

[Granddaughter Loraine had taken a couple of items that belonged to her grandmother back to Vancouver. The small crystal ball was set on the mantle and at night it glowed bright with an internal light. Also, the small green houseplant had died back but left in the pot – it sprung to life on the following Mother's Day and grew large for many years to come.]

THE DAY AFTER returning, Daisy was startled to walk into the yard of her home to find the landlord hanging upside down in the cherry tree. At first she wondered if he was alive. He was quite alive with legs wrapped around a heavy branch. From that position, he took a piece of white paper out of his jean pocket and silently held it out toward her.

This middle-aged man had in past acted weird and Daisy's reaction was always a twinge of fear since there was no telling what he was capable of.

The note was a scrawled notice to vacate the premises in favor of demolishing the small house to build several townhouses on the lot.

Within a few days Daisy fell off a balcony, crushing the 5th lumbar vertebra and breaking the right scapula as she hit the ground. The doctors at the university hospital told her that she had come within a tiny fraction of an inch to being paralyzed and, "Count your blessings." But with a broken back she also had to find another house and move again.

At the same time in Alberta, Daisy's brother Bill fell off the back of his truck and broke several ribs.

Ken explained that people are generally more accident prone when dealing with the stress and grief of a death.

THE MORNING AFTER her accident, Daisy was lying on the living room sofa because it was more comfortable than a flat bed. The pain had been excruciating all night regardless of the pills that were supposed to lessen the pain but instead just made her groggy. In a sleep deprived mind, she thought that all parents should have a broken bone before their children do, so that they can understand what it feels like and be all the more sympathetic. She felt bad about the times her children had broken bones and she had no concept of their pain.

The telephone rang. Lana handed the phone to Daisy. The administrator of the midwifery school was on the other end demanding that Daisy show up, "Right now! This morning! To write your exam."

Daisy tried to explain her situation by telling the woman that she broke her back last night and is too drugged with painkillers, foggy, and can't walk no matter what she is supposed to do, let alone write a midwifery exam. "And besides," Daisy tried to explain, "My mother just died!"

The administrator yelled, "I don't care!" She continued demanding, threatening, and insisting that Daisy get to school right now to write her exam.

Daisy felt beaten up by this woman who was not willing to take "no" for an answer even in these extreme circumstances. With no alternative but to refuse and hang up the telephone while the nasty woman was in mid sentence, a thought snuck into Daisy's mind that karma would probably take care of this woman and not to worry about it.

Ken hired their teacher of Chinese medicine to come to the house daily to do acupuncture for Daisy following the accident. With the treatments, she emerged from excruciating pain in lightening speed.

Two weeks later, Daisy went back to attending a midwifery class but by being out in public she realized something had happened to her that was not physical; she had shifted to being introverted. It was as though her mouth was glued shut. Participating socially with these women was difficult. She realized first-hand now how the shock of a physical injury can undermine the whole psyche. She better understood some of Ken's clients who had been seeking help after being severely injured, often finding no understanding elsewhere. Their faces now haunted her because they had held the same shock of becoming introverted in a world that expected them to simply get on with the big 'IT'. But more than that, she now had first hand experience of what Ken must be dealing with in his illness that knocked him off his feet, and why he described it as causing fogginess.

The gossip of this school day was that the same administrator who had yelled at Daisy, had just lost her mother to a sudden death.

Premonition? Intuition? Karma? Was this why the woman was avoiding her today? The questions were mind-boggling to a foggy Daisy.

At the end of the class, in conversation with one of the midwives who Daisy had thought of as a friend, Daisy mentioned that she and Ken had been talking about taking a trip soon to visit his family and a sister who was a practicing nurse-midwife in New England.

The woman walked away and took the head instructor aside. The two were in an animated conversation as Daisy watched from across the room, not realizing the conversation was about her. Daisy was surprised when her friend returned to tell her in no uncertain terms that she has not had approval from the school to visit with midwives around the country and she cannot do so.

What a surprise! These women were dictating that Daisy could not visit with Ken's own sister because she was a midwife. The question Daisy had was, who do they think they are and what kind of competitive jealousy is this?

Socially inept and not up for an argument no matter how unreasonable the women were, Daisy decided to leave. As she went out the door, the same woman and her midwifery partner (the midwife who had begged Ken several times for use of his office) offered Daisy a ride home. She accepted. The ride turned out to be a schoolgirl's worst ride. As the car moved through traffic, the two women harassed Daisy, accusing her of not believing in Homeopathy. Daisy had worked with both women and found them guilty of non-confidentiality; one had left the poopy diaper in Ken's office wastebasket. They seemed to have an axe to grind with Daisy and chose a subject that made no sense instead of what really bothered them. It was an immature game going on and it seemed futile to defend one's self in the situation; Daisy was glad to be leaving it all behind. But the question remained. Do we always revert to childhood behavior when in childhood settings – like school? Daisy reverted to her own childhood behavior of taking bullying silently and walking away.

She made a decision that day not to return to the school. Regardless of what had just transpired, Daisy justified her decision by realizing that continuing would be impossible anyway because the fees for this school were exorbitant. Under the circumstances she could not work for an income until she was sufficiently healed, not only in body but also emotionally if she was to work in the health field. Because the school had been moved out of where they had a free deal in Ken's office, there would be no way to negotiate a reduction in fees. Daisy knew she would not ask Ken for money because he had been ill and was now working only part time while financially taking care of three sons and Jane. Daisy believed the last thing Ken needed was for her to be another unnecessary financial responsibility.

She made the decision to continue low-key lay-midwifery and phase it out slowly, knowing now that she did not want to make a career as a licensed midwife if or when it would be legal in British Columbia, because the fight was all too consuming at her age. Her thoughts were that lack of money was making the final decision. But for a broken back, she might have continued. Fate pointed the way.

[Unknown at the time, it will take several years for her to phase out completely.]

THE NANNY HAD quit as Ken's receptionist. Son Stephen had quit university and replaced the nanny in Ken's medical office. By hiring his son, Ken hoped he could begin keeping his promise to himself to educate his sons in real life, and hopefully in medicine.

But on this day, Daisy just happened to be at the front desk when the midwifery school administrator arrived unexpectedly, telling Daisy that she wanted to talk with Ken. Politely, Daisy asked her to take a seat and wait while Ken was with a client.

Musing that the woman was obviously on a warpath as she sat like a large bull on the chair, Daisy could not imagine why she came to see Ken.

Ken had heard from Daisy about that last class and how this woman had treated her the morning following her accident.

The inner door opened. As Ken followed clients out of his office, the administrator jumped toward him aggressively. In a loud voice she said that the school had forgotten a couple of books in his office.

Daisy was surprised. The woman had not asked her for the two mislaid books that were actually in plain view on a shelf in the reception area. Instead, the woman exhibited deranged behavior like the morning after Daisy's accident; she had waited to attack Ken in front of clients.

Taken by surprise and smarting over what she had done to Daisy, Ken ushered the woman to the door.

A FAMILY CAME in through the door as Daisy's family was gathered in the living room. The young woman headed directly to the sofa to lie down. "Ken, I'm so sick. I think I'm dying." The words barely made it past her lips.

"Sick with what?" Daisy asked.

"I haven't eaten in a whole week. My doctor plans to order an X-ray and some other tests starting tomorrow. He says I might have liver disease."

"Oh, my god!" Daisy gasped, "Why does he think that? You're not yellow."

"He had another patient this week with liver disease and he thinks my symptoms are the same."

Ken said, "I think we can simplify this. Let's do the Chinese food test."

This was a surprising suggestion. Daisy asked, "Chinese food test?"

"Yes, we'll order Chinese food in."

He took Daisy aside and explained that he knows the woman loves Chinese food.

AN ASSORTMENT of Szechwan Chinese food arrived and a buffet was laid out on the large, walnut dining room table.

The woman's energy picked up as she ate. When she was refilling her plate, Ken made an announcement.

"I think you are pregnant."

Surprised, she looked up from her food. "Pregnant?"

"You haven't stopped eating since the food arrived," Ken told her. "I'm going to phone your doctor right now and ask him to give you a blood test that's sensitive to pregnancies only a few days old, and ask him to hold off on all other tests."

Ken talked with the woman's doctor by telephone immediately, explaining that he had just given the Chinese food test and he is sure she is pregnant. The doctor had never heard of the Chinese food test and Ken had a bit of fun with it.

It was confirmed a day later that a baby was on her way into the world.

Daisy was once again completely grateful to Ken for saving a child from what might have been disastrous tests that could have damaged or caused a complete loss of the developing embryo.

SIX WEEKS AFTER the accident, Daisy's daughter-in-law and son traveled a thousand kilometers to her home to have their baby. Daisy begged off because of her back. The daughter-in-law was in no mood to take no for an answer and would not consider a hospital. Normally a bossy person, she wanted to give birth at home, and furthermore, the birth was imminent. Daisy agreed only because Lana was able to assist. There was a flurry of activity in renting the oxygen equipment in case of need, and wrapping and sterilized sheets and equipment.

Though midwives like to work in pairs, for no explained reason while in labor, this mother suddenly got moody, just another of her distinguishing traits. She refused the assistance of another woman. Not wanting to upset the laboring woman by insisting on anything, Daisy relied on her son during hours of exhausting labor coaching.

Pope John Paul II had also come to Vancouver. His timing just happened to coincide exactly with the birth. A new grandson emerged from the birth canal on September 18th, 1984 in the evening just as Pope John Paul's helicopter was landing on Kits Point right outside the window. The scene was dramatic.

Daisy's son caught his baby, greeting his son amid the outside roaring noise and circling flashing lights. The baby was laid on the mother's abdomen. Baby's airways were checked. After pulsing of the umbilical cord stopped, with Daisy's guidance he clamped and cut the cord. The baby was wrapped in a soft blanket. Nursing was attempted but given up quickly. The father took the baby in his arms while the mother gave up the placenta. The uterus felt firm and good. No excess blood.

Without warning the mother suddenly wanted to stand up. Daisy cautioned her to take it easy and just rest for a few more minutes, but in one quick leap the mother was on her feet, only to turn an ashen grey-white and topple over in a faint. Daisy guided her fall softly to the bed.

What appeared to have been a good birth, a prophetic birth, suddenly took a turn. The mother immediately gained consciousness but started hemorrhaging, gushing large quantities of thick, bright red blood.

Loud footsteps bounded up the staircase and into the room. At lighting speed and without a word, Ken began the lifesaving massage of the uterus. Even though Daisy had been trained in the massage technique to stop a hemorrhage, she never had reason to use it in a real emergency. She watched in wonder at the sureness of Ken, his hands massaging so perfectly as though he had been doing this over and over all his life. The hemorrhage stopped quickly under his healing hands. No drug was needed by injection.

Daisy wondered how Ken knew when to make his appearance so fast that the air had moved. She thought he was watching television or reading on the main floor. He must have been listening and bounded up the stairs at the first sound of anything out of the ordinary. On entering the room he made a diagnosis and acted correctly in a flash.

While watching, Daisy analyzed what she knew to date about the patient, who was an extremely stubborn, headstrong person and Daisy wondered if she had been told everything about the family history.

Even though the daughter-in-law had been set up with a family physician that Daisy had worked with before, he had made it clear that Daisy would always be on her own unless in hospital, even in an emergency. Except for post-partum care in the days following a successful birth, his telephone would be the closest he would come to a homebirth because it was illegal in this province for physicians to be party to home births.

Ken, on the other hand, risked his medical license to be on hand for Daisy and did save a life in doing so. Once again, Daisy counted her blessings, feeling the protective comfort of Ken. She had loved this man since that first meeting in July of 1969. Then she became his student and loved the teacher. Tonight she was infatuated with his healing hands. She was in love with the man, the teacher and the physician.

OVERCOMING SEVERE POSTPARTUM difficulties with nutrition, vitamins and homeopathy, the new mother was pink cheeked and healthy on the seventh day and able to walk happily together with Daisy's daughter and their babies in the sunshine the few blocks to her doctor's office. It was a happy day with no foreshadowing of what was to come.

In his office, the doctor performed a lancing procedure on the new mother to alleviate the problem of large hemorrhoids. She was promptly sent walking back home.

Three days following the lancing, Daisy could see that her daughter-in-law had turned grey. This time the grey looked very sick, not temporary.

Daisy told her that she must see her doctor and have him take care of her. The mother stubbornly refused to hear it. An argument erupted and this time Daisy would not let this stubborn person have her way because she recognized it was a life and death situation. After several attempts to persuade the woman, Daisy shouted, "You need to see your doctor! Now! TODAY!"

Angry that her mother-in-law yelled at her, the new mother chose to pack her bags in a fury and call her own mother to come and pick her up.

Minutes later, Daisy answered a rage of banging on the front door. A large woman barged in, bowling Daisy over, causing her to lose her footing and land on the staircase. The woman angrily bounded past Daisy and up the stairs to swoop up her daughter and grandson. She paused only long enough to give her shocked son-in-law a mean tongue-lashing, accusing him of *making* her daughter have a home birth. As she departed out the door with daughter and grandson, she turned once again to call out several more insulting names.

This same daughter-in-law, within a few minutes of a first meeting with Daisy, had expressed how much she detested her own mother, giving Daisy the willies up and down her spine. Then within a few months, she who was the 'older woman' years older than Daisy's son who was barely out of his teen years, had convinced him to elope to avoid family involvement. Then, after eloping they handed a glass of champagne to Daisy who almost dropped it when hearing in the next breath that they were quickly moving north. The woman had applied to take a transfer of her job in a large company to the far north. By doing that, she was moving far from her own mother and pulling Daisy's son out of the close vicinity of his family. This woman's attitude came as a terrible shock to Daisy.

The mother, who this daughter-in-law had claimed to hate, took her daughter with the newborn baby to her own apartment where the family partied, not noticing that the new mother was sick until a couple of days later when she suddenly needed to be hospitalized and found to have blood poisoning.

At the hospital, Daisy and the home birth were blamed for the life threatening infection. Everyone had so eagerly wanted to blame the home birth, that it was overlooked that the woman had been rosy-cheeked and healthy at seven days after the birth, and that her health declined three days following the lancing of hemorrhoids that happened in a doctor's office. She only got ill a full ten days after the birth, and now it was two weeks after the birth.

Meanwhile, Daisy's son, who was in the doghouse with his wife and in-laws, had gone home with their dogs to the North. Ken arranged his immediate flight back to Vancouver to reconcile with his ill wife and baby.

[Sixteen years later in divorce proceedings, the daughter-in-law will tell her story in a British Columbia Supreme Court of Law and to the world, forcing Daisy to defend herself publicly about allegations that as a midwife, she caused the infection.]

30

Time for Healing

"CONSIDERING YOUR HEALTH and how you are struggling to keep going, you should consider bankruptcy." This advice came in January of 1985 from the accountant that Ken and his ex-wife had employed during their marriage. He had continued to know each story separately after divorce.

Based on that advice, Ken visited a trustee in a large well-respected firm to seek debt counseling, not bankruptcy. The Trustee made a clear statement that unless Ken wanted to kill himself over money, he should take time out to heal and simply go bankrupt. Daisy and Ken were sitting there, hearing words that felt like a slamming door.

Extremely reluctant to go the route of bankruptcy, Ken continued working for several more months.

Since the major illness in November of 1983 that had caused him to be bedridden, Ken had been struggling to keep working through constant relapses into disabling health problems. Concerning him was the possibility of the disabling and disfiguring illness carrying him away while continuing to be a frontline physician, a dangerous place to be for himself and for his patients. He was afraid of making medical mistakes because of the overwhelming weakness and tiredness that came with each illness. It was a dilemma whichever way he looked at the problem.

Consulting with the mother of his child continued to be important to Ken regardless of their divorce because they were co-parenting a son. He relied on and respected her legal opinions. It was a kind of companionship the parents had together that Daisy just had to understand and accept.

Besides personally advising Ken, Jane also sent him to her friend for additional backup legal advice for which the lawyer charged Ken Five Hundred Dollars and told Ken that he "CANNOT' pay maintenance during bankruptcy'". The Five Hundred Dollars he charged was steep for such a short visit because lawyers at the time were usually charging Two Hundred Dollars per hour and this appointment was not nearly that long. Ken had been willing to follow whatever Jane suggested and paid the bill without complaining. Neither Ken nor Daisy had reason to believe this to be a setup but in the following months, it would appear to be just that.

Ken's parenting responsibility for Andy had been steadily maintained for months. Andy was with Ken all the time except when the child was in school. Saturday afternoon until Sunday afternoon and usually one evening during the week was when Andy would see his mother.

If Ken was working, Daisy or Lana helped. And that was when a walk to school with Andy one morning caused a life-changing decision. It started out happily. Lana's small son rode his little bike with the help of being pushed most of the way. Andy walked alongside.

Later that afternoon, Daisy relayed a disturbing story to Ken. "Andy suddenly, with nothing precipitating it... just out of the blue, threw himself face first into a ditch beside the sidewalk. He lay on his stomach, crying out, "I'm going to commit suicide!" Then he just lay there. We physically picked him up. I asked him where he learned that. He told us he learned that from his mother. He said she does that."

Ken was silent while the significance of his son's behavior sunk in. He then made the decision to be with his son more fully and not let others, including Daisy, care for his needy child. With difficulty, he came to the conclusion that he needed to retire, temporarily at least, and take time to really heal if he wanted to be around for his needy children.

Life-long work ethics and family responsibilities had kept him going, fighting the idea of bankruptcy. He sadly closed his office, not knowing which was worse, a physician not trusting himself in his work or being out of work entirely – or even worse, ignoring his child's problems.

IT WAS A SUNNY Saturday afternoon at the end of May 1985. Jane arrived to pick Andy up, revving the motor of her BMW. The ground responded by shaking with a deep moan, as usual. She got out of the car as Ken walked toward her with Andy by his side.

Prepared for this meeting, Ken held a cheque in his hand for Jane.

Daisy had walked out with them and stayed back a few feet, watching and surmising – no! – knowing that Andy would be taken from Ken and driven directly to a friend for babysitting, as usual. That was the least of either Ken's or Daisy's worries right now.

Standing face to face with Jane, Ken spoke softly but firmly, "Jane, you know I've been too ill to work for several months now. I have had to close my office. We discussed that. There is no income. This is no surprise since I have consulted with you and you have advised me about going bankrupt. Your friend, the lawyer that you sent me to for advice regarding maintenance said I should not pay maintenance during bankruptcy. I don't feel right about that so I have cashed in my remaining Retirement Saving Fund to pay you maintenance for Andy and it has to be advance payments for the months of bankruptcy. In good faith between us, I trust you will accept advance payments for maintenance. Here is a cheque for Eighteen Hundred Dollars. I'll continue looking after Andy as I do now and I'll pay for other things as needed."

Jane's light blue eyes looked Ken straight in the eyes as she accepted the cheque in her white hand. Without a word she turned her back, clutching the cheque as she and Andy walked to the car.

The motor growled again. It always sounded angry.

Ken watched as once again his son left, but this time he was wondering why she had not said anything, just simply taken a cheque and driven off; after all, in 1985, Eighteen Hundred Dollars was considered to be a lot of money.

Daisy watched Ken watching his child leave. She ached for him and she was disturbed at how this event went. The memory of Jane's cool eyes devoid of emotion looking into Ken's eyes as she took the cheque burned into Daisy's brain. She ran through her thoughts that having been a single parent herself, if anyone had given her a cheque for Eighteen Hundred Dollars for no other deserving reason except that she is a female and a mother, she would have been ecstatic with joy. She thought about how she had never been given a cent for raising her children and never pursued it, preferring to be thankful to have the gift of her children. Having good health to be able to work to support her children was an additional gift rather than becoming entangled in bad karma. Seeing a woman take and take – and take, and at the same time be so blatantly ungrateful and cold was exasperating.

Neither Ken nor Daisy knew what to make of Jane's reaction as the car disappeared but it did not feel right.

As they climbed the staircase to the house, Daisy suddenly felt an outburst coming on, "Wow! She did not even thank you for the money! What strange behavior, considering your generosity! You look after Andy every day, feed him all his meals except for a couple of meals a week when she in fact takes him to a baby sitter just like I'm sure she is doing now, and then he is back again Sunday afternoon, the very next day."

Ken's answer was, "I'm fine with that so long as I have my son with me. The hard part is going bankrupt."

"Yes, but even that is for debts Jane helped to make. Oh well, I was sympathetic toward her but this somehow changes that. I just wish she would show some... *any* appreciation for all your care... all you do for her... at least for the extra money you've always given to her whenever she asks."

WITH THE REMAINDER of a few measly dollars in Ken's pocket, a couple of weeks later in June, Ken took Jane out for dinner in a French restaurant to honor her birthday. They had been there before and he knew she had liked it.

Later, Ken relayed part of the conversation to Daisy. "During dinner Jane made a remark that there must be something special about our relationship since it has gone on for so many years through all kinds of trouble."

Not pleased about the date but accepting it as part of Ken's way of caring for the mother of his child, she thought, what's new? But the idea of Jane trying to penetrate into the unquenchable depth of her relationship with Ken was accompanied by foreboding. It had not helped that Ken's oldest son had dropped by that evening with the news that Ken was having dinner with Jane in a French restaurant. Daisy had an idea about who sent him with that message but knew it was not Ken.

* * *

July 8, 1985

Dear Jane,

In accordance with our separation agreement, which allows for negotiation of the amount of maintenance depending on our relative incomes, I am writing to request that we negotiate a major change this month as we have done many times before.

At the end of this month, I will be making a voluntary application for bankruptcy for health reasons. I have paid maintenance to you out of monies received since I stopped practicing psychotherapy in May and from a de-registered R.S.P. (retirement savings plan). My lawyer tells me that this preferential treatment of you as a creditor is supported by law and that when I go bankrupt this preference is not supported because National Revenue would have priority on all my earnings. He has also told me I cannot pay maintenance in advance. However, I would incur a debt to you for arrears maintenance which would survive the bankruptcy.

For reasons of my health, and in hopes of being available to Andy for the next fifteen years or more, I have stopped working for the Medical Services Plan and have applied for GAIN so that I can care for Andy. He is doing well with the schedule you and I have worked out for his care. During the time he is at the Odyssey Bayview Day Camp, I am volunteering time for research with SPEC. I plan to continue this research schedule when he attends Grade 1 in the fall. This volunteer work may lead to a small amount of income in 1986 which will cover research expenses. Realistically, at my age, I do not expect to find salaried work and working for the MSP is hazardous to my health. It may take three to five years for me to develop an alternative career. During the period of bankruptcy and for an unknown time following, I will be making a substantial contribution to Andy's well being.

For these reasons, I believe it is necessary to stop all maintenance payments immediately while I am on GAIN, and for the duration of the bankruptcy, and then to negotiate a new *agreement when the bankruptcy is discharged. **If my assumptions are incorrect, or there is other relevant information I should consider with you, please advise me as soon as possible.***

Thank you.

[Signed] *Ken*

> [The only changes negotiated to date had been for Ken to give Jane extra money when she asked. He always complied.]

* * *

To Whom It May Concern:

This is to confirm that since September of 1984, Ken has assumed increasing responsibility for Andy's care from 8:30 a.m. until 7:30 p.m. Mondays through Thursdays and from 8:30 a.m. Fridays until noon on Saturdays. Overnights have been negotiated without difficulty. Andy is doing well on this schedule of shared responsibility by both parents which we are prepared to continue at least through the school year 1985/86,

August 1, 1985   K. Schramm

August 2, 1985   Jane Anderson

THIS SIGNED AGREEMENT was an outline of the bare minimum formal hours agreed upon but the message in 'overnights have been negotiated without difficulty' really meant Andy was overnight with Ken most nights; it was just not written in stone. Both parents seemed happy with this agreement.

BELIEVING HE HAD Jane's approval, Ken and Daisy went back to visit the trustee who worked in a distinguished downtown building. While sitting opposite him on hard wooden chairs, they heard the news repeated, "Bankruptcy is advised. Alternatives would not be helpful in your situation. Bankruptcies are not free. It will cost you..."

Ken interrupted, "I don't have any money."

"You do need to pay for bankruptcy. In your case I will accept monthly payments instead of a lump sum."

"Can I work a few hours to do that?"

"Yes. In fact, you may have to do something like that. Social Services doesn't pay enough for you to live on and pay for bankruptcy. People are allowed to work while in bankruptcy. However, you need to fill out a sheet stating all your finances, income and expenses, once a month. See that I get it on time. In other words, everything you do for the next few months will be scrutinized and everything you did in the past five years will be thoroughly examined."

Coming from a proud background, a family of financially self-sufficient people, relatives of the Woolworth fortune (that was not shared with the extension of family but never-the-less a family with respect for money) and knowing he will no doubt reap the wrath of his brothers and sisters coupled with disrespect from his grown sons, Ken made an agreement to go bankrupt regardless of extreme personal reluctance. In agreeing, he hoped his choice of life over money would gain him years with his sons. He hoped they would eventually understand.

31

New Start to Recovery

"Historians are asked to do what God is supposed to do: tell us true stories about our lives so that we can be healed and build with love and hope another world to live in. We are asked to tell these stories in words, music and drama in person and in writing. Speaking and listening and rethinking precede reading and writing. Reading presupposes listening, hearing, speaking and seeing. The magic of words with feeling, felt heard within mother – child."
Kehnroth Schramm [notebook]

JANUARY 1986. AFTER MONTHS of slow recovery and feeling somewhat stronger but with a heart that had been damaged over the years, it took great effort to muster enough energy to keep going. With determination and enthusiasm to be a father and not let his son Andy suffer because of his bad heart, Ken made the daily trek to and from school four times a day, every school day with Andy. Welcomed by teacher Mrs. Ma, Ken often stayed at school as a helper. One of Andy's schoolmates sometimes accompanied Ken and Andy home from school for after-school playtime. Through the boys' friendship, Ken gained a friend in the father, a professor at UBC who invited him to audit classes in History.

For Ken, this was an invitation to recreate a time when he was feeling at his best in life – his life at Dartmouth College. To recreate this now was a healing blessing because his stamina had been severely weakened inside and out, and from head to toe.

He hoped that auditing a class would be the stimulation needed to rebuild strength while Andy was in school.

After a few classes, he told Daisy, "They speak a different language. They look upon me as the old man in class." This was another time in history and not a recreation of 1950's New England.

Thirty-five years after Dartmouth, this particular group of the new generation had little or no time for in-depth philosophic discussions like Ken had experienced at Dartmouth. They were in a hurry, running here and there. Never the less, it was an exciting time and Ken was delighted to be in the university environment again. Wanting to share it all with Daisy, he invited her along to as many classes as she was willing to attend.

After being so ill, Ken was overjoyed at being able to write short papers again. He wanted so much to share ideas that he excitedly read every word to his sounding board, Daisy, his best and worst critic. She challenged him daily while enjoying his newly found happiness more than his papers and told him she wanted to hear more – more of *his* ideas. She teased, "He's a poet and doesn't know it!" And actually, she meant it.

Then he expressed the wish to complete the Medical Anthropology PhD that he had been close to earning before suddenly having to leave it all behind in the United States.

Completely understanding that Ken had unfinished goals, Daisy encouraged him to apply for a student loan as soon as the bankruptcy was discharged. The idea was that he could commit to becoming a registered student to complete the expansion to his career that he needed. Ken loved teaching and had taught at some of the best universities. Daisy understood that Ken was a teacher as was his great-grandfather, who was a physician and an accomplished educator and that Ken would follow in Charles Kehnroth, M.D.'s footsteps; Ken had his name and his genes.

Now that Ken had fulfilled his side of the promise to educate Jane by paying for her education and helped her financially and physically even after divorce to finish her articling and to become ensconced in her chosen career as a lawyer, Ken wanted to make his career change – the change he believed they had both agreed to.

As usual, regardless of a divorce, Ken discussed everything in his life with Jane. In preparation for when the bankruptcy would be discharged, he turned to Jane again for help in filling out forms to apply for student loans.

Afraid of having a stroke behind the wheel of a car like his mother had done, Ken had completely given up driving during his illness in November of 1983. So determined was he to not be tempted to drive again, he had given the car to Daisy back then for all the volunteer work she had done and not been paid for. And she had turned the car into a computer because she could not drive. Without any car, Ken often was a passenger in Jane's car in the comings and goings of their son. They appeared to be getting along just great as a family separated but caring for their child together.

During this time Ken took Andy out of the country to visit the child's ailing grandmother in Vermont. Jane drove them to the airport and picked them up on return, showing her trust and approval.

All seemed peaceful.

AN EXPLORATORY VISIT to the Anthropology department proved challenging. The head of the department said to Ken, "Just because you're a physician, doesn't mean you can waltz in here and take up where you left off. I would insist you do statistics for a year to prove yourself."

There was no mistaking the deliberately insulting deterrent. It was for no apparent reason because the guy did not know Ken and had no academic transcript from which to make such a decision. Daisy was appalled but not surprised at the slur.

True to his nature, Ken refused to grovel and kept his dignity by walking out. He gave up the idea of pursuing a PhD in Anthropology at UBC.

Outside he told Daisy, "I have done statistics in the past. I'm not doing that again, especially for a year of my life."

Daisy had been silent in the meeting, feeling it was not her place to butt in, but it always bothered her to the core that anyone could be that mean to Ken. As they left the building, she offered a statement meant to sooth his feelings. "I'm a little bit familiar with the anthropology scene here. He has never impressed me."

Before they had left the building, a female PhD candidate had invited them to the social gathering of the anthropology department that evening and they did attend. While Ken made friends with students, Daisy decided to talk with the guy who had put Ken down earlier. He was sitting with his wife. Since it was a social gathering, Daisy intended to break through his veneer. After light conversation with his wife, Daisy turned to him with a story out of her midwifery bag that any anthropologist might be interested in. He listened in silence and when the story was finished, he just continued looking at her with vacant eyes and then turned away. Not the conversation Daisy expected. They never spoke again. She regretted wasting her story and wasting time she could have spent with Ken. Though Ken would harbor no hard feelings and did audit some of the guy's classes, Ken did not give over power to that man or pursue completing his PhD in Anthropology at UBC.

KEN'S NOTEBOOK – 16th October 1986:

History Makers: Healing With Words

As a physician, I have studied history through the lives of individual children, parents and families: bodies who learn and use languages, as Kenneth Burke might say.

When I was in medical school in Vermont in the fifties, I was called 'the writer' by my teacher of surgery. I wrote as I read to understand the lives of the people, the patients who were teaching me medicine.

My mother threw away all my notes from high school, college and medical school, the only record I had of my peoples' history of the worlds I lived in. I think I have forgiven her because I am rediscovering that history now.

In 1957 or '58, as I was graduating from medical school, I discovered Kenneth Burke's The Philosophy of Literary Form: Studies in Symbolic Action where I read of "literature as equipment for living". Writers like Kenneth Burke saved my life by helping me rediscover it, perspectives through incongruity. I think in words, feelings, impassioned conversations, prayers and conversions, with occasional soft images in contrast to the colours of my night dreams. Perhaps that is why I am called to be a healer with words and a maker of history, of true stories to repay my debt to my teachers and to discover another world to live in with children and grandchildren.

I have been in the process of a career change from physician-anthropologist to physician-historian since coming to Canada in 1967 when I was expected by my draft board to go to Vietnam despite my conscientious objection to war. My dream, then and now, was and is to build a home-farm-school in which refugees from the colonized worlds of North America could learn together how to build another world to live in for our children and grandchildren. Knowledge of our own histories is crucial to that process of education or paideia as Lewis Mumford calls it. Students are history, in Page Smith's words, following our teacher Eugen Rosenstock-Huessy.

I have in mind a cooperative effort of those ultimately and vitally concerned with independent scholarship, home schooling, home labor, home birth and home centered living and healing. I believe that the hospitals, schools and other bureaucracies of our lives are essentially defunct without our living and often loving support. So I am asking others and their families to withdraw part of their support for bureaucracy, so that we can put that energy into building a teaching-learning community for people of all ages. I want to work and write for this voluntary association of independent scholars so that I can share my knowledge of healing within a community of at least two generations working together.

In order to complete my knowledge of history, so that I can be clearer about what I want to share with my friends, my children and grandchildren, I want to study and write about the lives and rethink the thoughts of my teachers: Kenneth Burke, Page Smith, Stanley Diamond, Paul Radin, Herbert Marcuse, Tom Szasz, Ronald Laing, Christopher Lasch, Francis L.K. Hsu, Lewis Mumford, Edwin Burtt,

Eugen Rosenstock-Huessy, Bernard Lonergan, Alice Miller, Catherine and Harris Coulter. What these people have in common for me is their individual commitments to loving life as an ultimate concern in a world of technology and narcissistic relativism.

I was lucky to have teachers like Eugen Rosenstock-Huessy, Francis Gramlick, Philip Wheelwright, Maurice Mandelbaum, George Wolf, Fred Berthold, George Kalbfleisch, Paul Tillick, Ernie Becker, Brad Starr.

I want my families to have teachers like these, too.

* * *

A FORMER CLIENT with a wife and baby was determined to find Ken and ask for help regardless of a closed office. They were the first possible clients after closing the office, and as a result, Ken consulted with Social Services. Ken was told that within their rules, anyone could continue a small business and receive income, and that he could bill the Medical Services Plan; it was also approved by Social Services that paying rent for an office space and someone to manage the small practice could be paid out of gross income. A small personal net income of One Hundred Dollars per month for service provided was allowed over and above Social Services Assistance and anything over that would be clawed back. With that advice and safeguards built in, Social Services gave approval that this would allow Ken to be able to give Andy an allowance and extras to benefit both Jane and Andy.

Ken consulted again with his Trustee of bankruptcy. The Trustee assured Ken that fees for going bankrupt could also be paid out of that net income. The only reminder was the stipulation that all income and expenses were to be reported monthly to the Trustee.

Daisy quipped to the Trustee, "It is an irony that people have to have *no* money to go bankrupt but are required to pay a large fee to do so."

Her comment had been met with a wry smile and a nod. "That is why I take payments spread over a year during bankruptcy."

All had given permission and encouragement to do a small practice.

Ken was in constant communication with Jane over his finances and daily life, keeping her informed about every decision and every move.

A second former client found Ken. One afternoon she waited for Ken with her small son on the staircase by the front door of the house. When she was brought into the house, she explained that they had just been to their family physician because her son had a nail puncture his leg right to the bone. They had been given an antibiotic prescription and because Ken was the only doctor she trusted, she had come to ask if she should give it to her son. She wanted to use Homeopathy or something holistic. Ken was quick to explain the necessity of the antibiotic because of the seriousness of the wound but she could include Homeopathy. This surprised the woman but Ken explained that allopathic medicine was sometimes necessary – better to be safe, and in this case the two medicines would not interfere with each other.

Another former client and her four children embarked on a search to find Ken. They had lost their home to a fire and a divorce followed in the year before Ken had become involved. While the mother spent time with Ken, Daisy kept the children occupied in the kitchen with jars of tempura paint and rolls of paper spread across the tables. Walls became stained from happy splashing colours. They took turns with Ken separately and as a family.

The tiny practice was made up only of families who searched and found Ken on their own.

ALWAYS IN THE PAST, contributing to society as a volunteer had been a way of life for Ken. Now was no different so long as he can get out of bed and put one foot in front of the other. While Andy was in school, he and Daisy volunteered in a church food bank for single parents one morning a week. The large lawn that no one used caught Ken's attention; he wants to turn it into a vegetable garden for the food bank. The hierarchy of the church rejected the idea but it resulted in a fenced outdoor play area for children.

Ken offered to lead a philosophical discussion on Love in the church setting for a few weeks on the evening that Andy was with his mother. Daisy worried about Ken's health in taking this on.

Only women with strong opinions turned up each week to argue loudly about the meaning of Love. It seemed to Daisy it was a healthy outlet for women to let off steam once a week. Since the discussions were not personal attacks on Ken and he did not have a responsibility to fix anything, Daisy learned to relax. She decided Ken needed the stimulation as part of getting well, kind of like getting on a horse again after being dumped.

DAISY HAD A WORRISOME premonition and for many months had been keeping a wall calendar marked with the hours that Ken looked after Andy. Most of the time, Andy continued to be with Ken, except for the Wednesday evenings and the hours between Saturday afternoons to Sunday afternoons. Ken continued to be at Andy's school where he read to groups of children and helped wherever he could. Regardless of Daisy's uneasiness, all seemed well between Ken and Jane.

Ken's older sons, now in their twenties, had moved on to live with friends. Because no one wanted a small child in their building, Ken had moved a couple of more times and heard complaints from Jane that he moved around too much. Daisy also had moved several more times, not finding any stable housing since she had moved from the housing co-op. Once again, a landlord has sold her home out from under her after only a few months. As a result of the bankruptcy and Daisy's financial difficulties following her broken back, it had made sense to rent together to ease their housing problems. Ken and Andy had been spending most of their time at Daisy's home anyway.

The newer problem was that by sharing accommodation with Daisy, Ken had no separate space for dealing with his own family problems. The evening came when Andy was upset that he could not play on the Commodore computer because an adult family member was trying to make the disappointing thing work. Being a Wednesday evening Jane arrived to pick Andy up. Out he went but a few minutes later, Andy marched back into the house. He went toward a smaller child who had been quietly playing under a table and he kicked her. Then he turned and marched toward the door to leave.

Ken stopped him. "Why did you do that?"

Everyone was stunned when he answered, "My mother told me to get back in and get even."

KEN HAD WORKED hard to build a good father-son relationship with Stephen and Peter and they did have a few good years since 1981. Before Ken's bankruptcy but soon after the house of the marriage sold and Ken had given his share to Jane, there should have been a lump sum of many thousands of dollars in her name in a bank somewhere, but Ken's oldest son announced that Jane was too broke to pay her Hydro bill. Regardless of the questionable situation, Ken became concerned and made an effort to pacify his ex-wife. At that time, Stephen let it be known that he was diligently looking out for Jane and Andy.

Ken explained to Daisy, "Stephen believes he is standing in for me in my failure. He doesn't understand how Jane had been fighting me and pushing me out of her life. I am pleased that Andy's brother is taking an interest in him."

Concern was written on Ken's face as he continued, "Jane has made a point of telling me that she and Stephen have been attending parties, sitting in hot tubs, and going to movies and concerts together."

Now in 1986, Jane would sometimes arrive with Ken's oldest son on Wednesday evening to pick up Andy, but oddly, Stephen waited in the car instead of acknowledging his father.

Daisy questioned, "Ken, what is that about?"

Ken was sad about it, explaining to Daisy, "Stephen believes that he is filling in for me. He won't listen when I try to talk with him."

Stephen's strange involvement left little doubt that there was an undercurrent. Something was brewing and bothering Andy; he was showing new aggravation by hitting and kicking, not only the children, but also Ken. The notion that everything was peaceful between Ken and Jane was being eroded by something not yet out in the open. Ken and Daisy were both uneasy.

After one of the strange pickups when Stephen waited in the car, Daisy blurted out, "I believe your son is being groomed to be a witness. I believe he is being set up to think she is spending more time with Andy than she does. And Andy is really unhappy about something going on there and is lashing out."

It bothered Daisy that the sons continued to believe their father abandoned them and Andy, and that they did not seem to understand their father's generosity and constant care.

True to his daily writings of hope, unconditional love and wishes for strength to deal with his problems, Ken was loyal to all members of his family regardless of the hurts. His adopted family did provide family life that he was not able to have with ex-wives and children of broken marriages.

The Sunday family dinners were Ken's salvation in keeping with the childhood memories of making the trip to his grandparents' home Sunday afternoons and paralleled Daisy's childhood in the tradition of Sunday dinners. Her parents had always made Sunday dinner special and sometimes the family made weekend trips to family gatherings at her grandparent's farm.

Ken and Daisy found companionship outside of any problems as they shopped for the family dinners in the Granville Island Market where food was stacked high in stall after stall. Fresh seafood was in abundance, and the bakery sent out smells of freshly baked goods.

Sometimes they rode their bicycles to the market. In rainy or cold weather, they took the bus for lack of a car. They often sat and relaxed for a half hour on the docks, feeling the fresh sea air on their faces while watching the boats, before going home for Andy's return and to cook for the family gathering.

While preparing the dinners together, they shared memories and ideas about cooking food, and occasionally had to sort out differences in ideas about cooking. Ken had changed his diet for health reasons and found it difficult not to indulge in some of the family favorites. Then the families would arrive, sometimes in large numbers and sometimes only a few. The invitation was open to all. Daisy's family had multiplied with spouses and grandchildren who arrived with enthusiasm. The children had never known life without their grandfather Ken. He was always caring and available, giving of his time as though he had no other problems.

Ken's loyalty to caring for Jane and their son, his children by his first marriage, while maintaining a relationship with Daisy and her family was admired by Daisy. His divided loyalties had not deterred her; instead she saw in Ken, a good man who wore himself out by trying too hard.

LIKE CLOCKWORK, Jane was in hospital again. Andy had been ill all night, loudly panicking with worry about his mother while projectile vomiting on Ken, into his bedding and around the small apartment. It stunk. No one was getting any rest. There was no laundry facility in this apartment. After a sleepless night, a march down the street to a coin Laundromat would be necessary, costing more of the scarce money, not to mention the hassle of carrying the stinking, sour laundry for blocks. Daisy was fed-up with the child's suffering over what she assumed were unnecessary cosmetic surgeries. She bundled up a vomit sheet for safekeeping.

I'm no saint! Daisy mused over the thought. Knowing how ill Ken became under the years of stress that started long before 1981; seeing how relying on the wrong physician had led to a cumulative allopathic medicine reaction to bring Ken's health down to collapse; seeing his struggle to regain his strength; seeing his ex-wife playing games around not only one son, but escalated to two; seeing how the youngest son mimicked his mother by threatening suicide any time his mother was in hospital or fell ill which was often; seeing how this very small boy projectile vomited every time his mother went into hospital every few months; watching Ken clean vomit off his child and himself; often washing vomit bedding; seeing Jane in the credit union with obvious scars around both blackened eyes after one of her "emergency" hospital visits; knowing that there were many of those kinds of emergencies over the years and Andy had been sworn to secrecy but told his story anyway because he was scared; overhearing the Saturday late night phone calls to Ken to tell him that she was having fun at a party which was followed by fairly regular Monday morning illnesses; through all this Daisy had been a silent friend to Ken, never saying anything to Jane one way or another because she had not wanted to cause Ken additional problems. Sympathy for a troubled woman had always been Daisy's foremost sentiment, but inevitably after five years there came a point of reacting.

Without prior warning one evening, Jane's friend Leslie arrived to pick up Andy because Jane had been released from the hospital.

While Leslie stood inside the kitchen doorway waiting for Andy to be ready, Daisy did the unthinkable. She handed Leslie the bundle of white sheet with vomit and told her, "Give this vomit to Jane to clean. She should be aware of what she is doing to her son."

The artist in Daisy often surfaced in the most awkward moments. She saw the dramatic picture of the dark-haired woman dressed all in black with a typical lawyer's long black coat, standing on the bright red rug with her red rimmed mouth open, producing a dark hole in her white face with wide open shocked eyeballs, holding the white bundle in both hands in front of her.

Daisy could feel Ken's shock through her back. Ken had been helping Andy get his things together and now that the child was ready, Ken was taken by surprise at Daisy's bold move. Daisy had never reacted like this before.

Ignoring Ken's reaction, Daisy was determined that the mother of Ken's son should finally get a graphic, stinky picture of how her antics were affecting her child.

After the sheet went out the door, Daisy realized that she had given up an expensive, top-quality, king-sized sheet that she has had for years. Somehow, she had imagined she would hand it directly to Jane and insist it be cleaned and brought back. In the reality of the moment, there was sudden knowledge that she would never see the sheet again and worse, she could not afford to replace it. On the other hand, she was proud of herself for finally standing up to Jane. The sheet was the price to do this.

Yes, I am no saint! But maybe something will change for Ken and Andy, she told herself. Then she had doubts about it all.

Over the years, Ken had tried to explain Andy's problem to Jane to no avail. The events of this night came as a terrible surprise in many ways. He thought Daisy had a right to her own thoughts and actions but he also knew those women were capable of larger conflict than Daisy could ever imagine and in the long run, Daisy would be no match. The last thing he needed was conflict with his son being in the middle. He said nothing and went to bed.

While straightening up the kitchen, Daisy had time to think about how Ken allowed her to be herself and react in her own way. He never tried to impede her freedom.

Daisy thought back to the day former partner Saul criticized her for always trying to change things by sticking up for underdogs. At first she was surprised he even noticed and even more surprised that it bothered him, but he was so disgruntled with her and disapproving in his remark that it bothered her all day. When she went to the elementary school later that day to pick up her youngest daughters, she did something she could not forget. A teacher was having a group of children practice for a concert in the hallway. A small Greek boy was not singing to perfection and the teacher was bullying the boy until the boy was in tears. Normally Daisy would have intervened to defend the boy but this day, because of the earlier criticism, she tried out non-interference and walked away. That little boy was on Daisy's conscience years later and would not leave. She worried about the long-term effects of the adult bully on the small boy and whether he would ever sing again. How she wanted to make it up to the little dark-haired boy with tears in his brown eyes that she abandoned in a situation that he was trapped in with no escape and no protection.

So here she was, determined to defend a small boy and his father.

32

Peace to War in 1987

SINCE MAY OF 1985 when Ken had to close his office and through the most of 1986, everything seemed relatively calm between Ken and ex-wife Jane. Ken had been trustingly taking Jane's personal and legal advice about his financial situation and what he should be paying for regarding their son. He was happily looking after Andy as the equivalent of a full time parent. He was making the walk to and from school four times a day and spending time in the classroom. He had consulted with Jane all the way about Andy's care and schooling. He was keeping Jane up to date about the school adventures. During the last couple of years, Ken had been with his youngest son for breakfast, lunch and dinner usually six days out of seven, and he had been involved with Andy and his friends for school activities.

Ken had managed to get his son into the elementary school by the university campus where together they were in the university environment. Walking through the forest after school hours was an important time for father and son to talk while under the green umbrella of trees emanating peace and reminiscent of Ken's childhood forest.

During this time, Ken had been under intense scrutiny by having to report every penny of his income, or lack of it, and expenses to both the Trustee and to government social workers. Even though it had been tight financially, sharing accommodation with Daisy and her family was a bonus for everyone. Andy was like an older brother to multiplying grandchildren who were around a lot.

They had moved again and now had more space. There were lots of painting sessions. Daisy mixed big jars of tempera paint and stretched out long rolls of paper on the extra long table made of two tables together that doubled as dining tables for large family gatherings beside large windows across a whole wall in the spacious old-fashioned kitchen. Weekend afternoons were usually filled with children making the walls their art gallery. The house also housed cats and a dog, castoffs from other homes. The painting sessions were often punctuated by a comedy of Daisy running out of the house, into the garden, to yell at a cat not to be a cat and demanding that it leave that poor bird alone – to Ken's amusement.

Andy was with his father and the children for regular Sunday family dinners, and celebrations of birthdays and holidays. Baking birthday cakes happened often. Daisy sculpted fairy tale characters and trains out of the home baked cakes – whatever the birthday child would choose. Then the children would help to decorate the cakes with brightly coloured icing, red and black licorice, and an array of candies. Andy would participate fully.

Started as a baby, Andy continued to spend hours sitting on his father's knee or curled up under Ken's arm with his head against Ken's chest, listening intently to his father's soft voice running through words of many books of stupendous imagination, describing ideas and events. Through the years Ken had read to Andy at least once a day when together, and then they would share thoughts about the stories. The look on Andy's face as he was read to, was always of being totally connected with Ken's voice and intently involved in the story while cradled in the warmth and protection of his father's body. It was Ken's way of instilling the love of books and learning while sharing the father/son bond. This time shared by father and son was a time when no one interrupted or interfered.

Finally Daisy had become legally divorced from the marriage she refused to remember. Now she was free to marry Ken.

JANUARY 1987, Ken read a letter as he paced among the orange kittens playing with their shadows in the sunlight spilling across the kitchen floor.

Ken was obviously bomb shelled! "Daisy, look at this letter from Jane. She is claiming I paid no child maintenance during the bankruptcy and she intends to take me to court. It states that I am discharged from bankruptcy *today*! I don't even know that yet. My Trustee hasn't informed me."

Daisy was shocked but her worst fears about her intuitions to not trust the ex-wife had just come true. She wanted to reassure Ken but the first thing to escape her mouth was, "She has obviously been planning this by keeping track of dates from within the court system and pounced."

Then she tried to ease Ken's shock. "She's lying about non-payment of maintenance so all we have to do is prove it. You have a cancelled cheque for the lump sum payment. And you have receipts for regularly paying other things that she did approve of and expected each month. So, no problem! And besides, what does caring for Andy seven days out of seven amount to? Even on Saturday and Sunday you have him part of each day. I am a witness to all of that. She should have been paying you!"

Daisy took the letter from Ken and what popped out immediately was Jane's name, which waved a red flag pointing to deceit. "She has been using her maiden name since she divorce you and is a practicing lawyer as Jane Anderson but she's doing this action as Jane Schramm, obviously hiding her lawyer name. Is that legal?"

What Ken and Daisy did not yet realize is that this was the beginning of a legal tearing down of a man, and the attempt through legal means to rid Ken of his companion, Daisy.

Games began in full force.

Ken found out that Jane had changed Andy's last name at school to her maiden name and this was followed by a request that Ken agree to a legal name change for his son. Ken refused a change.

"Beware!" Daisy warned, "I think this may be the beginning of Jane asserting herself to make you disappear from Andy's life."

Jane had moved back into the same housing co-op that Ken and Jane had lived in years before; the same housing co-op that Daisy moved out of, supposedly to please Jane. Regrets for not defending her home were significant under the circumstances. Daisy was reminded of the psychic's advice to hold onto her home and to not give it up regardless of outside forces. She remembered the dream about being attacked by a vicious dog with long red hair.

When Daisy was told of Jane's move into the co-op, she said to Ken, "I thought Jane said False Creek was not suitable for her precious child. It's almost impossible to get into that co-op. They have a closed wait list. She must have had someone pull strings, just like the letter I received from the board that she knew about in advance of it being mailed."

Ken was at a loss for an explanation. "I'm sorry, Daisy. I feel responsible for you losing your home."

"I don't blame you. Remember, you thought she was one kind of person but after marriage you found her to be a different person. She's deceptive. This letter is proof that she can never be trusted. The more I see, the more I believe your life was in extreme danger when living with her. I see that you could never be sure of what she was up to behind your back. I wonder how we will ever know if she has a life insurance policy on you even if you don't know about it. I am now more worried about you than ever before. I want her know you have no life insurance."

HARASSMENT FOLLOWED that letter in the form of a torrential flood of Affidavits written by Jane and signed by the lawyer she shared an office and letterhead with. The papers arrived sometimes daily, sometimes weekly, and usually on Friday after 4 p.m. It soon became obvious that this was intimidation tactics so that Ken and Daisy's weekends were taken up primarily by anxious worries and in turn writing Affidavits to answer outlandish twists of imagination of an ex-wife. To think of Jane's writings as an unhealthy imagination was the only way Ken and Daisy could make sense of her writings because her written reality did not make any sense in the world of facts Ken and Daisy knew.

On the surface Jane's focus looked like it was to get money but it also appeared that the subject of money was simply a means for another agenda, and that was to insult and hurt Ken in the public domain.

Ken and Daisy still believed that a Judge would see through the sham and set things right.

Daisy tried to put a perspective on the situation by telling Ken, "It is like we are being sent repulsive evil gifts from Pandora's box... or jar. As the myth goes, we are being sent the most horrible illnesses of this world in these messages from the dark side."

Ken said, "I know what you mean."

"And remember in the myth, I think the husband of Pandora was warned that she wasn't what he thought she was, but he married her anyway. And a male gave her the jar of the world ills but even though she was warned that opening the jar would cause her marriage to fail, she opened it anyway and released the ills into the world. The parallel to that myth is uncanny."

THEN THE UNFOLDING farce took a sinister turn.

They had tried to hire their next-door neighbor as their lawyer. He was someone Daisy had known for many years under different circumstances, long before he became a lawyer and head of his own firm, but because they both lacked sufficient funds to pay top legal fees, he quickly offered another young man working in his office.

As usual, on Friday just before offices closed for the weekend, they received word that another Affidavit arrived. They trekked several blocks to pick it up. As they opened the door to his tiny office, it was obvious that the young lawyer was stiff with fear, his face drained of blood as he listened to someone on the telephone. He did not look up from his desk.

They took chairs and waited, not realizing his fear had anything to do with them.

He slowly hung up the telephone and looked at Ken. "That was Bruce Katz, Jane's lawyer. He just told me he wants you in jail or out of the country."

Ken was shocked as the threat sunk in.

Daisy jumped in, irate, "But Ken didn't do anything wrong!"

The lawyer face was still white. All he would answer was, "Never the less, that's what he is fighting for."

Daisy was determined to make him understand. "I believe they want to cause Ken to die! Jane knows Ken has been ill! She knows he had a damaged heart when he lived with her. Ken has no life insurance policy so there is no insurance money for her to collect if he dies. I want her to know that! I want you to tell her that!

Ken has looked after Andy full time plus paid some maintenance for the bankruptcy period and he has paid all after-school childcare as Jane asked him to do. And she does this? She had better not have taken out an insurance policy on Ken's life! Is there any way to find out if she has?"

Daisy had hoped that a fire could be lit under his behind but the lawyer was unresponsive. He was clearly disturbed and out of his depth. Angry and frustrated, Daisy wanted to lash out but there was no way to lash out, especially at a young lawyer who she surmised saw his own career threatened by an older lawyer.

"Did you hear me?" Daisy continued. "There is no insurance policy! Can you let her know that? The only thing Ken ever did wrong in my view was that he relied on her legal advice to lead him down the garden path to get him here. He treated her like a needy child and answered her every whimper. He gave Jane all the assets and continued to give her more. The motive has to be vengeance! There is no other reasonable reason for all this. Ken has always responded to give Jane what she asked for... Always! Katz and Jane share a letterhead but she's doing this in her married name, not her lawyer name on their letterhead. What does that mean?"

There was still no response as the lawyer's head hung, nearly touching his paper in front of him on the desk, not raising his eyes to look at either Ken or Daisy.

Ken was more composed and asked, "What should I do?"

The lawyer remained vacant, shaking his head.

Ken repeated himself, "What should I do? Should I be paying more maintenance while we are going through court?"

The lawyer made his second clear statement in this meeting, "No. Wait for an amount of maintenance to be settled by the Judge. You are already paying for childcare and other expenses. That should be sufficient for now."

ON THE WALK HOME across the green park that separated the lawyer's office from the street they lived on, they carried the nasty late Friday Affidavit. It was a neighborhood park with a Community Centre and indoor skating rink on one end, and a park where Daisy and her children had come in years past to skate or attend community festivals because they had lived in this Kitsilano neighborhood before False Creek. If she looked up, she could remember the happy faces of her small children over there.

Ken's sadness was palpable. He was trying to find reason to defend the mother of his child – and the child within the mother. "I'm sure Katz is putting Jane up to this. I can't believe she would do this."

Daisy did not want to hurt him more but he had to stop defending Jane once and for all. "Ken, I wish you would just get it through your head that it is her! She signs those outrageous Affidavits. She is a lawyer and knows how to read. She even goes so far as to say in one of her Affidavits that she should be believed because she is an 'Officer of the Courts' and then she continues to fabricate stories that you have been a deadbeat dad even though you have witnesses to that not being true. I notice that she never brings up what you did for her in the divorce and after; and that she is a lawyer because you paid her way through school and even helped her get through articling after the divorce. I mean all the money and assets she got and you got nothing and you still cared for Andy while she did her own thing. She's trying to lead everyone to believe that you ran away, leaving her destitute. I just hope a Judge catches her up on perjury to teach her a lesson. After all, there are separation and divorce documents that tell a story. I think she should be punished for lying to the courts because, as a lawyer, she knows better. I think she should go to jail. What worries me is that she seems to know she can get away with it and that worries me about our judicial system. Otherwise I can't imagine why she would take such chances with her career and her life. ...Ken, you need to stop finding reasons to make excuses for everything she does. She is a grown woman, not a child. She is a lawyer. I am sure she knows exactly what she can get away with. She is not out to lunch."

Ken was clearly hurt beyond measure by this day's revelations. He had left the marriage for reasons he felt were life threatening, but at times when things seemed peaceful between Jane and himself, he had suffered terrible remorse over breaking his marriage vows. Now he had become the focus of treachery brought out into the open and made public. He had to accept the fact that fears for his life that caused him to leave his marriage were well founded.

Walking beside Ken, Daisy could feel his overwhelming pain. Real fear for Ken's life was uppermost in her mind. It was a known fact that Ken was vulnerable with a weakened heart – in fact, abnormal – and because there was a longstanding medical record, Jane knew. This very fact convinced Daisy that Jane's motive was in trying to get rid of Ken by way of a heart attack and that the threat from Katz to get Ken out of the country or in jail was to make sure that if Ken did not die first, then he would be taken out of his son's life another way. Jane and Katz were now out in the open with full force to completely destroy Ken one way or another.

Daisy thought about how the sound of his heart continued to frighten her. And how the gushing sound and uneven heartbeats like she had never heard before in a living person was obviously an abnormal heart. Ken was in trouble with his heart and it had not started the day Daisy entered his life. His blood pressure was explosively high even though he had been under a physician's care and on allopathic medication that was supposed to correct it, but only caused extreme side effects on top of not making any correction to a damaged heart. He had a ticking bomb in his chest.

It had been with sadness that Ken had explained to Daisy the reasons he left the marriage to Jane, and he had described his fear of Jane – real palpable fear that she would kill him or herself and set it up so that he would be blamed for her murder. With each outlandish affidavit written by Jane, Daisy was reminded of Ken's fears for his life and now they had become hers.

Daisy remembered her first instinct about Jane – just an intuition – was that Jane would try to cause Ken to die with emotional abuse. Regardless of his sorrows about leaving his marriage, Daisy had been secretly convinced that she was saving Ken's life by offering him another life – a safe haven with her family. This whole scenario had started in False Creek when Ken and Jane had first walked by as Daisy was watering her flowers. Daisy had an odd feeling about the seemingly sullen red-haired woman and asked her children what they knew about her. The response from them was that the woman was someone they would rather stay away from. Then at Christmas, Daisy had knocked on their door to collect funds for gifts for co-op children and Jane answered. Daisy had been unprepared for what she perceived as a dark void surrounding the woman in the doorway. No other home in one hundred and sixty-seven gave her that kind of feeling. The experience left a lingering fear for Ken. That same worry for Ken occasionally surfaced in the years following and peaked again when she heard that phone call between Ken and his wife in his office. The day Daisy dared to profess her love to Ken and then walked away was accompanied by hope for his future but also by a worrisome feeling that she was abandoning him.

Jane's present blatant public display of viciousness toward Ken emphasized the truth of the reasons why Ken had to leave Jane and their marriage to save his life. It was all crystal clear.

Daisy was absolutely convinced Ken's ex-wife had a plan that was to cause Ken to die of natural causes. Daisy was fearful that Ken would have a heart attack over these latest threats and intimidation tactics. She knew that the thought of going to jail is very frightening for any Psychiatrist who would have to defend himself against inmates who are possibly predisposed to getting even with the Forensic Psychiatrists who may have helped to put them or keep them in jail. The alternative of leaving the country would mean leaving all three of his sons and the newly adopted family. Even though, he had dreamed of going back to Vermont, Ken would not run away.

Daisy suggested, "Ken, all we have to do is think of the most awful thing Jane can think of to do next and we will be able to anticipate and be ahead of her in her game."

Ken said he could not go there.

Daisy was on her own in thinking along that line and acknowledged it was not in keeping with Buddhist thinking. But what would Jane's next step be?

She said, "I have to change that statement. I think that would be wrong. I was at the Abbotsford air show one year. As I was watching a plane leave the ground, I saw it in flames, crash landing. I saw it before it happened and then it happened right there in front of everyone. For years I struggled with whether or not I caused the crash with my thoughts or had I just been clairvoyant and seen what was about to happen before it happened."

"Knowing you, I don't believe you caused it." Ken consoled Daisy, "In case you are blaming yourself for Jane's bad behavior, don't. I left the marriage because of her behavior. Not yours. You did not cause the marriage break-up. I would never have left her if she had been treating me differently. I was hoping you could help me with my children and mend my damaged heart. That was a lot to ask of you considering the trouble I was in."

Daisy tried another tactic. She elicited a half-hearted agreement from Ken that in future he would simply be careful about any friendly gesture from Jane that could be a trap. Even that, was only partly agreed to because as Daisy knew only too well, Ken would always keep the door open to the mother of his son and take his chances in hopes of coming to a truce and raising their child together in harmony – just as he did on the Christmas morning when Jane offered him a drink and a talk.

Warning Ken, Daisy said, "Considering the pattern being established by Jane, you must expect that she will suddenly take Andy away entirely from you prior to the big court battle because she will want to be portrayed as the best parent, and you portrayed as though you do nothing."

Ken responded, "I will have to rely on my son being determined to see me."

"Yes, he is old enough to demand time with you if that should happen."

Ken was wistful. "On the other hand, he tries so hard to be part of his mother's life that he will do anything to get there."

"Do you think he would betray you?"

"Maybe. She does play the push-pull game with him. It makes her more enticing. In some ways no different than she did with me in marriage."

"And after, too."

"Yes, I know. ...She pushes him away and he talks about the treats of sleeping with her. I think he is a little too old to be sleeping with her for a treat."

Ken told Daisy that when he had gone to Jane's house to be with Andy on occasion when invited, he continually had to see a picture on the refrigerator in which Jane was sitting on Katz' knee.

Daisy expressed herself. "God! I can't understand why any self-respecting woman would sit on his knee. There are other lawyers to choose from in this town. Why would she pick someone like him? It must be a match! And Andy is being taught that Katz is his friend while Katz is destroying Andy's father! The question is, has Jane been lying to Katz and he doesn't know the truth or is he manipulating lies with her. I'd be willing to bet that the photo on the fridge is there for you to see in the hope of hurting you, just like she flaunted dating your oldest son in your face... and for Andy to know she likes Katz more than you, which will cause major conflict in Andy."

KEN AND DAISY BELIEVED that they had to answer each and every statement in Jane's Affidavits because they believed that every Affidavit would end up in front of a Judge who would then read every important word. They wrote truthful Affidavits while believing that telling a lie in an Affidavit is against the law and punishable in a court of law by a jail term.

The weeks and months were punctuated by court appearances where nothing seemed to get done. Nasty, insulting Affidavits kept arriving.

A focus of accusations appeared to be that Ken had been hiding money with Daisy regardless that his income had been scrutinized by a Trustee and Social Services, and regardless that Ken had hired the nanny Janet to work in his office only two years after the divorce and following her, he hired his oldest son Stephen to manage his office and money affairs during the many months before bankruptcy. And prior to that, it was all in public court documents that in divorce, Ken had given all marital assets to Jane and kept the debts of the marriage for himself. Between his illness and the people looking after his finances, Ken had no way, no time, and no reason to hide money with Daisy. Furthermore, Daisy was extremely broke and had no money or assets except old furniture after breaking her back and having had time out of work. She had also been a single working parent and had collected no child maintenance from ex's to help her. She had used up her retirement savings plan and the money paid back from her co-op housing years before. She had no money stashed anywhere on earth.

LIFE DID NOT start and stop with Jane Anderson even though she was like a mosquito buzzing around, trying to sting with a constancy that lead Daisy to question whether the woman had anything going on in her brain except the desire to cause harm.

During this time, life at home was busy with other life and death matters; Daisy's children had been having babies. Both Daisy and Ken were involved in the births.

In a lucid dream Daisy saw a woman in labor on an island. In the dream, the umbilical cord was too short for the baby to descend normally.

The following day, Daisy burned candles and was in constant prayerful meditation, doing midwifery by psychic means this time. The baby descended and was born normally, attended by a midwife on the island. Through the midwifery grapevine, Daisy then heard about the birth.

The baby had a severe congenital heart malformation, which is why there was a malformed cord. At ten months of age he needed open-heart surgery in Toronto because no one in Vancouver could do it at the time. A request arrived for this family to leave their older son, the three – soon to be four-year-old child to stay with Ken and Daisy for the coming weeks.

Heart surgeries and transplants were in the experimental stage in the mid 1980s. A heart of a baboon was being experimented with and transplanted into a human child. Various man-made apparatus were experimented with. Any heart surgery done was considered successful if the patient lived even a few hours or a few months.

Daisy and her sister raised funds through the Lions Club of Regina for the family to travel and stay in a Toronto hotel. The child left behind clung desperately to both Daisy and Ken as his lifeline, but he suffered extreme nightmares about his baby brother being cut open.

The surgery in Toronto, considered successful was followed by failure and was repeated. Then there was the treatment plan to keep the baby alive and it ran into trouble.

While the mother was constantly with her baby, her husband, who was a stepfather to the older boy, lost touch with reality. He was convinced the son left behind in Vancouver, who just had a fourth birthday, should travel by himself in an airplane across the country to Toronto to join them. He informed the child by telephone that he must do this. The child panicked with fear. His face turned white as blood drained, leaving blotches of red with blue eyes turning into wide horrified saucers.

Daisy took the telephone and offered to fly with the child. The stepfather freaked out, insisting his son make the trip by himself because, "What will we do with you here?"

Daisy offered to get on a return flight and come right back. In a fury, the stepfather rejected the offer. He repeated the demand to his child on subsequent phone calls.

The child reacted by ripping arms and legs off dolls. On a shopping trip to the supermarket, the child got hold of a plastic produce bag and pulled it tightly over his head in a smothering gesture. Daisy saw the face of a wildly disturbed child smiling at her out of the bag. She rescued him.

The Robson Square outdoor skating rink had been kept open regardless of the warm Spring weather, extending its season because of Daisy's personal plea to the manager. She had explained the circumstances of the boy's emotional turmoil and that she had been teaching the child to skate on that rink. But on the way home from one of the evening skating sessions, he wailed loudly; his heartbreaking sobs echoed through the buses and dark streets so loudly that some people opened doors to see what was going on.

The stepfather persisted through continual angry phone calls. He sent his own parents to take the child out for a few hours and the frightened child fought going with them. The boy refused to get dressed. He hid under the bed. He locked the door when they knocked. The father's father believed it would go better if the boy was delivered to him on Granville Island.

The child reluctantly went onto the little sea ferry with his step-grandfather. As soon as the boat left the wharf, the wails began. He wailed, calling for Daisy. The water carried his cries back to Ken and Daisy on the dock. The child's heartbroken call could be heard echoing over and over across great distance as he crossed the inlet. The cries would become ingrained on Ken and Daisy forever. They left for home on their bicycles with an empty bike trailer. No sooner did they get home than the child was delivered back to them by the grandfather, who made a hasty retreat.

The four-year-old was in trouble and the stepfather was off the wall. The baby in Toronto was relapsing regularly.

Behind the scenes, the pediatrician side of Ken had been on the telephone daily with the medical team in Toronto. After the several severe setbacks and near failures, Ken was convinced that there was a question about the follow-up treatment. Enough was enough! Ken consulted with Children's Hospital medical team in Vancouver and he then spearheaded the airvac to bring the baby and parents back to Vancouver.

Bringing the family home solved a problem. The baby was quickly stabilized. But the stepfather, now back home and reconnecting with the four-year-old boy continued to agitate and cause trouble.

The mother phoned to say her husband and son needed to come to the house for a bath. Daisy timed their travel from Children's Hospital and prepared a bath for the child, placing rubber ducks in the tub so that he could jump right in – assuming that the father would have a shower after the child's bath.

They arrived. When the stepfather saw the tub with water ready for the boy, he freaked, angrily yelling so loud that the boy hid behind Daisy in fear. He insisted his son must shower with him or not at all. The child was crying and shaking with terror. The stepfather reached around Daisy and grabbed the boy roughly by the ear. Leading the boy by the ear, he shoved the boy to the front door and threw him outside onto the porch, shutting and locking door. Outside, the boy cried a kind of sickly wail that was nothing like Daisy had ever heard before and would never forget. Now the terrible secret of this child's life was out in the open.

Daisy went out to be with the child on the porch. The stepfather followed in a rage and made loud insults and threats for the neighbors to hear. It was a nightmare for the boy again hiding behind Daisy.

Meanwhile, Ken got on the phone and made a crisis referral to the psychiatric team at Children's Hospital where the baby was now a resident and where this whole family would hopefully be looked after.

News of the referral angered the stepfather even more. He vowed revenge.

In a next minute, two-faced Jekyll and Hyde got on the phone to his wife in hospital and was as sweet as pie, twisting the story so that his wife had no idea why a referral to the psychiatric unit was made, except that any trouble was Daisy's fault. She got Daisy on the phone and blamed her for upsetting her husband. The man clearly had two faces.

IT WAS NOW in the hands of the psychiatrist at the hospital. Ken hoped that the small boy would gain protection from abuse at the hospital where the family was going to be for some time to come.

Daisy was called to the hospital and was shocked to find herself the butt of what the child psychiatrist called an inquiry. The stepfather was deflecting attention away from his abuse of the child by turning the table and blaming Daisy as being the abuser. The stepfather had done such a good job of protecting himself and deflecting onto Daisy that her final statement to the psychiatrist was that she had better take care of the child, to which she added, "I would turn that father over to the SPCA. Actually most animals are better behaved."

At that statement, the psychiatrist who let it be known that she was determined to believe the father, lost her cool manifestation of a person in charge. The woman's face gave her away. She was used to being in charge but she had met Daisy and Daisy was not frightened of her or about to take her crap. The woman looked stunned as Daisy stood up and walked out the door.

Walking away from the hospital, Daisy thought she had blundered by making such a stupid remark. After all, she was a health care worker herself. Silent laughter bubbled up inside her anyway. But she could not help wondering why that stupid woman could be so blind when it was Ken who made the referral.

[In future: This man was protected for years by this child psychiatrist. The couple did eventually divorce. Reason? Husband and stepfather abused his wife and son, leaving years of emotional scars on the son for him work through. Daisy would find herself sitting beside the man's mother in one of Ken's discussion groups at the church. The woman apologized to Daisy for having experienced her son's behavior.]

33

The Joke's On Us:
Earth Is Our Only Home!

[*Written by Ken Schramm, September 15, 1988*]

Why are human ecologists like anesthesiologists? Both are professionals half awake tending patients half asleep. Justice Tuchman-Matthews, ecologist and strategic planner, Washington, D.C., told Bill Moyers' Tuesday night prime time public television viewers that human kind is waking up to realize Earth is our only home. We are waking up because we can see the greenhouse effect on climate: record-breaking temperatures, drought, hurricanes, floods, tornadoes. What we can't see, what scientists were surprised to find because we were not looking, is a continent-size hole in the ozone layer over America. These changes have accumulated like the effects of cigarette smoking over the past twenty to thirty years. In the next generation, the time for historian Barbara Tuchman's granddaughter to come to university, changes will come much more quickly, dramatically, and unpredictably. Invisible gaseous residues of fossil fuel burning from industrial, airplane, and automobile motor emissions will accumulate more rapidly, trapping reflected solar heat within our home atmosphere. On present projections of automobile industry sales by 2000 A.D., Earth will heat up 2-3 degrees Centigrade causing polar icecaps to melt, flooding coastal cities while temperate zones become tropical drought areas. In 75 years the world could be uninhabitable. Her worst news is that catastrophes will come suddenly, unpredictably without warning because scientists are just beginning to be able to study this relatively new phenomena compounded by fluorocarbon omissions which destroy ozone. The good news is that like Finnegan, Northern

Hemispheric Man is waking to discover Earth is our only home. Dr. Tuchman-Mathews is optimistic that North Americans and Russians can make the conversion to more fuel-efficient engines of transport and industry before the End of the World. The difficult problem is educating the educators, leaders, and general public to be more energy efficient and responsible. This is not a simple solution to a complex family of environmental problems...

* * *

[ks notebooks]

"...Ecology derives its root meaning from the Greek **eikos** for household or home and **logos** for word, truth or study: literally the study of the home..."

"...What professional and personal forces provoke or prevent us from speaking and teaching honestly and truthfully with others in our daily lives in our "free country"? Within such truthful discussion in "places of refuge" I hope we develop the academic community..."

"...We can continue to work for change that will require at least 3 generations or 100 years. The past 100 years were devoted to protecting interests in petroleum and other fossil fuels of industrial society. For the next 100 years we need to recover from the toxic effects of fossil fuel pollution while building on solar, wind, organic gardening, and human powers..."

"...Healing, making us whole again, requires constant rebuilding of communities as safe places for growing fully human beings who can make our living and dying into sacred play so that our grandchildren will have a future..."

EXCERPT FROM PAPER: **To Make Things Better: Community Development for Healthy Housing and Home Care. A Research Prospectus, July 1, 1988, by Ken Schramm, M.D.**

...Making things better for our children and grandchildren is an essential human need often disregarded in the name of progress...

...Anxiety interferes with exchanges of love. Anxiety reflects the chaos of an untrustworthy universe, incompletely ordered and differentiated by our kind. Mothers and fathers as caretakers need to live in a world which can be relied upon, or we cannot know and meet the real needs of our children. The development of one single individual presupposes the work of many more who have ordered and are maintaining a universe of discourse as a living body able to transform humans into divinities, mortals into immortal ghosts. Without the human power necessary for immortality, we are paralyzed by our fears of death. Alienation and anxiety are inseparably linked. The distance experienced between people mirrors our emotional communication in the times we lived together. One is hungry and is fed – the world is living, good, and reliable. One is hungry and is not fed – the world is predictably hateful and evil. One is hungry and is randomly beaten or fed – the world is predictably unreliable and unjust. One wants to be loved and is not – our skin is the wrong color, or gender is wrong, our sexual body taboo, we have no right to be alive as we are. Mother Earth, parent as caretaker, is the world, present or absent, reliable or unreliable, just or unjust, touchable or untouchable, systemic rhythms of self, other, and world development together in anxiety, pain, pleasure, and repression. Relationships among these communicated exchanges as gifts are reflected in the familiar, conceptual, and bodily skills of individuals who live in worlds, ordered, made and found by nature-cultures, human-machines, body-minds, and kind-their kinds. ...

34

Affidavits

CHRISTMAS EVE, DECEMBER 24th, 1988 was the last day Ken was allowed to see his son Andy. A few days later and without prior notice, Jane cleaned out Ken's entire bank account containing the student loan that had just been deposited.

Ken questioned his whole married relationship with Jane Anderson. 'Sleeping with the enemy' took on a clear-cut meaning – a reminder of his reasons for leaving her. Fear for his son's wellbeing became a focus because Jane and her friends were now raising him in secrecy.

BELIEVING IN THE true meaning of writing an Affidavit – that it must be a true, sworn statement signed by the declarant and witnessed by a qualified person for use in court, and that making a false statement must be considered perjury with consequences of criminal charges that could be large fines and a jail term, Ken wrote and continued answering truthfully to allegations and insults that Jane (Schramm) Anderson made in her Affidavits. His ex-wife's versions of past and present events had no resemblance to events in Ken's world, nor did they to witnesses not influenced by Jane. Ken believed a Judge would read all his answers and put some common sense to it all. His biggest hope was that a Judge would do what he did in his medical practice and that was to care for the child and help parents parent their child together regardless of their differences.

IT WAS NOW 1989. Two years had passed since that morning when bankruptcy ended. Nothing had a conclusion after two years of Affidavits and court appearances. It appeared that the time had been used to simply harass Ken and make him as uncomfortable as possible.

Getting no help from his lawyer, Ken had been on the telephone each morning trying to get a court counselor to help with re-establishing some communication with his son. He sought help from a government office connected to the court system where women sufficiently blocked him. The more he was blocked and grew frustrated, the more the women seemed determined. He experienced first-hand the same fate as other men who, over the years, had been referred by Ken to various government offices for help and would come back saying they got no support from the women in those offices, and in fact discovered it was a woman's world when it came to their children.

FEBRUARY 2ⁿᵈ, 1989, Ken wrote a list and briefs for his lawyer:

- *Removal of the charge of contempt of Court for non-payment of maintenance against me;*
- *Variation of Separation Agreement of April 1, 1982 to allow me: regular access at my home to my son Alexander Kehnroth Anderson-Schramm (Andy) every Wednesday, Friday, and Sunday, overnight as needed, and every other weekend from Friday to Monday when I will bring Andy to school;*
- *respect for my continuing rights and responsibilities as joint guardian and caretaker of Andy since his birth so that I can know where he is at any time of the day or week and therefore, I am able to participate in decisions: about his health, where he lives and goes to school or child care, especially respecting my right to communicate directly with him;*
- *variation of paragraph 8, page 6 to permit resolution of access and maintenance disagreement, when there is a change in circumstances, by arbitration before the Court Registrar or mediation with a family court counselor;*
- *variation of regular monthly maintenance payments to zero beginning immediately because I will be caring for Andy on a half time to full time basis and the costs for doing this are equivalent to those of full-time custody;*

- forgiveness of arrears maintenance from 1985 to present because during this period I cared for Andy regularly half to full-time despite my illness which necessitated: my retiring in 1985 from full-time medical practice, supporting Andy and me in 1985-87 by GAIN, resulting in bankruptcy due to illness; and my half to full-time care of Andy including his day care fees from May 1987 – December 1988;

- Return funds garnished unnecessarily from my account.

BRIEF: *I, Kehnroth Schramm, of [address], am a single parent and full-time student in Community and Regional Planning at U.B.C., specializing in emergency preparedness planning. Since May 1987, after discharge from bankruptcy due to illness, I have provided for myself and my son, Alexander Kehnroth Schramm, solely from funds obtained from student loans and bursaries. I made the decision to make a career change from primary care physician to researcher, writer, and consultant in community health on the basis of recommendations in 1985 from my family physician [name], and from professor [name] based on my work in his 1986 graduate seminar in History of Science and Technology. Since my illness and retirement from medical practice, my professional life insurance policy lapsed because I could not pay the premiums. At the time of stopping my practice in 1985, I deregistered an RRSP [retirement savings plan] which I paid to Jane Anderson in lieu of maintenance. I do not now have any insurance on my life because I cannot afford the premium required of any physician with a history of high blood pressure. I also do not have any malpractice insurance because I do not need it as a professionally inactive physician. As my health has gradually improved, I have responded to the requests of former clients and their friends for family health consultations on a totally different basis than I had done before bankruptcy. I take limited responsibility as a consultant because I am teaching medical self care with families who want to take responsibility for their own health, the education of their children, and care for their pregnant, sick, or dying members. I could not do this consulting work without the help of Daisy Heisler who has special training and skills in art, music, conflict resolution,* *negotiation, and mediation. Ms. Heisler manages the office along with her other business responsibilities. I do not need nor do I take any income from this work. In January, I had to pay the business rent and expenses out of my student loans because the MSP payments were delayed. My bank statements, reviewed by my lawyer [name], are the basis for financial statements in the appendix which show clearly that I am living at a level of income less than that I had while I was an undischarged bankrupt, and that I am going into debt for my student loans...*

BRIEF*: see attempt July 18, 1985 to vary maintenance order. When I was accepted for GAIN (guaranteed annual income for need), I understood (explained by a social worker) that any person is entitled to receive GAIN and maintain a business so long as there are no assets and no net income. When I applied for bankruptcy after a year of GAIN, I understood that my financial affairs were monitored by a trustee, that any creditor, including my ex-wife had a right to meet with the trustee and to insist on limiting my discharge from bankruptcy so that she could be sure I was meeting my responsibilities as a bankrupt. So far as I know, no complaint about my behavior was made about my very limited work as a physician preceding and during the period of bankruptcy. My gross income, like that of all physicians paid by MSP of BC, is published yearly. I had no assets during, nor following bankruptcy and I have no new or hidden assets now, nor prospects for any future assets. The life style changes I have made in managing my life stresses do not automatically protect my health. I have regained my health sufficiently to continue to care for my son Andy regularly, providing for his emotional needs, day care, food, shelter and clothing, as I have since his birth, especially during the frequent periods when my ex-wife has been ill or recovering from surgery. My health permits me to work part-time (less than 12 hours per week) as a consultant in child, family, personal and community health with the help of other people and to be a full-time graduate student applying for Ph.D. in community and regional planning before I am 60 years old in Nov.'92. I do not expect to find a salaried job. I will have to compete, as a consultant in child, family, personal and community health, for contracts to work as a member of a* *planning team assisting families and planners to prepare for emergencies such as earthquakes and other health risks. This career change, begun when I was totally unable to work but able to care for my son Alexander Kehnroth (Andy) Schramm, provides the best chance I have to continue to meet my responsibilities as his parent and joint guardian. Toward that end I request regular access to Andy at my home... I believe an effective method of mediating or negotiating problems or differences between his mother and me regarding his care, education, and support, such as arbitration by the Court Registrar, is urgently needed. I request that arrears in maintenance should be forgiven because of my bankruptcy due to illness and my care of Andy in lieu of maintenance, as well as my regular and generous maintenance payments to Jane Anderson prior to my bankruptcy. I request that the amount of monthly maintenance be set at $100 because of my circumstances as a student and my willingness and ability to care for his needs on a half to full time basis.*

* * *

KEN'S AFFIDAVITS showed his complete bewilderment at the accusations used against him considering his complete generosity in the Separation and Divorce, and following in the years when he paid many thousands of dollars in excess of the maintenance agreement and in time spent caring for both his ex-wife and his son Andy. Even though Ken had been frightened enough of Jane to leave the marriage and had believed wholeheartedly that she wanted him gone, he found it difficult to believe Jane could be devoted to vengeance against him. Believing that some sense of justice and honesty would somehow be recognized and prevail, Ken continued trying to explain and provide proof of his situation under oath.

SINCE THE THREATENING phone call from Bruce Katz, Ken's lawyer ceased to be helpful to Ken and Daisy in writing Affidavits. He was working for small fees, so they chocked his lack of help and saving time up to that. They brought typed pages to the lawyer, who glanced at them and then registered the as-is Affidavits with the British Columbia Supreme Court.

AFFIDAVIT REGISTERED FEBRUARY 7, 1989, in answer to the many Affidavits received late on Fridays, Ken wrote:

No. D141314 VANCOUVER REGISTRY
IN THE SUPREME COURT OF BRITISH COLUMBIA
BETWEEN:
CAROL JANE SCHRAMM   PETITIONER
AND:
KEHNROTH SCHRAMM   RESPONDENT

I, KEHNROTH SCHRAMM, graduate student and professionally inactive physician, of [address] MAKE OATH AND SAY AS FOLLOWS:

1. That I swear this Affidavit in response to the Affidavit of Carol Jane Schramm, now Jane Anderson, sworn the 23rd of January 1989, and filed in support of her application to be heard by this court on the 7th Day of February, 1989.

2. That I am the Respondent herein and as such have personal knowledge of the facts and matters hereinafter deposed to, save and except where stated to be made upon information and belief, and where so stated I verily believe the same to be true.

3. That the Petitioner and I were married in Vancouver British Columbia on the 7th day of February, 1972.

4. That there is one child born of the marriage, namely ALEXANDER KEHNROTH SCHRAMM, known as Andy, born [date].

5. That on or about May 13, 1981, the Petitioner and I separated. At that time I left the matrimonial home and we have neither resided nor cohabited together since that date.

7. That a Judgment by way of Decree Nisi was pronounced by the Honorable Mr. Justice Andrews on the 7th day of June, 1982 and entered on the 9th day of July, 1982. This Judgment incorporated the aforementioned terms, namely, that the Petitioner have custody of the child, that I would have reasonable access to the child, that the Petitioner and I retain joint guardianship of the estate of the child, and that I pay $500.00 per month for the child of the marriage commencing July 1st, 1982 and continuing thereafter until the child is no longer a child of the marriage as defined in the Divorce Act of Canada.

8. That since that date of the Order until August 1985, I have complied with the child support payment provision and, in fact during the 1983 calendar year voluntarily paid the Petitioner $1,000.00 per month in Child Support to assist the Petitioner during her period of unemployment. In the calendar year of 1984, I paid the Petitioner $600.00 per month in Child Support and that this monthly sum continued until August 1985.

9. That in September 1984 the Petitioner secured a full-time position as a lawyer with the law firm of Mulholland and Webster, of [address], at a salary unknown to me.

10. That after a year of treatment for a work-stress related hypertensive illness, which had incapacitated me from November 1983 through to February 1984, I learned in September of 1984 that my blood pressure was dangerously high. My family physician [name], recommended that I stop working entirely or at least drastically reduce my workload for one to three years to avoid a stroke or heart attack or both.

11. That I followed my doctor's advice while continuing a reduced workload until May 1985 when I reluctantly gave up my office as a physician. At the age of 53 years, after twenty-seven years of work as a physician and teacher, I retired to do research, teach and write.

12. That due to my health and financial problems I was unable to pay the Petitioner child support from September 1985 until May 1987. The Petitioner was aware of my financial circumstances at the time and noted it in her Affidavit of January 23rd, 1989.

13. That in lieu of the child support payments I assumed increasing responsibility for the personal care of our child Andy. Since September 1984 until April 1987, I cared for the child from 8:30 am to 7:30 pm, Monday to Thursday, and from 8:30 am Friday until noon on Saturday. Overnight stays were negotiated without difficulty in addition to this schedule. In addition I cared for Andy full time when the Petitioner was ill or in hospital. Attached as Exhibit "A" to this my Affidavit is the Petitioner's written confirmation of this schedule of shared responsibility dated August 2nd, 1985.

14. That on or about May 31, 1985, I de-registered an R.R.S.P. valued at approximately $1,800.00 net, and shortly thereafter paid this amount directly to the Petitioner as child support for the months of June, July and August 1985. I explained to the Petitioner the source of the funds and that they would be the only support monies available for an undetermined time because of my impending bankruptcy.

15. That a Modification to the Separation Agreement of April 1ˢᵗ, 1982, was not signed by me, upon advice by my legal counsel at the time, due to my impending bankruptcy and lack of provision in the Modified Agreement regarding arrears. The Modification Agreement was drafted by the Petitioner and was not in accordance with all my requested terms.

16. That on or about the 18ᵗʰ of July 1985, I applied, without counsel, to vary the order of Mr. Justice Andrews, entered the 9ᵗʰ day July 1985. Attached hereto as Exhibit "B" to this my Affidavit is the Appointment to vary the order before the Supreme Court of British Columbia.

17. That my attempt to vary the maintenance provision of the order was blocked by counsel for the Petitioner. Due to financial reasons I was unable to retain legal counsel to proceed with further actions to vary the maintenance order.

18. That I believed and assumed that in view of my generous maintenance payments during the years of 1983, 1984 and part of 1985, and my increased responsibility for the care of the child in lieu of support payment, the Petitioner and I would negotiate Andy's maintenance in good faith.

19. That due to my ill health and increased debt load, primarily to Revenue Canada, I was advised by my accountant [name] to apply for personal bankruptcy.

20. That due to my illness, my son from my first marriage, Stephen Schramm, handled my financial transactions during the latter half of 1985 in preparation for the bankruptcy.

21. That I have not filed income tax returns since filing for bankruptcy and have asked my accountant to prepare financial statement to rebut allegations made by Jane Anderson in her affidavit sworn the 23ʳᵈ day January, 1989.

22. That due to the garnishment, by the Petitioner, of my personal account at the Vancouver City Savings Credit Union, containing the latest Student Loan installment, on or about mid-January 1989, I have insufficient funds with which to pay my rent or living expenses.

23. That I have maintained my membership in the College of Physicians and Surgeons. At no time did I inform the Petitioner I had resigned from the College. That I did not resign from College of Physicians and Surgeons because it was my understanding and belief that retired Physicians could maintain practices which reflected their abilities and needs. It was also my understanding and belief that unless I continued to use my Medical Services Plan billing number, I would lose it with little chance of regaining it later.

24. That it is my understanding and belief that the British Columbia Medical Association dues structure defines a professionally inactive physician as one who is under the age of 65 and earns less than $40,000.00 per annum.

25. That I began a part-time consulting practice on or about April 1986. There was no net income from my consulting practice.

26. That in order to maintain my status as a professionally inactive physician and to maintain my qualifications for graduate school and subsequent student loans, I restricted my practice to less than twelve (12) hours per week. ...

27. That on or about the 9th day of July 1986, I voluntarily assigned myself into bankruptcy. Attached hereto as Exhibit "C" to this my Affidavit is the Notice to Creditors of my voluntary assignment.

28. That my ill health was not due to "serious psychological problems" as was misleadingly claimed by the Petitioner in her Affidavit of January 23rd, 1989, but due to physical illness and financial stresses of impending bankruptcy.

29. That on or about September 1986, with the permission of the professors, I attended history classes at the University of British Columbia. With the encouragement and sponsorship of Professor [name] of the University of British Columbia, I subsequently applied and was accepted in May 1987 to pursue the full time study of the history of science and the human sciences.

30. That I am currently a University of British Columbia full time graduate student in Community and Regional Planning.

31. That since May 1987, my personal income has consisted solely of Bursaries and Student Loans.

32. That on or about January 21, 1987, I was granted an absolute discharge of my bankruptcy. Attached hereto as Exhibit "D" to this my affidavit is the Notice to Creditors of my application for discharge.

33. That on or about June 1, 1987, our child Andy was enrolled in the University Hill Elementary School "After School Care Program". I paid for this daycare from monies obtained for this purpose through my Student Loans. Attached hereto as Exhibit "E" to this my Affidavit are copies of cancelled cheques totaling $2,324.75 in day care payment for the period June 1, 1987 to August 31, 1988.

34. That during this period, at no time did the Petitioner ask me to pay the maintenance arrears, in writing or otherwise, in addition to the day care payments which I made directly to the day care. I continued to care for Andy regularly on Wednesdays 1:30 pm to about 8 pm and on Sundays with overnight stays and longer periods of access when either the child or the Petitioner was ill.

35. That on or about September 1988, without consulting me as co-guardian, the Petitioner withdrew Andy from University Hill Elementary School "After School Care" and made private arrangements for his care. I advised the Petitioner at this time that I would pay $150.00 per month, commencing September 1, 1988, for the child's private after school care. Attached hereto as Exhibit "F" to this my Affidavit are three cancelled cheques in the amount of $150.00 each dated September 14, October 1, and November 1, 1988.

36. That in December 1988 I was only allowed access to Andy on two occasions and have been denied access since December 24, 1988.

37. That I do not have a common-law spouse. Since my separation and divorce from the Petitioner I have lived alone or at times with one or both of my older sons from a former marriage. For the past two years I have resided at [address] in separate accommodations with an adjoining room for my child, in a house managed by Daisy Heisler.

38. That I operate my health consulting practice from an office with a separate entrance also located at [address].

SWORN BEFORE ME at the City of
Vancouver in the Province of
British Columbia, this 7th day
of February, 1989.
[signed by lawyer]   [signed]***K. Schramm***
A Commissioner for taking Affidavits
Within the Province of British Columbia

* * *

THE WRITING WAS briefly interrupted. While it seemed that Jane was determined to be the centre of the universe, a tragedy happened. Granddaughter Maria and her mother Loraine waited at the rink for Maria's skating coach, Scott, one afternoon. Scott was the tall, good-natured young man who had hired Loraine to teach figure skating along with him. He had just bought a new tape player for music at the rink and was on his way north, having just crossed the Knight Street Bridge when at the end on the

Vancouver side of the bridge where many accidents had happened, a truck with wheels the size of his little white car crossed the centre line and drove over his car. Scott was crushed.

Everyone was in shock and grief for the young man who seemed too good for this world. Ken and Daisy took time to visit with Scott's family along with Maria and her family.

Then it was back to writing. Ken and Daisy were seated side by side at the long desk in their office. She started to write when she became aware of Scott's strong presence in the room. He was visiting people, wanting to make his continuing life on the other side known. Daisy was aware. She told him to come back later because she really needed to concentrate on this affidavit and get it done. Scott faded away.

Scott never returned. Maybe there was no need to return because his survival was acknowledged, but sadly, Daisy had not followed her own rule of social behavior, even with spirits, that was to give Scott the time for whatever he needed to say. Regrettably, she had allowed Jane to be the centre of the universe.

* * *

AFFIDAVIT REGISTERED February 8TH, 1989
No. D141314 VANCOUVER REGISTRY
IN THE SUPREME COURT OF BRITISH COLUMBIA
BETWEEN:
CAROL JANE SCHRAMM   PETITIONER
AND
KEHNROTH SCHRAMM   RESPONDENT

I, DAISY HEISLER [address] MAKE OATH AND SAY AS FOLLOWS:

1. That I swear this Affidavit in response to the Affidavit of Carol Jane Schramm, now Jane Anderson, sworn the 23rd day of January, 1989, and filed in support of her application to be heard by this Court on the 8th day of February, 1989.

2. That I have known Kehnroth Schramm for twenty years, first meeting in Regina, Saskatchewan and then living as neighbours in the False Creek Housing Co-operative. When my family was experiencing problems, I asked Ken for professional help. We mutually terminated the therapy. We did not have an affair. I was not a patient of Ken's when he terminated his marriage to Jane or left her home. Ken left his wife and marriage and took with him no money or cheques. He called me as an old

friend and I offered him my home to stay in. That within months Ken obtained his own apartment and continued for many years to maintain his own apartment while supporting his sons which included his two older sons by his first marriage.

3. That I am a qualified Medical Office Assistant, with 35 years experience in secretarial and business management skills. I am trained in Conflict Resolution, Mediation, Negotiation, and also have training in Art Therapy, Family and Child Therapy. I have always had and do have independent income. That if I do not work with Ken in his medical practice, he would need to hire someone else or fold the practice just like any doctor with a medical practice.

4. That I am not Ken's common-law wife. Recently we have shared housing on a co-operative basis. We each maintain our private and separate bedrooms. Ken has a separate part of the house with two adjoining rooms, one for himself and one for Andy with a door on the outside closing the area from the rest of the house. There is a bed in each room for them. I have my private bedroom. We pay separate rents.

5. That the medical practice is in an office which is a separate suite rented at the same address, and the only access to the office is from the outside of the house. The rent is separate, based on market rents for equal space.

6. The present medical practice is new and small, having started up on or about April 1986. The practice sustains itself and no more. The practice merely allows Ken to keep his license and billing number which he worked hard to get in the first place and does not wish to lose. The blue book income is public information about medical doctors' incomes in B.C. The blue book publishes GROSS incomes only which differs from Net income. I receive money for the work I do from the practice. Ken cannot do the practice without help and if I were to quit working in the practice, Ken would have to hire another assistant. We follow the rules and regulations of the Medical Services Plan exactly.

7. That Ken has no net income from MSP. Ken's student loans and bursaries are his only moneys and he is careful to keep within the guidelines of the rules for obtaining these moneys. He is allowed 12 hours work a week under the guidelines and he does not exceed this.

8. That there is no concealed income. That it is illegal for a physician in British Columbia to extra bill.

9. That Ken is a full-time student and has professionally inactive classification with the British Columbia Medical Association. Under the BCMA guidelines, any physician who is under age 65 and earns under

$40,000.00 a year is considered professionally inactive. The College of Physicians and Surgeons of B.C. has only two categories, a member fully registered or a member fully retired. Ken has always been fully registered.

10. That we have been advised several times since the year 1985 by the British Columbia Ministry of Social Services and Housing that a person can own and/or operate a business and receive social assistance so long as there are no assets and no net income. When Ken needed assistance because of ill health, there was no net income and no assets. He was in bankruptcy also.

11. That until Ken was discharged from bankruptcy on or about January 21, 1987, his financial and living situation was scrutinized by a trustee.

12. That when I was on welfare as Jane states in her Affidavit of 23 January 1989, I was suffering a broken back. This had nothing to do with Ken's medical practice or his bankruptcy or with Jane.

13. That about 2½ or 3 years ago, Jane told Ken that she wanted to make a career change and that the law had changed so that she could force Ken to pay for her to go back to school to make a career change. I did the research to find out that Jane had lied to Ken and that because Ken had already paid for her to go to school to become a lawyer, he was not obligated to do it again.

14. That Ken has gone to the registrar in 1985 to ask for variance of the order for maintenance. I remember Ken coming away from the Registrar's office and telling me that he had been surprised that someone had shown up to represent Jane's interests to block the variance. Ken was then told by the Registrar to go to Supreme Court. Ken had no money to pursue the matter since it would obviously involve legal costs.

15. That I believe maintenance payments made directly from the Medical Services Plan of B.C. is ensured disruption of payments for maintenance. The MSP gross income depends on the hours worked in the months and year. Interruption of work means interruption of payments. The billing cards are not automatic and depend on when they are sent in, when they are received by the computer and sometime they are lost in transport. The cards are often stopped for payment because clients may not have paid their medical plan or they might be held up for manual investigation. There are seasonal disruptions, especially over Christmas and the Government employees have been known to go on strike. There have been several rollbacks in fees where Government collects money back. MSP should not be depended on for regular payments.

16. That most reliable monthly payment of maintenance would be from Ken himself. Ken has demonstrated that he cares about his son and when he had no money, he cared for him physically. When Ken had money, he both cared for Andy with money to his mother and cared for Andy physically.

17. That I have been witness to much of Andy's care and who cared for Andy since he was a baby. Even though Ken and I lived in separate residences, Ken chose to have Andy participate with my grandchildren and my children in my home over the years. I also met with and talked with Andy's nanny, Janet Strickland, who looked after Andy while Ken was at work so that Jane did not have the burden of motherhood to herself. A Nanny looked after Andy from during his first years of life until Andy went to the Montessori Day Care at age three where he was in full day care. Jane was not always working even though Andy was cared for by the Nanny or in day care.

18. That I have been witness to Ken taking responsibility for at least half of Andy's physical care since about September 1984 until about April 1987. That during the autumn of 1984 until Spring 1985, Andy ate most of his meals with Ken and slept over several nights a week. Jane claimed she was working and was often found to be in the exercise gym instead.

19. That when Jane signed the letter providing written confirmation of shared responsibility dated August 2nd, 1985, I was witness that these were in fact the actual hours Ken looked after Andy during that entire year. I was witness that Ken in fact looked after Andy longer hours than stated in the letter and fed him almost all his meals during the week. My own daughter helped Ken cook the meals Andy ate. I believe Jane to be most mistaken when she claims otherwise.

20. That I have been witness to the full-time care Ken gave Andy when Jane was in hospital having cosmetic surgeries or when she was ill, about twice a year for several years. I have also witnessed Andy upset at his mother's cosmetic surgeries and other illnesses.

21. That I have been witness to Ken caring for Andy when he was ill and Jane would ask Ken to take care of Andy.

22. That the reasons for Andy staying overnight have not always been for work reasons. I have been witness to Andy staying overnight with Ken when Jane asked for time with boyfriends. Andy was upset over this because he told me he always slept with his mother when he was at home. That this happened in 1988.

23. That I have seen Andy cry when he has not seen his mother for days and his mother informs him they are going straight to a babysitter.

24. That I have seen Andy inadequately dressed for weather even though Jane was getting regular maintenance. That Ken has often had to buy Andy extra clothing.

25. That Ken has paid for prescription drugs for Andy and personally taken him to other physicians during the summer of 1988. That Jane is mistaken when she says she does it all herself.

26. That I have been witness to Ken paying Andy's bus fares.

27. That I have been witness to Andy's Christmas presents from Ken. Andy spends Christmas Eve with Ken and my family at my home wherever I live and Andy always receives gifts from Ken and my family.

28. That Jane does not give a true picture of Ken's contributions to the care and support of Andy in her Affidavit of 23rd January, 1989. That Jane did not give Ken credit for his financial care of Andy when Andy at age three started demanding money from Ken for his mother. Andy said Ken owed his mother lots of money and she wanted it now. We could not take Andy near a bank with us because he would demand money for his mother. This was at a time when Ken was over-paying the maintenance voluntarily and gave up all his assets to Jane in the divorce. I was of the opinion the child was being lied to by Jane about Ken's monetary care. Andy continued this demand through ages 3, 4, 5, and 6.

29. That when Ken began receiving student loans, he budgeted day care for Andy because that is allowed in student loans and to call it maintenance is not allowed. To keep things honest, Ken paid that money for Andy's day care and Jane benefited by not having to pay the day care. Jane would telephone to make sure Ken was paying it on time.

30. That I witnessed Ken giving Andy cheques to give to Jane in the months of September, October, and November 1988, in the amount of $150.00 each, totally $450.00 instead of two months at $300.00 as Jane states in her Affidavit of 23rd January, 1988.

31. That Jane has made it difficult to pay the cheque for December, January, and February by withholding Andy and refusing to talk with Ken. That in my opinion she deliberately stopped receiving cheques from Ken.

32. Jane often withholds Andy from Ken and refuses to let Ken know Andy's whereabouts or what care he is being given. Since September 1988, Jane has withheld information about Andy's after school care. Ken tells me he does not know if his child has adequate care or if Andy is a latchkey child at age nine.

33. That I believe there is reason to worry about Andy's wellbeing...

34. That the conduct of Kehnroth Schramm has been overly generous to Jane. Ken has been extremely reliable in payments to Jane and in his care of his son. Ken in my presence has been overly open with Jane about all his personal and business matters considering that she has chosen to be less than truthful about the facts.

35. That I am concerned about Andy's wellbeing because of the precedent set over the years. Andy has been in the care of his father for major amounts of time and it is a sudden change for Andy to be withdrawn completely from his father for such a long period of time. Andy is heading for puberty and early teens, and it is my opinion that he and his father should be together as they are in the habit of being.

36. That my grandchildren miss Andy and want to see him regularly, as they are used to and consider Andy part of their family.

37. That all financial transactions will be audited by an accountant and income tax statements prepared for the Court.

SWORN BEFORE ME at the City of Vancouver
in the Province of British Columbia,
this 8th day of February, 1989.

[signed by lawyer]   [signed] ***Daisy Heisler***
A Commissioner for taking Affidavits
within the Province of British Columbia

* * *

NEARLY EVERY AFTERNOON or early evening, the tenants in the bedroom over Ken and Daisy's heads made love. He was a PhD student and she a concert vocalist whose voice carried to fill whole concert halls. While Ken and Daisy wrote Affidavits, they and the whole neighborhood were being serenaded through open windows by long arias of O-o-oh-h and Au-au-h-h in happy cadenzas that rose to fever high pitches and fell into lullabies.

35

Affidavits Continued

AFFIDAVIT REGISTERED FEBRUARY 27, 1989
No. D141314 VANCOUVER REGISTRY
IN THE SUPREME COURT OF BRITISH COLUMBIA
BETWEEN:
CAROL JANE SCHRAMM   PETITIONER
AND:
KEHNROTH SCHRAMM   RESPONDENT

I, KEHNROTH SCHRAMM, graduate student and professionally inactive physician, (address), MAKE OATH AND SAY AS FOLLOWS:

1. That I am the Respondent herein and as such have personal knowledge of the facts and matters hereinafter deposed to, save and except where stated to be made upon information and belief, and where so stated I verily believe the same to be true.

2. That in several affidavits, the Petitioner claims that I lied to her to avoid paying the maintenance for our son, Andy. As teacher, student, physician, and father, I have a reputation for being honest and generous, especially with my sons. The Petitioner knows the following to be true: I left the family home because I was no longer welcome, replaced by a nanny to care for Andy, and by Jane's friends. We had been arguing a great deal and I feared for my health, which was not improving despite the prescription medication I took for hypertension.

3. That I attended professional counseling sessions with the Petitioner to attempt to reconcile our differences over Andy's care, money, and life style.

4. That I separated from the Petitioner first within the family home, and even after leaving her, in May of 1981, I attempted on every possible occasion to resume communication and our friendship which had been the basis for our marriage.

5. That I sought the Petitioner's legal advice on every matter she now claims to be contentious: terms of our separation agreement, variation in maintenance payments, bankruptcy, and even about applying for student loans.

6. That I have been more open with the Petitioner regarding my finances than she has been with me regarding her earnings as a lawyer. She managed the business side of my medical practice. She is thoroughly familiar with the frustration I experienced, especially when I was ill, in being totally dependent on Medical Services Plan, my sole source of income as a family psychiatrist.

7. That the amount and timing of payments is unpredictable because they depend on the number of services provided to clients whose insurance is paid up to date, and the number of cards key-punched and processed during the pay period. Everything I learned to do to improve my effectiveness in counseling families is considered part of psychotherapy, insured services for which I cannot extra bill. General practitioners and dentists, with whom I attended training sessions in hypnotherapy and acupuncture, are allowed to extra bill for these same services. If I decided to opt out of Medical Services Plan, I would then have to compete with physicians, psychologists, social workers, nutritionists, massage therapists, and laypeople in the health promotion and life style service industries. I believe health and medical care are human rights: people should not have to pay for health services, especially when they are ill.

8. That because I taught anthropology, human ecology, and health science courses in the past, my best alternative to provide for my sons' education is to return to university for a career change which would allow me to complete graduate education, to teach and to consult about community health.

9. That in 1980, when Andy was 1 year old, I took a course in Self Help Housing at U.B.C. School of Community Planning to develop my knowledge and skills as a builder so that I could work cooperatively with other families to build solar heated homes. I also studied Mandarin Chinese with a tutor [name] who introduced me to Professor [name] with whom I later studied History of Chinese Thought.

10. That in the Fall of 1980, Jane and I discussed our future with a financial consultant and I spoke of my plans to study and teach Chinese Medicine when Jane was able to work as a lawyer part-time. When I supported her undergraduate and law school education, I believed that we had agreed to a partnership in which both of us would share the work and opportunities for further study.

11. That during the first week after birth, our Paediatrician told me to get help to care for the baby or he believed the Petitioner would end up in Riverview hospital. I took over care of Andy and have been actively involved in his care ever since.

12. That after we were divorced, I continued to care for Andy half to full-time as I had since his birth, so that Jane could complete her articling position, and establish herself in her chosen career. When she was depressed enough to seek psychological and psychiatric help, or when she wanted an overnight free for socializing, or if she required surgery, I took responsibility for Andy's care half to full-time as needed and enjoyed caring for him, except when it led to confrontations with Jane.

13. That I believed, on Jane's advice, that our legal separation agreement supported joint guardianship so that I would be consulted about everything that concerned Andy's well being: that maintenance and access agreements could be negotiated easily with the Registrar of the Court. These beliefs encouraged me to take full-time responsibility for Andy's care when needed because I believed that we had achieved a de facto equivalent of joint custody.

14. That when I found that I could not reconcile the conflicts between Jane and myself even with professional help, I did the best I could to meet my responsibilities as a separated and divorced parent of a two-going-on-three-year old son. Maintenance payments covered the monthly mortgage and the nanny's salary. I assumed the practice and personal debts and Jane received all assets and the proceeds from the sale of the house.

15. That I have refused to become an every other weekend father, but have arranged my working schedule around Andy's needs and Jane's schedule as much as possible preparing for the days when he would be with me full-time. I am proud to be a single parent because I have worked hard to enjoy my three sons.

16. That I am living cooperatively with Daisy and her family in order to provide my sons with as healthy an environment as I can. Andy enjoys the company of her grandchildren and children with me and I want to have him with me at least half time, sharing our own separate rooms in the house which is managed, but not owned by Daisy.

17. That Andy picked out his own [new] bed in November and when I asked his mother if she would help me pay for it by forgiving the day care payment, she refused so I gave the cheque to Andy which she later cashed, but failed to acknowledge in her first affidavit.

18. That I did not pay her in December because I did not have the money and in January, without warning, she garnished my entire student loan for January through April 1989. That the Petitioner's lawyer not only threatened to make trouble for me about the student loans, but did so through his telephone calls.

19. That the Petitioner continues to make access impossible. I have requested that we both consult a family court counselor together voluntarily in order to resolve our differences for Andy's benefit, as we have done in the past.

20. That I made no secret of my illness before or after being divorced from Jane. When I was too ill to work, I deregistered my last RRSP and gave it to her for maintenance. Since then, and until Jane garnished my personal account and student loans, I have lived first on GAIN and later from Student Loans and Bursaries, with no illegal or immoral income from MSP. I doubt I would have survived the financial, physical, and emotional stresses of the past 8 years without the friendship and hard work of my friend and co-worker, Daisy Heisler.

21. That the amount of money earned in my professionally inactive medical practice is barely enough to meet costs. I have no life or malpractice insurance; but in order to keep my license and a consulting office in which to establish my career change as a teacher and researcher in community health risk management, I am fortunate to be able to work up to 12 hours a week to assist families in making their own health care plans.

22. That because my practice is a referral practice from general practitioners and friends of former clients, I have no way to guarantee that there will continue to be any further income.

23. That my only secure income was the student loans which Jane has garnished.

24. That attached to this affidavit and marked Exhibit A is a true copy of my curriculum vitae which clearly illustrates my varied background.

25. That attached to this my affidavit and marked Exhibit B is a true copy of a Verification of Full Time Status form the University of British Columbia, Department of Community and Regional Planning, dated February 9th, 1989.

26. That attached to this my affidavit and marked Exhibit C is a true copy of a letter from the Office of Award and Financial Aid at the University of British Columbia dated February 8th, 1989.

27. That attached to this my affidavit and marked Exhibit D is a true copy of my Medical Services Card with my son Andy Schramm named as a dependent.

28. That attached to this my affidavit and marked Exhibit E is a true copy of Samples of the Hours of Care given to Andy by myself, taken from my daily appointment books and prepared by Daisy Heisler.

29. That attached to this my affidavit and marked Exhibit F is a cancelled cheque for my rent at [address].

...31. That attached to this my affidavit and marked Exhibit H is a true copy of the Canadian Association of Planning Students Annual Conference Program in which I presented a paper on Planning Education for the 1990's.

32. That I am requesting an access investigation with access in the interim on a fifty-fifty basis.

SWORN BEFORE ME at the City of Vancouver
in the Province of British Columbia,
this 27th day of February, 1989.
[signed by lawyer]   [signed] ***K. Schramm***
A Commissioner for taking Affidavits
Within the Province of British Columbia

* * *

JANE'S FRIENDS, Gail Davidson and Leslie Baker, both lawyers, had each taken advantage of Ken's services and expertise for their personal or professional needs in the past. Now insults from these two women became part of the equation again. Gail's simply written Affidavit came without much detail, except to backup Jane as a single parent and to insult Ken by resorting to childish name-calling. Based on Gail's statement under oath about the care of Andy, it was obvious she had no true, first-hand knowledge.

Leslie Baker's Affidavit outlined details of Jane's medical condition in November 1986. Instead of remembering that Daisy gave her the sheet that Andy had thrown up on in November of 1986, she stated in her Affidavit that Ken gave her a 'bag of dirty laundry'. Leslie complained in her Affidavit that when Ken and Daisy brought Andy to her apartment, they were 'over one hour late'. She also wrote that in 1988 when Andy was staying overnight with Ken, that 'Andy telephoned his mother at 4 A.M. on a Sunday to say he was frightened and alone in the house and intended to walk home'.

Leslie's version of events had little match to real life adventures even though she was under oath, and she did not mind using hearsay and left out a few dynamic details.

Leslie Baker's Affidavit was a reminder to Daisy of the event when they arrived late at Leslie's home. Both Ken and Andy had been reluctantly following Jane's orders to deliver Andy to yet again another babysitter instead of to his mother. Daisy had accompanied them because she did not want Ken to go there and have to leave alone. After traveling by bus for lack of a car, they were late. Leslie opened her door in a screaming rage. Daisy was shocked that not only did Ken face an angry tirade from Jane if he was a minute early or late delivering Andy to her door, but her friend spewed hostility and anger in his face in front of the children as though it was her right, and she did not care that Daisy witnessed her behavior.

Ken had responded by speaking gently in his soft voice and he did not rise to the bait. Ken had calmed the spewing woman enough so that they were all invited in for a few minutes to settle Andy who was showing stress.

It always amazed Daisy that Ken did not retaliate but continued to be kind, maintaining calm in response to hostility, even though Daisy knew he felt a deep hurt. She also worried that the hurt caused more damage to his already damaged heart and she wondered when these women would actually cause him to have a heart attack and die. She had seen Ken respond with kindness to dissolve antagonism over and over and even sit on the floor to be lower than a threatening person.

Watching Leslie Baker was another sad reminder that Ken's stories were true about the people and their behavior that had been affecting his life. Also, Leslie's behavior was a reminder that for all of Andy life, the child had been witness to women verbally beating up on his father. Daisy worried Andy could grow up with a tainted idea of manhood – if he was being allowed to grow up at all under the tutelage of these women and the example of a man his mother approved of being Bruce Katz. Daisy was always astounded that these women were so out of control but thought it their right to act out in front of children; it was all so foreign to Daisy. In

Daisy's upbringing, real women would never behave the way these women behaved.

Never the less, the Affidavits of these two women had to be answered.

Ken wrote again, spelling out his frustration in the differences between himself and Jane over the years.

AFFIDAVIT REGISTERED March 6th, 1989.
No. D141314 VANCOUVER REGISTRY
IN THE SUPREME COURT OF BRITISH COLUMBIA
BETWEEN:
CAROL JANE SCHRAMM   PETITIONER
AND:
KEHNROTH SCHRAMM   RESPONDENT

I, KEHNROTH SCHRAMM, graduate student and professionally inactive physician, [address], MAKE OATH AND SAY AS FOLLOWS:

1. That I swear this Affidavit in response to the Affidavit of Carol Jane Schramm, now Jane Anderson, sworn 2nd of March 1989, and filed in support of her application to be heard by this Court on the 6th day of March 1989.

2. That in Jane's Affidavit sworn March 2, 1989, paragraphs 3 & 4, Jane argues that the first and most important issue to be resolved is money, not Andy's care by both of his parents. We have often disagreed about money and medicine. Just as I offer my emotional support, intellectual insight, and moral judgment to my clients instead of pills, I have shared my life and myself with my son Andy since his birth. I came to Canada in 1967 as a conscientious objector because I refused to accept money for a civil or military position in the U.S. as a psychiatrist to provide medication and hospitalization in violation of civil rights or in support of the Vietnam War. My refusal to make monetary success the highest priority of my life is a major reason for my two marriages ending in divorce. In both instances, I continue to provide care for and with my sons.

3. The issue of maintenance arrears is intertwined with the issues of access and custody to such an extent that they must be resolved together. Otherwise, the affidavits from Ms. Davidson and Ms. Baker presenting their views on Andy's care by his parents would be irrelevant. Because of my experience in court as a child and family psychiatrist in disputed custody and access cases, I am concerned that prolonged disputes over money and custody are harmful as well as stressful to children and their parents. Instead of barrages of conflicting affidavits back and forth between Jane and me, I believe a professional custody and access investigation would be a way to settle what is the appropriate custodial arrangement for Andy's best interest as he grows into young manhood.

4. That in response to paragraph 6 of Jane's affidavit sworn March 2, 1989, I am concerned that my access to Andy has been made and still being made impossible by arrangements his mother had made for his care with friends like those who now provide affidavits in support of her claims for money. I left the matrimonial home because of being displaced by a nanny, Jane's friends, and conflict about her money demands. The $500 maintenance payment now in dispute, was agreeable to me in 1981 because it was the exact amount paid to Janet Strickland, Andy's nanny, who was very important in his life at that time. I also paid the mortgage on the matrimonial home and later gave Jane full title. I do not intend to relinquish my right to provide nourishing physical and emotional care for and with Andy now or in the future. Jane has moved to a more convenient location for her friends to care for Andy instead of allowing me to do so. She denies me access and then uses my lack of access as evidence I should pay more money for someone else besides his parents to care for him. Summer of 1988 when, for reasons unknown to me at the time, Jane began to withdraw Andy from University Hill After School Care. I have found it increasing difficult to know who is caring for him, when, and where. Since December, my telephone and direct access has been blocked by Jane and her lawyer while she claims in her affidavit, paragraph 12, she is not denying access. I believe there is no way to resolve the question of my access without raising the question of joint custody of Andy and requesting an access investigation.

5. That Jane accuses me of an elaborate scheme to conceal income which is published in the Blue Book annually. I resumed a professionally inactive family health consulting practice because of repeated requests from former clients, assurances from the Trustee who supervised my bankruptcy that I must do so in order to pay required fees before being discharged from bankruptcy, and because I found a way to consult with a selected few families by negotiation and mediation that did not interfere with my care of Andy, neither compromising my principles nor my health. I believed that the purpose of bankruptcy is to allow people a new start and that by slow and careful steps I could regain my health, resume my studies, and make a career change to teach others to plan for healthy communities, families, and children. I told Jane every step of the way what I was doing to plan for meeting Andy's needs and recognizing her needs for security. I have treated her honestly and respected her informal legal opinions because I believed that despite our differences we both wanted to provide for Andy's education by making our own unique contributions to his development as a person. In her barrage of affidavits, I see no sign of respect for me or for the truth which is bigger than either one of our positions. I believe knowledge of truths relevant to the arrears maintenance and present legal custody requires a full access investigation.

6. That regarding Jane's conspiracy theory, I repeat I have taken no illegal, immoral, or hidden monies from MSP or any other sources. Nor have I diverted money to others to avoid paying maintenance; nor have I paid for inflated rents or office services. I have slowly and with great difficulty recovered my health sufficiently to return to full time study and to care for Andy half to full time. With the help of my friends, I am barely maintaining an office without malpractice, property, or life insurance, in a rented house in Kitsilano. I have frequently looked for less expensive accommodation and office space, or housing cooperatives, and have not found anything. The amounts of money provided by MSP payments are low for both office rent and services.

7. That Jane waited to take legal action until early January when I was legally discharged from bankruptcy. I have no secure tenure here in Kitsilano and I am unlikely to find a better situation for Andy and me to live together. If Jane and her lawyer are allowed to continue harassment, I doubt that I can afford to practice medicine in B.C., but certainly not in Kitsilano where I have a reputation for honesty among my friends and clients. MSP is an erratic source of payment at best so I wonder if Jane's motive is vengeance rather than regular maintenance payments. In any event, she has not provided any income information to cover the period when she has endured economic hardship while working full-time with Bruce Katz, and denying me access by arranging for her friends to care for Andy while she works. I fear Andy is becoming a latch key child and I want to know who is caring for him daily, how, where, when, and why?

SWORN BEFORE ME at the City of Vancouver
in the Province of British Columbia,
this 6th day of March, 1989.

[signed by lawyer]   [signed] **_K.Schramm_**
A Commissioner for taking Affidavits
Within the Province of British Columbia

* * *

EXPRESSING HER ALARM at inaccuracies in Leslie Baker's Affidavit, Daisy complained to Ken, "It seems that Jane has surrounded herself with friends and lawyers who don't mind twisting the truth to suit themselves, even in Affidavits. I had always thought that the fear of being caught lying would keep lawyers honest, but they seem to be void of any fear of perjury. What does that say about our legal system? Our judicial system needs to be revamped so that lawyers winning cases at all cost is not the goal. And Judges! I really wonder if Judges are always clear about justice for all."

Daisy spent another weekend writing an Affidavit, going over all the details and attached to it a copy of a letter she wrote to Jane's doctor in 1985.

AFFIDAVIT REGISTERED March 6th, 1989
No. D141314 VANCOUVER REGISTRY
IN THE SUPREME COURT OF BRITISH COLUMBIA
BETWEEN:
CAROL JANE SCHRAMM   PETITIONER
AND:
KEHNROTH SCHRAMM   RESPONDENT
I, DAISY HEISLER [address] MAKE OATH AND SAY AS FOLLOWS:

1. That I swear this Affidavit in response to the Affidavit of Carol Jane Schramm, now Jane Anderson, sworn the 2nd day of March, 1989 and the Affidavit of Leslie Ann Baker, sworn the 2nd day of March, 1989, and the Affidavit of Gail Y. Davidson, sworn the 3rd day of March, 1989.

2. That I wrote the letter marked Exhibit "A" and attached to this my Affidavit as a plea for help in September of 1985. That I wrote the letter to a physician and hand delivered it to the physician who I knew was seeing Jane and Andy, in hopes that he could have better insight into their problems and do something to help Jane and Andy. ...I would also like to say here that Ken was and had been renting an apartment for himself and Jane knew that, and he was not actually living with me and my family but was doing the care of Andy in my home most of the time so that Andy had a family life instead of a lonely life of single parent with single child. ...

3. That the Affidavits of Leslie Baker and Gail Davidson are based mostly on what Jane has told them, and not on first hand witnessing the care I have witnessed. If Leslie Baker has done as much child care as she claims and the other babysitters have also done as much child care as they seem to have done, and Ken has done as much child care as I have witnessed, then I wonder when Jane has looked after Andy at all.

4. That in answer to the "vomit on sheet" matter, I would like to say I was a witness to Ken trying for years to convince Jane that her many surgeries and her long absences from Andy under mysterious circumstances were very upsetting to Andy. I witnessed Ken trying to convince Jane to give up any unnecessary surgery for Andy's sake. I heard first hand the many pleas Ken made to Jane that Andy was getting ill and vomiting and would she please think of him. ...So I sent the sheet to her. ...

5. That in answer to Leslie Baker's statement regarding Andy leaving our house in the middle of the night with his mother, I would say that Leslie was not here so she does not have first hand information. However, there was a time when Andy did telephone his mother to pick him up in the middle of the night and we did get upset with him about doing this and later had long talks with him about it. The reason Andy did that is because he knew his mother was sleeping with other men in "his" bed. Andy told us that he was still sleeping with his mother and when the other boyfriends were around he mostly had to stay with us or someone else. Andy told us he resented this and was insisting no one else would sleep with his mother. Then, according to Andy, his mother was having an affair with a "married man". Andy told us outright that he would break up this relationship. The night in question, he was calling his mother all evening trying to get home so that her boyfriend would not sleep with his mother instead of him but at about 11 pm Andy fell asleep in the living room. We covered him with blankets and left him there instead of moving him to his bedroom. When he woke up, he quietly went to the telephone and called his mother to pick him up and snuck out of the house, hoping he would not wake us up. The telephone is right outside my bedroom door, in the kitchen, and when a child is in my house at night, I always sleep with my bedroom door open so that I can hear the child. The fact that I had my door open, Ken was in his own room, and I did not hear Andy, meant to me that Andy was deliberately not making noise. I have had thirty-two years practice at listening for children in the night. When that particular boyfriend and Jane broke up, Andy told us he was sure he had made them break up and he was very proud of himself. Andy also told us that Lesley was "mad at Jane' about this married boyfriend and would not speak to her, so Leslie apparently does know about this incident but not first hand.

SWORN BEFORE ME at the City of Vancouver
in the Province of British Columbia,
this 6th day of March, 1989
[signed by lawyer]   *[signed]* **Daisy Heisler**
A Commissioner for taking Affidavits
within the Province of British Columbia.

Exhibit A: (letter attached to March 6, 1989 Affidavit)

August 5, 1985

Dear Doctor...

After remaining the silent observer and often active caretaker of Andy for over four years, I can no longer remain silent. Thank you for allowing me this opportunity to speak up.

Our present schedule of caring for Andy is... I am trying to point out that Andy is with us most of his waking hours. He eats most of his meals with us. ...

Jane complains so much about having to see him at all that she in fact hires a babysitter for him on Saturday afternoons so that he goes from us directly to a babysitter (he waits for her, then the tears roll again when he is told she will not spend time with him), then often again a sitter Saturday night and again Sunday she often parks him with friends. She tells Andy outright that she "needs a break". ...

...There is nothing unyielding about Ken's willingness to negotiate with her. Ken's attitude is that Andy is better off with him instead of her but is willing to help in most any capacity. He even did her laundry and vacuumed her floors since I've known him, anything to help out...

Andy is her PAWN.

It is not my objective to take any child away from his/her mother. ...I do not have an answer other than to treat his mother and by doing that perhaps all our lives will be easier. Ken's health might improve. ...

I fear for Andy's future... I see a mother who only wants power, money, and control but one who does not actually want to be with her child. She uses every excuse to not spend time with him but last I heard he still sleeps with her. Therefore, he is constantly in a tug of war. He is pushed away and brought in on an unconscious level where he is extremely attached but daily feels rejected.

So he blames his father that his mother is so far away and hard to reach, but in fact his father is the one who gives him personal attention and care. It is heartbreaking to watch that child expecting to spend time with his mother finally, only to be rejected the moment he steps into her car.

In all sincerity,

[signed] *Daisy*

[This letter was submitted complete and unedited with the Affidavit. The letter has been edited for this book, deleting some descriptions of perceived behavior and health concerns.]

WHEN DAISY BROUGHT this affidavit to the lawyer at the same time that Ken brought his latest one, the lawyer suddenly woke up to say he did not like her Affidavit. She asked him why and how to change it. He offered no answer but simply went ahead and registered it as-is.

AGAIN IN COURT, lawyers Jane Anderson and Bruce Katz sat together in a front row. Jane swung her chair around so that her back was toward the Judge. Her hard, beady eyes bore into Daisy, who was seated at the back of the room. From that angle she smirked at Daisy with an "I've got you!" look. Facing away from the Judge, he could not be the wiser.

Daisy tried to respond with an "I'm not afraid of you." look. Unknown yet to Daisy, this would be the day of the inevitable attempt to get rid of her legally.

On this day, out of Katz' bag of tricks, he was bringing to Judge Scarth's attention the Affidavits written by Jane's friends, Leslie Baker and Gail Davidson, and he added an extra frill of telling a fabricated story that Andy was supposed to have told that Daisy physically assaulted her own daughter in front Andy, and therefore Daisy was not fit to be around Jane's child.

Ken's lawyer was extremely still and quiet, not responding at all, making no argument – no attempt to offer a counter-argument nor to bring up Ken's and Daisy's responsive Affidavits, nor did he ask questions throughout the proceedings. Their Affidavits were being ignored. Their presence was being ignored by their lawyer.

It was a one-sided argument all the way. No one bothered to ask either Ken or Daisy about the allegations. Neither one was brought to the stand to speak for themselves. Ken's lawyer would not look Ken's way, avoiding communication with him even though Ken was seated beside him. Rooted to his seat with eyes locked on Katz, Ken's lawyer acted like he was just an onlooker with no part in the case happening around him.

Ken had named a particular male psychologist he wanted to do the child custody investigation that he in fact had been begging for by requesting the custody investigation through phone calls, letters to his lawyer, and through his Affidavits registered with the Court. Through Ken's work as a psychiatrist in the courts, he knew the man to have a reputation for being protective of children regardless of the fight between parents. In front of Judge Scarth, Katz suddenly asked for the same psychologist to do an investigation; that's when Ken's lawyer sprung to action, actually jumping to his feet to argue loudly against using the named psychologist.

Ken was stunned. Daisy was so shocked that she jumped to her feet, wanting to take action but squelched an outburst and sat down. They could not believe what just happened but were silenced by court rules that people remain silent unless asked to speak.

Judge Scarth made no attempt to speak to either Ken or Daisy. Instead, he bore his eyes into Daisy at the back of the room and muttered, "Andy should not be around a person like that." It did not sound like an order, just a mutter, but Daisy's face burned with shock. Until now, she had not known that the Judge knew who she was because she had always been at the back of the room.

Hiring of the psychologist Ken had wanted to do the child custody investigation was quickly dismissed after what appeared to be a ruse.

[Ken's Journal] June 3, 1989

Andy, I am writing this book for you and me because I want you to understand what this Supreme Court business is about. The reasons I have asked for a family court counselor are: first, to help your mother and I talk together about what is happening to you and for you because we have not been able to talk together since she became ill after you were born; and second, to hear from a counselor what you want us to know about what you have to say to both of us; third, to ask the counselor to talk with you, your teachers and other people who know you and us, so that she can report to the court what she believes would be best for you during the next few years. Whatever the report says, your mother and I will both be caring for you, sharing the expenses by paying our shares of the costs of your education and growing up. I hope that we will learn to talk with each other about the decisions which affect your life.

My lawyer [name] tells me that we will be going to court in September to give Judge Scarth the opportunity to decide what is best for you during the next few years. I hope that he will decide that your mother and I will both participate in all the decisions that affect you: where you live, where you go to school, how much we should save for your future needs, and that we learn to discuss without criticizing each other.

Your Dad

36

Child Custody 1989

LETTER WRITTEN MARCH 21, 1989 by Ken's lawyer to: *Trial Division...*

> Please find enclosed a copy of the Order of the Honourable Judge Boyd in which $1,000.00 from the sum of $3,733.05 paid into Court, pursuant to the Garnishing Order after Judgment issued on behalf of the Petitioner and date stamped the 19th day of January, 1989, was applied to maintenance for the months February and March 1989. This sum of money represents the Respondent's sole source of income in the form of student loans. This assignment order by the Honourable Judge Scarth on March 15th, 1989 completely eliminates all potential sources of income for the Respondent and effectively forces Dr. Schramm to discontinue his practice. I am not sure the Honourable Judge was aware of the existing monies paid into court when he ordered the Assignment.
>
> Yours truly...[signed by lawyer]

* * *

KEN DECIDED THAT since he loves books and libraries so much he would offer to work in the local Banyen Books store that devoted shelves to books on spirituality, philosophy, and self-help books. It was healing work for the allowable twelve hours a week work. It was at the minimum hourly wages meant to top up his student loan. Since Jane had cleaned out every cent of the student loan installment from his bank account and also had taken money directly from the government offices of the BC Medical Services Plan, resulting in an overpayment from MSP that Ken must now pay back, and he no longer had any other financial help, the bookstore was his only income on which to survive and do a payback. His lawyer had advised Ken to quit seeing clients.

DAISY HAD BEEN working at St. Helen's Anglican church as secretary, something she had always thought would be fun to do in the religion she had been brought up in. She was looking forward to all the celebrations this job should bring. Her Buddhist experience had not hindered the joy of being in her Christian church; she embraced all religions. Regardless, inner unrest started in her first weeks on the job when a movie crew rented the church for a few days. Daisy was surprised at feeling like a church mouse while watching the excitement of the artistic crew working to transform the church into a movie set and knowing she could do any and all their jobs.

The Reverend had been in the habit of bossing women around as demonstrated when he emptied a senior parishioner's purse and insisted that she use the 'new second-hand' purse that he wanted her to use. He transferred all personal contents of her purse against her objections. Daily, he grilled Daisy on her spiritual beliefs and Daisy had given information she began to regret. He nearly flew off his chair in anger when she admitted to believing in reincarnation. He insisted that Daisy put her mother's ashes in the little garden by the front door of the church regardless of what her family wanted. It did not take long for this place to feel like a mistake.

Daisy was suddenly fired from her job for no obvious reason. She could not figure it out but before leaving the church, she paused to take one final look at the row of past Ministers' portraits on the brown wood paneled wall. The current Reverend's picture was nearest to the front door. She was taken aback by the evil look of the face and his hair appearing to make horns over his forehead. He was not the compassionate Reverend Crouther she grew up with in St. Peter's church in Regina.

She stood in front of his picture remembering how he gave her hell for going into the church before work one morning, which in her mind defied any rationalization; and how the newsletter and church notes that she had been working on for the last Sunday's service mysteriously disappeared from her desk drawer over night.

She had suspected he had taken the notes but after calling him up about it and getting no decent response, she relied on her excellent photographic and audio memory to reproduce every page exactly as it had been. She had noted his not very well hidden shock when she handed the finished pages to him with copies already printed in time for the Sunday congregation. Because of his response, she knew without a doubt that for some strange reason he had tried to engineer a reason to fire her.

Walking out of the church, past the small sparsely planted flower garden out front, she was relieved that unlike some parishioners, she had dared to defy the Reverend's insistence to have her mother's ashes put there.

Out on the street, she paused to look up at the large stained glass window. Jesus held a lantern just like the picture in the book her mother had read to her children at bedtime. "You owe me," Daisy silently shouted – followed by, "Sorry, no you don't. I guess I have been paid back for all the times I raced around the church hall with other kids instead of going to church and then spent the offering quarters that my mother gave me on ice cream."

Walking down the hill above Jericho park overlooking the ocean with the North Shore mountains in the distance, she looked forward to the comfort of visiting Ken at his work in the bookstore, and sorry to give him the news that she was now out of a job.

When he saw her walk in, Ken's eyes lit up. They talked for a few minutes in a bookstall where they could be alone and then she walked the few blocks to home. The store was near home.

Within the hour, Ken came through the door with a wry smile on his face.

"I've been fired!" he announced, still in disbelief.

"What? Why?"

"I was fired by the psychiatric nurse who works there. She told me I am not fast enough with the cash register and that I should be doing more surveillance on the patrons. I took the job to be helpful to people and I am fired for not being a fast policeman."

"Oh, Oh! It is the first time I've come in to talk with you. Odd you should be fired within minutes of my visit. And it's odd that we should both be fired in the same hour. I wonder if my presence had something to do with it. Jealousy maybe? I've spent years shopping and reading in that store, in fact, since it first opened and I have known the owner. I was never aware of surveillance being a top priority. It was always a place where people could spend hours just holed up in a corner reading books. It has always been customer oriented – though I have noticed that the two women working there recently have changed the atmosphere."

"Daisy, I may have been fired by a psych nurse because she had a chance to stick it to a doctor finally, and preferably a psychiatrist."

"I bet you are right. I think the owner should be told about what's happening in his store."

"I'll talk to him but I don't expect to get the job back as long as those two ladies work there."

"Ken, on the other hand, neither of us had any warning and we were both fired in the same hour. Isn't that extremely odd? Maybe interference from an outside source?"

KEN WROTE IN HIS NOTEBOOK:
"June 17th, 1989. This week I was retired from Banyen Books; discussed a consulting role with Kolin, and began meeting with Mary Murray...

"Mary [Murray] told me about parental alienation syndrome and the priority given to the parent who encourages access to the other parent. She said she will make a copy of the relevant chapter from Richard Gardner, The Parental Alienation Syndrome: How to distinguish truth from falsity in child abuse. I believe Mary can handle both mediation and investigative roles. She said she would ask another person in her office to mediate access if she could not. I kept my discussion to my concerns about Jane's lying re my guardianship and her restricting my access while being unable (working or sick) to care for him herself. I emphasized her withholding of love as a manipulation combined with giving favors in a well-planned scheme to revenge herself on

me. I used her relations with Andy and Stephen as examples. I indicated my willingness to have full custody of Andy and encourage access to Jane when she can be with him. My work as a student and family health consultant-mediator permits me a flexible schedule to be with Andy. I am attending his school regularly as a teacher's aid, helping the children with writing.

This week we worked on dialogue for a puppet show about sexual abuse. Andy seemed to want to use Zenith 123 after one try at talking to a trusted adult, the mother. He seems to need physical contact, wrestling and resting."

* * *

MARY MURRAY HAD been appointed to investigate and make a child custody report for Court. Ken had not been consulted about her appointment.

The first problem noted was that Mary Murray was Jane's neighbor. Since the False Creek Housing Co-op townhouses are only fourteen feet wide attached in rows, their homes are only a few feet apart and they probably see each other regularly as they step outside their doors and go to their cars via the same staircase, or attend the same co-op meetings. Mary was also a single parent of a boy about the same age as Andy. As neighbors in the False Creek Housing Co-op, the women and the boys will supposedly have ongoing relationships to contend with for years to come.

Having feelings of misgivings, Ken asked Daisy, "Do you think Mary can be objective and do this job?"

She answered, "It is extremely odd that of all the many people doing custody investigations in the lower mainland, that Jane's neighbor would be chosen. Well, Mary and I had the same friends and attended a couple of the same social gatherings when I lived in the co-op. I know her as a musician entertaining us with her guitar and singing. I think we can give her a chance." While saying this, her fond memories of Mary turned to a foreboding as the memory crept in of Mary and a few other musician friends coming to the door the first Christmas that Ken was living with her. An eerie feeling lingered.

Daisy would soon regret ignoring her gut feeling of doubt.

Ken questioned Mary's competency to be objective. Mary made a promise to Ken that she can and will be objective. Because he would keep his word to clients, he tried to believe Mary.

Both Ken and Daisy were basing their trust on wishful thinking and a belief in basic goodness in people.

Ken wrote answers to Mary Murray's questions.

QUESTIONS ARISING FROM LEGAL PROCEEDINGS & CONCILIATION:
Why are you asking for a custody and access report now?

I did not ask for custody of Andy until now because I believed I had accomplished the equivalent of joint custody and there was no need for further court action which would be more stressful than helpful for Andy. I have been daily involved with Andy's care since his birth and I believed I continued to have the same rights and responsibilities as his parent following my divorce from Jane in 1982. When Jane made decisions about holidays or babysitters which limited my access to Andy without consulting me, I believed she chose not to follow the terms of our divorce. I believed Jane had agreed to accept my care of Andy, and daycare fees from my student loans, as equivalent to maintenance. I spoke with her often about my graduate study in community and regional planning as a career change so I can provide more for Andy's education by participating in his daily life, and when I am successful in securing a research or teaching position, reduced tuition fees at school or university are possible. Only after Jane had garnished my entire student loan account did I discover that she has been lying to me since the Separation Agreement when she led me to believe I had retained parental guardianship and a means of resolving problems of access and maintenance. Since I cannot rely on her good faith to be sure that Jane is caring for Andy adequately, I asked for an independent assessment of what is best for Andy as he grows to manhood. I do not believe that Jane is well enough to care for him full time and that is why he has become a latchkey child in her home and she has placed him with her women friends for childcare instead of with me as I have asked because she no longer wants me to have the "liberal access" specified in our divorce, nor to be accountable to me for her care of Andy.

I believe that she has been planning this court case for the past 3 years and that she consulted Joyce Bradley about bringing a court action against me in 1988. Last fall, Andy told me he was still sleeping with his mother as a "treat". In January 1989, he told me that he is home with his mother only on Saturday afternoons and during the rest of the week he is with Jane's friends, mothers of his friends. His older half brother, Stephen takes Jane to dinner, the ballet and to concerts, rarely including Andy who "sleeps over" at a friend's house. I believe that Jane is manipulating both Stephen and Andy by using her sexuality and her illnesses for sympathy and support. Andy seems afraid of losing her love to others or her life to illness. If he were to spend more time with me, he risks being unavailable or disloyal to his mother and may lose his "treats". Jane needs him as her caretaker and insurance policy for continuing financial support from me. Under the stresses of her continuing illnesses, I believe I am the better parent and could more reliably care for his needs and support his access to her. I am 12 years older than Jane. The eldest of 5 children, I have cared for children all my life as elder brother, family physician, pediatrician, family psychiatrist, and teacher. Since Andy's birth, coincident with Jane's illness, I have been preparing myself to be his full-time parent with or without her participation. I work flexible hours as a consultant in child, family, personal and community health, while being a full-time student in community and regional planning, researching and writing about families as partners in planning healthy communities. This work allows me to participate directly in Andy's schooling as a volunteer and to be available for him when he is ill or needy.

I refused to become a part-time or weekend father and have cared for Andy full-time when Jane was unable to do so because of illness or her work. I separated from Jane because, as I told her then, "I believe I am killing myself trying to live up to what I think are your expectations." I hoped I was wrong to believe that she simply wanted me to provide her the means to be wealthy. But after many attempts on my part to reconcile with Jane, I found she did not want to negotiate or to be reconciled with me, but preferred to live the life of a single woman with my financial support. I was shocked when she told me sex and intimacy are separate. Despite our differences, I believed that we both cared for Andy and that Jane would not prevent me from continuing to be his full-time father.

Our lawyer, Wayne Powell reviewed the Separation Agreement written by Jane in 1982, confirming that my parental rights and responsibilities as Andy's father and guardian continued; and there was a mechanism for arbitrating conflicts over access and maintenance without expensive litigation. On that basis, I gave Jane the house, the car, and all our joint assets, while I assumed all the debts. I would not have agreed to this unequal settlement without those legal safeguards for Andy's care. This decision led to my bankruptcy due to stress-related illness, and to the present court action which Jane initiated as soon as [name] trustee for my bankruptcy, was discharged. Her timing has the consequence that no other creditors come before the payment of any maintenance arrears and current, not past, income tax. Because I believed I was still Andy's guardian, I paid the salary for Andy's nanny before and after I separated from Jane on May 13, 1981. Her salary was the basis for the $500 monthly maintenance now under review by Judge Scarth. I also paid more than the required maintenance when Jane told me it was needed.

What do you want to accomplish by this investigation?

I want an investigation into what is actually happening in Andy's life with his mother as custodial parent and how she is affecting his development as a human being so that we can learn what is best for Andy beyond the conventions of single parenting. As a result of your work, I hope to learn how to negotiate with Jane about what is best for Andy. Whatever the Judge decides, we will have to make it work. Your investigation is needed to answer the questions: What are the "facts" of Andy's life? What does Andy need now and for the next 10 years of his life? Who is the best custodial parent? What plan of custody, access and guardianship will provide for his needs? What can we do to make sure his needs are being met? What can the Court do to insure that problems affecting his life are quickly resolved or mediated?

Why are you studying full-time and not practicing medicine?

I am using my family health consulting practice and my full-time studies in community and regional planning to make a career change to researcher-teacher in emergency planning for healthy communities. Since immigrating in 1967 to teach at McGill University when I was not yet licensed to practice medicine in Canada, I have continued to teach and study healthy communities. I met Jane while doing fieldwork in the intentional community in which we lived on Lasqueti and Calvert Islands. As a result of this work, I earned my license to practice medicine in B.C. After I was married to Jane and supporting her education, our plan was to begin my career change after she was established in legal practice.

Since our separation and divorce, I continued to provide financial, emotional, and physical support for Andy so that she could complete her education and begin her law practice. I often paid more than the required maintenance to cover rent and living expenses when Jane was unemployed or ill. During the past 4 years since illness required me to stop my medical practice, I have been studying at UBC and kept Jane informed of my progress while providing childcare for Andy myself and by paying his daycare fees at U-Hill After School Care or directly to Jane. She advised me about how to apply for student loans. As explained above, I believe my decision to return to graduate study is the best way for me to continue to care for Andy now and in the future.

KS 6/22/89

* * *

EXCERPT from KEN'S UBC Student Loan application July 1989:

I am applying for student loans to continue my graduate studies. I transferred from anthropology to a pre-doctoral program in Community and Regional Planning in December '88, and in January '89, my ex-wife garnished my student loan account. Since then we have been involved in complex litigation over custody, access, and maintenance of our son, Andy, now 10. A family court counselor's report regarding custody and access will be completed by September 1989 and the trial is scheduled for December '89. I have applied for custody of Andy and I continue to provide a full-time home for him.

Through her lawyer Bruce Katz, Jane Anderson made allegations which led to restrictions on my eligibility for student loans. My lawyer had provided Ms. Dean MacLeod with information requested by her office regarding my previous student loans. In order to care for my son and myself, I found temporary work and applied for three related research grants which were all denied to me... Despite these difficulties I have continued to do well in my studies which I plan to continue full time at least until September '90. Without student loans I will be unable to continue my studies in the research and planning of family health services and housing in Vancouver.

* * *

DOUBTS HAD ACCUMULATED for a lot of reasons about Mary's ability to do the job. It had also come to light that Mary Murray worked as a counselor for the Corrections Branch of government. She was neither a Psychologist or Psychiatrist qualified to do a Custody and Access Report under Section 15 of the Family Relations Act of British Columbia. She, in fact, was a loose cannon somehow placed into a position of authority to decide Ken's son's fate. Even though Mary Murray had made promises to Ken that she would hand over the job to someone else if she could not do it, she hung on with a firm, steely grip.

Ken made frantic phone calls asking for a qualified person to take over. Everyone ignored his requests.

Mary soldiered on, disregarding Ken's professional knowledge of what kind of credentials were needed to do the custody and access report. She obviously had strong backing from somewhere.

One afternoon, for the home visit investigation in Daisy's home, Andy arrived with Ken. Mary then arrived. Though Daisy smiled and greeted her as a guest, Mary was unresponsive; her eyes were hard. She was not the person Daisy had fond memories of.

Andy had not been able to be in the home with his father or around the grandchildren for many months and was obviously delighted to be back. Mary watched Andy in the sunny kitchen while he painted pictures along with the grandchildren and ate and talked in a relaxed happy way. Mary wrote furiously in her notebook without revealing what secrets she was writing. Daisy had invited her into the inner sanctum of her home to experience the warmth of her precious grandchildren but had no idea what Mary was making of it. But seeing Andy so happy and well adjusted with Ken and the children made Daisy think Mary had to be writing about that.

While the children were busy with each other, Mary surprised Daisy by looking straight across the table into her eyes and said, "Jane is cold! No feeling! She doesn't keep any food in her fridge."

Confiding this kind of information struck Daisy as odd. She thought Mary might be enticing her to say something negative about Andy's mother. Instead, while she had Mary's attention, Daisy took the opportunity to explain to Mary in detail that she and Ken had met in another province twelve years prior to 1981, long before Jane had come into the picture; that Jane is spreading false information about them meeting as doctor/patient. Daisy reminded Mary that Ken, Jane and Daisy had lived as neighbors only a few feet apart in the same co-op while Ken was married to Jane and that Mary was fully aware of this because she also lived there at the same time. She reminded Mary that verification could be gotten that from the co-op administration office.

MARY DISREGARDED obviously provable truths. In her written report, she repeated Jane's blatant distortion of the truth, and stated that Daisy and Ken met in 1981 when she became his patient. That alone was proof that Mary was willing to commit perjury for her neighbor, Jane Anderson, by lying to Judge Scarth in a Court of Law.

During Mary's home visit, Andy had been visibly happy and relaxed being back with his father after being withheld for so long, and he was thoroughly having fun with the grandchildren. Of Andy's own volition, he had gotten on the telephone in the same room and only about four feet away from where Mary sat, and dialed the numbers by himself to inform his mother and the next babysitter that he was staying with his father for the night. Mary watched and heard Andy's refusal to leave.

Daisy had watched Mary scribbling notes as Mary watched and listened to Andy on the telephone.

Mary had assured Ken that she knew all about Parental Alienation Syndrome but in writing her report, she completely disregarded it. Mary disregarded the alienation of the child by the mother that was taking place right next door to her – the alienation that Ken had been complaining about daily. Instead, in her report, Mary recommended drastically reducing Ken's access to his son, completely disregarding the fact that Ken had been Andy's main caretaker since birth.

Mary had completely disregarded parental alienation and mind control. She disregarded the fact that this boy child was still trying to get close to the constantly disappearing mother and might say anything his mother told him to say in order to please her – something any novice should have picked up on.

Mary recommended that Andy never see his father with Daisy's family; that any access should be just Ken and Andy. Mary claimed Andy wanted nothing to do with Daisy or her family. She disregarded the fact that Andy insisted on staying the night on her visit to the home.

Regardless of Mary's promises to Ken, when she produced her written report, it was obvious she had clearly taken Jane's point of view in every aspect of the case and disregarded truth. Mary was clearly without a thought or opinion of her own about Andy, Ken or Daisy.

It was questionable about how Mary got the job in the first place. Now she had accomplished her mission with a damning finished written report ready for court.

KEN WROTE A REBUTTAL FOR MARY, giving her the chance to rethink and correct her myriad of mistakes.

Tuesday August 17th 1989 re Custody-Access Report:

1. David Sellars and Peter Swayne – confirm Andy's improvement in past school year due to my participation in his life at school. ...

McArthur (Jane's counselor) – has never met or seen me professionally, nor has he responded to my written and telephoned requests to speak with him regarding advice he gave Jane about Andy's care. Yet he supports Jane's statement that I harass her.

Stephen Schramm dates Jane regularly.

Gail Davidson and Leslie Baker: voice Jane's complaints vs. me without having seen or talked with me for more than one year.

#1 – does not mention: Janet Strickland's care of Andy 1980+. Jane was supported thru' 2-3 years of University as well as Law School. I had a half time family psychiatry practice so I could help with chores, Andy's care, and have time for study toward independence of Medical Services Plan as my sole employer and opportunities for becoming researcher.

#2 – I met Daisy in 1969 in Regina, Saskatchewan, not as a patient. I left the marriage because as I told Jane, May 13, 1981: "I am killing myself trying to live up to what I think are your expectations." I hoped that Jane would discuss this with me and we could live without an increasing demand by her for more "things". Since her years in law school, she had replaced me with her lawyer friends Leslie Baker and Gail Davidson, a nanny to care for Andy, and a gardener, urged me to seek sex outside the home, and removed my office from our home.

Under these pressures to care for her material-emotional needs, and later hers and Andy's, I experienced a series of health crisis which paralleled hers. ...[Ken's friend/former colleague] stayed with us during my first health crisis in False Creek. We then moved away from a damp basement of the Co-op to our first home in Dunbar where after we both began an exercise and Yoga program, we got pregnant and had Andy.

The closing down of my practice and bankruptcy were the direct result of assuming the debts of the divorce and my work to provide more than maintenance requirements and child care for Andy until Jane established her law practice. I supported Jane's work with Gail Davidson, even providing informal unpaid medical consultations to Gail and Jane re their legal cases. In turn, Jane advised me re: bankruptcy, student loans (and wrote our separation agreement to include shared guardianship of Andy, not just his estate).

Page 4 #2 – As explained to Mary, my work in Community Planning is a continuation of my studies begun before I met Jane where we were building a ranch community with 60 adults and 20 children. My small practice in Vancouver and move to False Creek Co-op, and tutoring in Chinese language, were all part of my effort to build a community of families as friends who would help each other raise our children.

Since 1967 when I came to Canada, I have worked to build a Farm School Community like the Peckham Family Health Centre in England. In 1982-83, I founded the Pioneer Health Centre (Vancouver) which was disastrous for me financially and emotionally but led to my becoming a Founder-Member of Pioneer Health Centre Canada 1986. My small family consulting practice, work at the Food Bank, and my studies at UBC, are all part of this project which began for me at Dartmouth College where I studied with Rosenstock-Huessy, a founder of the American Peace Corps idea in 1940. I am writing about his work, and Lewis Mumford, and the Peckham Experiment in my studies of family health planning in Vancouver.

Page 4 #3 – I supported Jane, Andy, and Janet Strickland through the articling and after through Jane's unemployment and further surgery and suicidal depressions. "I'm going to kill myself" was Andy's cry whenever he thought he could not do something his mother or he expected of him. Alternatively it was: "Jane's going to kill me." This statement resonates for me because I had nightmare Jane was going to kill herself or me before I left in 1981. She has alternately pushed Andy on me or held him ransom over the last 8 years, continuing the withholding pattern of our marriage where she controlled me by withholding love except for good behavior. This is all the more galling because in *the community where we lived together, Sidera's Place (MacLean's September 1970), we learned about love together as more basic than sex in a drug free working community which supported physical love only as part of marriage. She projects her instability and unpredictability onto me. I have paid maintenance regularly except for my bankruptcy when I was forbidden to do so, right up until September 1989, and when I could not pay money for maintenance or daycare, I provided full-time care of Andy while Jane worked. Often I did both! Jane also knows that it is not easy for me to provide family consultations when she and Bruce have so damaged my reputation and garnished my earnings. As a discharged bankrupt, I cannot borrow money except for student loans to re-establish my standing in Vancouver. My goals are obscured by Jane's effort to hide the fact I made my career choices so I could and can be available to Andy and meet his needs.*

#4 is a totally inadequate presentation of the reasons I asked for this investigation – I believe Andy's needs would be better met by my care, full-time, because I believe it is dangerous for him to live with Jane who farms him out to friends who then leave him alone, rather than allow me to care for him. A year ago when left alone with Robbie (child), he was severely burned because both boys were playing with the hot coals of a barbeque. I took care of him (while Jane worked) and helped him heal the burn on his foot.

I made it clear to Mary [Murray] that I am concerned about the way that Jane has alienated Andy from me over the past 10 years for her own emotional reasons. Even during this investigation, with regularly ordered access, she has continued to hold Andy hostage, reducing the hours I can see him to 2½ from 12 hours!

Daisy and I documented this process for Mary who refused to allow someone else in her office to mediate access because she thought she could do it. Andy's access to me is not dependent on his participation in Daisy's family – I often do things with him alone and have frequently lived separately from Daisy and her family.

TO HIS LAWYER, KEN WROTE:

> *I will review the details of this report further as needed. For now, I want to ask:*
>
> *What can we win and what can we lose by further legal action?*
>
> *Could we accomplish enforcement of the access order and lowering the interim maintenance by returning to court in September?*
>
> **Can we have an objective or at least professional evaluation by a psychiatrist or psychologist to put this report by Mary in context?**

* * *

KEN'S LAWYER ignored answering any questions.

MARY MURRAY ignored Ken's rebuttal.

* * *

IN COURT, Mary Murray made her appearance in front of Judge Scarth. The person who had seemed like the gentle, singing hippie sporting a guitar with friends interested in co-op housing and ecological farming, now showed up in court still looking like a hippy on the outside with her long flowered skirt, ill-fitting blouse topped by a jacket to bring a bit of formality to the outfit, and that loosely flowing red curly hair. Red hair! Red curly hair like Jane's red hair, same length, same style, same white skin—the resemblance was suddenly uncanny, except that Jane managed a neat look and Mary did not. Other than that, they looked like sisters.

Mary's appearance belied a clenched fist. In Mary's presentation to Judge Scarth, she made her intentions clear: that was to reduce drastically and as much as possible, Ken's ability to father his son, Andy, and to get rid of Daisy entirely. Mary gave absolutely nothing to Ken, completely ignoring his corrections. She backed up Jane's point of view entirely.

Even though Mary had spent hours with Andy and Ken, and watched Andy interact with Daisy and her grandchildren while he acted completely comfortable and refused to leave, she stated to the Judge that Andy told her that he did not want to spend time with Daisy and her family ever again. Mary had written in her report that she had read Daisy's letter regarding history of relationships and care of Andy, but at the same time Mary completely disregarded the provable truths even though she was under oath.

Mary emphasized that Andy must stay with his mother, not his father.

Then looking unsure of herself, not knowing where to look and not knowing where to put her feet as they crossed over each other, Mary slowly walked backward and tried to fain a bow to the Judge without tripping. Mary stole a peek at Ken but pretended not to look at him as she slithered backward out of the courtroom. A door slammed and the demolishment of a father was left in the courtroom.

Ken was stiff with shock as he grasped the reality of Mary's report to the Judge. Ken had poured his heart out only to have these women stomp all over him, tell lies, ignore provable truths, commit perjury and still they took the righteous road in court in front of Judge Scarth who looked hard as rocks.

JUDGE SCARTH ACCEPTED the opinions of a social worker without professional credentials to do the child custody report of this magnitude. Scarth did not speak with or examine the father at any time before making a permanent decision about the child's life. He reduced Ken's time with his son to Wednesday after school to 8 p.m. and Sunday 2 p.m. to 8 p.m.

In Affidavits, Jane had obvious trouble doing math regarding money she had received from Ken by various means. Money she did receive over and above ordered maintenance, she alleged that it was only for Ken's tax benefit that he gave it to her. Judge Scarth apparently believed her. He allowed no reduction in maintenance.

Judge Scarth accepted allegations made by Jane and Katz that Ken had hidden assets with Daisy even though he never spoke to Daisy or reviewed her assets. Scarth ignored Ken's real contribution of assets and maintenance given to Jane during separation and since divorce, and in child maintenance, childcare fees, and thousands of dollars in garnishments. Scarth ordered Ken to pay $21,700.00 to Jane and to sign the order immediately.

Judge Scarth completely ignored Ken's fatherly concerns about his child and his history of physically caring for his son. Instead, Scarth varied Ken's liberal access to Andy as had been outlined in the 1982 Decree Nisi, to two brief visits a week, no overnights.

Judge Scarth stated that he was unable to make a determination of whether or not Ken's conduct was "contumacious" because of conflicting Affidavit evidence and ordered a Trial to be held before him so that he could hear from the parties' witnesses in open court.

The only good news was that Judge Scarth had apparently peeked at Affidavits that were not brought to his attention in any Hearing. As a result, he wanted to hear from witnesses before the obstinate disobedient element could be decided. The fact that now there would be a Trial came as a shock after the harsh judgment already made. And for what purpose was a Trial being held when the Judge had already stolen a father's son from him, made a mess of the money situation and without proof accused Daisy and Ken of things they never did while ignoring things they did do? In other words, Judge Scarth had given Jane and Bruce Katz everything they seemed to want – except the one thing Katz had told Ken's lawyer he wanted, and that was to get rid of Ken entirely – in jail or out of the country. Ken had not been criminally charge by any law enforcement and had broken no law. What further punishment did Judge Scarth want to give and why? Why was Judge Scarth determined to carry this child custody and maintenance case to another level?

IN SHOCK over Mary's report and wanting to leave the courthouse, Daisy and Ken were in the hallway when their lawyer, the same guy who had been catatonic and pasted to his seat with his mouth pasted shut, was now in high gear, racing after them. His large black shoes flapped loudly on the stone floor while his coat tails trailed after him.

Out of breath after the chase, he called out, "You need to sign papers."

In Ken's quiet voice, he asked the lawyer why he had nothing to say in court.

The lawyer responded, "I was listening and learning."

Daisy confronted him, "Learning! You were just listening and learning? Why did you *not* have anything to say?"

The lawyer's face looked like a little boy caught with his pants down but had no answer.

"I guess you are afraid of Katz!" Daisy accused.

The lawyer just looked stupid in silent embarrassment. Then, like a little boy following orders with anxiety written in his face, he wanted Ken to sign papers without discussion.

Ken refused to sign on grounds that the ruling was made under false testimonies. The courts put the paper through without him.

BEING DUPED BY Mary Murray had been a shock. Ken and Daisy had ridden their bicycles to the Granville Island Market. Ken was busy choosing some vegetables as Daisy wandered a few feet away when she suddenly saw Mary Murray watching Ken from behind a vegetable stall. The observer was now being observed. Daisy's first instinct was of wanting to protect Ken from Mary's eyes. Mary's eyes were dark in a face like a frozen mask.

Since Mary completed her job and could no longer do harm, it was clear to Daisy that Mary was not looking at Ken, she was looking at damage she had done; her soul knew it and showed up in her face.

Daisy glanced over to Ken and when she looked back, Mary had disappeared into the crowd.

Opportunity missed? By pausing, Daisy missed an opportunity to confront Mary about what she did in court, but quickly decided that she did not have to do anything – Mary would reap her own harvest of karma and live her own future as she made it.

But... Mary Murray was not finished; she would surface again.

As Ken, innocently and out in the open, chose vegetables with absolutely no hidden agenda, there were people skulking around who belonged to a different human order. More than that, Daisy could see clearly how vulnerable a man like Ken is in a woman's world and she was more determined to try to protect him.

37

The Trial

THEIR LAWYER RAN AWAY. The last Ken and Daisy saw of him was when they arrived to receive another Affidavit late on a Friday afternoon and were planning to discuss the Trial looming in December. He had graduated to an upstairs office with a reception room. He acted strange as he shuffled papers around his desk with exaggerated movements, glancing up from his papers through an open door at Ken and Daisy several times, then ignoring them. They waited – and waited – until it seemed obvious that he hoped they would go away. Knowing there was another nasty Affidavit, they continued to wait. He could not escape his room without walking past them. He seemed to give up and quickly handed over the latest papers with no advice even though they asked, and he was never to be seen again. There was no explanation.

The only thing they knew about him was that he was an ill-fitting person in the cast of characters of this saga. He was a lawyer by day and a musician by night and weekends and his mind was on music and his new romantic interest, a vocalist who had recently separated from her physician husband. For some time, it had become an underlying concern to Daisy that the music venues he was known to play were tied to the same ethnicity as Katz and it was easy to imagine, whether true or not that the younger lawyer depended in some way on being in Katz' good books.

Ken and Daisy visited the head of the law firm, who told them in clear statements that the preceding lawyer had given Ken wrong advice when he said to not pay additional maintenance while the courts sort things out and that all the other things Ken had paid for and given to Jane one way or another, like after-school childcare, clothing, healthcare fees, prescriptions, bus passes and allowance given to Andy, totaling more than seven thousand dollars was not considered maintenance. Also, this lawyer now told Ken that the preceding lawyer should not have told Ken to stop billing MSP for seeing a couple of patients a week which had resulted in Ken seeing a family with children for free over several weeks rather than quit on them.

Once again, on the advise of a lawyer, Ken had been duped either by ignorance or purposeful intention. It was a question of whether the threats by Katz had anything to do with the lawyer's incorrect advice and then his disappearance from the case after severe damage. That would never be known but the result was that Ken would be compromised for the coming Trial.

The head of the law firm refused to finish the case regardless of the mess his younger lawyer left behind. He gave the reason that Ken had not enough money to hire him.

IT HAD BEEN YEARS of stress – years of an ex-wife's steady stream of abusive Affidavits and court appearances.

On Ken's two afternoons a week allowed by Judge Scarth, Ken continued attending Andy's school and meeting Andy after school for walks through the forest of Spirit Park. During one of the walks, Andy informed Ken that his mother did not want Ken involved at school. Andy asked Ken to stay away.

Torn between his son's fear of an angry mother and to stay away from the school, Ken chose to abide by his son's request and only attended parent/teacher conferences.

Jane had arranged for another neighbor, Marie Brooks to pick up Andy from school instead of allowing Ken to do so.

The relationship Ken and Andy had enjoyed was now reduced to rare hours after school, if at all, mainly to accompany his son to meet Jane where she often waited with a witness – like returning Andy to a Pizza parlor where girlfriend Gail Davidson waited with Jane.

The mystery to Ken was what could they possibly be witnessing. Daisy waited and watched from the street, also witnessing the delivery so that Ken could not be accused of wrongdoing or being late, but she could only wait and meet Ken afterward because Andy had been cut off from her and her grandchildren.

An earthquake had hit the father/son relationship because the son expressed fear of upsetting his mother. The infrequent and brief afternoon walks as father and son to a bus after school were better than not seeing his son at all. The craziness continued as they headed toward court again.

With the disappearance of his lawyer, Ken consulted a lawyer he knew in years past when Ken's work took him into the family court system. The older, experienced lawyer could not take the case himself because he was on the verge of being appointed as a Judge. He recommended a young woman, Marnie Dunnaway.

ANTICIPATING A NEW beginning, Ken and Daisy entered Marnie's office to find a woman with short blond hair sitting behind her desk. An open file was on her desk.

"Hello. I'm Ken Schramm and this is Daisy, my..."

"Daisy! Get out of my office!" Marnie shouted angrily, interrupting Ken.

Shocked and standing midway between the door and her desk, Ken and Daisy asked in unison, "Why?"

Marnie was livid, looking like a rabid animal, spewing at Daisy, "I don't like the Affidavit you wrote."

"I wrote the truth! I only wrote about what I have experienced."

"Get out! Get out of my office!"

Daisy left with her face burning, expecting Ken to come right out with her but he stayed. Daisy imagined he was taking time to calm the woman like he had done with Leslie Baker.

Outside, the day felt like it should be happy as the fresh air molecules filled with sunshine refreshed her burning skin, cooling it. She waited for Ken, pacing the concrete of the city – sitting, and pacing again. It was hard to believe what just happened. If ever there was a time for a cigarette, she decided this was it. She bought a pack at a corner store and ran back to smoke and wait.

Eventually he came out to sit beside her on the concrete. Now she stunk of smoke and knew he hated it.

"Ken, I am your best witness. Why would she eliminate me as a witness if she's working for you? There's something wrong here! And how did she get your file ahead of you? You hadn't even met her yet but she had a file on her desk!"

"She's been recommended by an older lawyer who is going to be a Judge – a man I trust. I have to rely on the Justice system to be fair and look after my child regardless of a fight between Jane and myself, or whether Marnie likes you or not. I expect the Judge to be fair and look after my child."

On one hand Ken made sense that the child was most important. On the other hand, Daisy felt impending doom. She tried again to convince Ken, "I think it's a set up. I think Marnie is not good for you. I think her sympathy is with Jane – not you! Even her age makes me think that."

"Daisy, I have to follow through with Marnie because she works for legal aid and I have no money. I'm just grateful she will take my case. I think she is doing it as a favor to Tom and I trust his judgment."

Ken continued to believe it was all about the care of his child and he was not advised otherwise.

REGARDLESS OF JUDGE SCARTH writing in his Reasons for Judgment that this trial should be held in front of him in open Court with witnesses of both parties because of conflicting Affidavit evidence, the case was suddenly in front of Judge H.A.D. Oliver.

It was a mystery as to the reason for Judge Oliver suddenly taking over Judge Scarth's case. Always looking for something bright to hold on to, Ken smiled as he told Daisy that he thought the Judge looked like Rumpel in the made-for-television detective stories. Always wanting to believe people to have a core of goodness, Ken tried to convince Daisy that a man looking like Rumpel would be fair and most importantly, that he would look after Andy.

Daisy thought Ken simply fantasized that Rumpel would be fair and good – just like Ken, always putting a positive take on everything! And he was still under the illusion that it was all about his child. He had not understood that this trial had nothing to do with his child but had been escalated to criminal status and Marnie had not corrected him.

Then Ken told Daisy that Jane's friend Leslie Baker had worked in Oliver's office.

"You mean she *articled* in his office?"

"Yes."

"Well, isn't that a conflict of interest? That makes me not trust Oliver!" Daisy continued complaining, "A handpicked Judge? In fact, if Leslie articled in his office, and considering the closeness of the three girlfriends, a social connection to Jane is not out of question. Of all the many Judges in this large city, I wonder how someone so close to these women has been chosen to do this Trial. It smacks of another Mary Murray story."

"I want to trust the judicial system to look after my son regardless of the players."

DURING THE FIRST day of the trial, Ken who was always the physician, was now concerned about his pregnant lawyer. At day's end, he spent his own money, even though he had next to none, on expensive good quality vitamins and minerals for her.

Daisy asked, "Why? Why would you spend money on Marnie?"

"I'm a physician. I don't need any other reason. But she is working for Legal Aid to represent me and they pay very little. I talked with her about her health and I thought the least I could do is get her proper vitamins and minerals for a healthy pregnancy."

"Ken, I know you mean well, but at least you could wait and see how she does represent you."

"I'm a physician. I saw a need."

"I know... I know."

THEN THINGS WENT BADLY! Everything that Ken produced was turned upside down and disregarded. The doctor, who had prescribed medications and taken Ken's blood pressure for years, provided a file to Katz that deleted all blood pressure notes. It was a false medical file presented as evidence.

Daisy could not help but wonder about cultural ties that bind... she did not want to think what she was thinking... that even a physician could be persuaded.

During a break while waiting in the lounge area, Daisy saw a woman who at one time was married to her musician friend. This woman had eaten dinner in Daisy's home during a musical evening. By her clothing and sleuthing around the hall with lawyers, it was obvious she had become a lawyer. She spotted Daisy, who assumed the woman was coming to say hello as her long legs galloped in her direction. Daisy smiled, eager to greet her but the tall, gangly woman suddenly veered off awkwardly to talk with Katz and Jane. Within earshot, she wanted to know what was going on. Katz had the opportunity to tell his nasty version of why they were in court while Daisy and Ken could hear and obviously would be insulted.

In amazement, Daisy watched the woman, who used to be sweet and shy but now had taken on the persona of a black vulture who would do anything to be part of the scene, making friends in a social climb.

The woman turned away after talking with Katz. She seemed satisfied and pretended not to have seen Daisy.

How strangely awful! Daisy thought. She knew the woman could not have forgotten who she was. Daisy had made an East Indian dinner from her cookbook and where the soup called for farm cheese, she had put in the wrong cheese, so they had string soup along with a lot of laughter between sessions of playing musical instruments. Daisy thought about her conversation a few months ago with this woman's husband when they met on the skating rink with their kids. He had divorced her and had laughed when he explained to Daisy that he hired the dirtiest lawyer he could find to deal with her. This had all come as a surprise because Daisy could not understand why he would need to hire a dirty lawyer to deal with the sweet woman. Now the conversation with the ex-husband made a bit of sense.

AFTER A WEEK of court, Ken emerged from a severe beating and denouncement while Jane emerged completely victorious again. It had been like a housewarming party of lawyers and Judge with Mary Murray and another neighbor, Marie, joining the party. The outcasts were Ken and the discredited doctor who dared to be a witness for Ken, and Daisy who was never allowed to testify.

Ken was told he owed thousands of dollars to Jane. He came away with a clear understanding that he had been told by the Judge to take allopathic blood pressure medicine and get back to work as a physician because he had no health problem.

Bruce Katz immediately held a press conference, publicly crowning himself as a winning lawyer.

OUTSIDE THE COURTHOUSE, Daisy asked, "Ken, do you understand now that Jane is behind all this? I saw her take the $1,800 cheque as advance payment for Andy at a time when you cared for him six days of every week. Ken, I saw her face when she took that cheque in her hands; there's no way she forgot. I was witness to Jane leading you down a garden path to destroy you. Not only that, she sent you to her friend who charged you five hundred dollars and he gave you wrong advice and said you don't need to pay maintenance during bankruptcy. She didn't tell you the law even though she's a lawyer and you repeatedly followed her advice and even asked in writing for her advice."

Ken was distraught. "I heard Jane lie in a court of law. She denied receiving the eighteen hundred dollars. It was only when I produced the cheque that was cashed by her that she admitted it and claimed she "forgot". I thought the Judge would take care of my child regardless of the parents' feud, but that has not happened. Instead of figuring out what would be best for our child and at least coming somewhere down the middle, he took one side only. A black and white decision."

Daisy knew that her anger was the last thing Ken needed right now, but she needed to spout off. "Jane is a lawyer telling the court to believe her because she is an officer of the courts and she tells lies – not only in Affidavits but under oath *in court*! How can she forget a cheque so large? How come she wasn't charged with perjury? Instead, the Judge completely overlooked it. And how can she deny that you looked after Andy the way you did? I was witness to all that. Your lawyer did not defend you."

"I apologized to Jane for any hurt I caused her. I apologized publicly in court."

"You did nothing wrong to apologize for. Nothing at all! Even when you were ill in bed, you looked after Andy. And Jane knows that! We all know that! But you weren't allowed any witnesses. Marnie even managed to discredit your doctor, your only witness."

Ken's sympathy was evident again, "If Jane thinks she needs an apology, she got it."

"Jane does not deserve an apology! I believe she framed you out of vengeance with the intention of making you into a criminal because she lost her control of you and her prestige as a doctor's wife. She worked at ruining your relationship with your sons and your mother and brother. That woman is not deserving of you or the child she has. I keep wondering why the universe gives such a beautiful child to such a person."

The painful look on Ken's face stopped her. Daisy realized once again that to continue down this road was destructive. Regardless of all the care he gave Jane and Andy with good intentions, his ex-wife had destroyed him in a public arena.

Daisy changed course. "Ken, it's against the law for any lay person to diagnose illness and suggest treatment, yet in court, Judges and lawyers do it all the time without having any training or knowledge of medicine. But if a person were brought into court for doing what they do, they would have the law thrown at them – like midwives who have more training than they do. What does that say about our judicial system and the rights of the public?"

Ken acknowledged her statement. "That's why medical files in court are so dangerous. They go through interpretations by any lawyer or Judge, not to mention the first interpretation written by physicians or nurses who made entries into the file. In my case, the doctor rewrote the file that my ex-wife and her lawyer brought into court."

"I know. I saw the original file. I think there is more to social connections here, too, than we know. I'd be willing to bet on that. The lawyer who ran away plus the doctor who produced this thin rewritten file and Katz have obvious cultural connections. There is no question about that. On top of that there is the long-time connection of the three girlfriends and this Judge. And then there is Marnie Dunnaway who refused to follow Judge Scarth's orders to hear from your witnesses."

THAT EVENING while Daisy was in a lineup to pay for groceries, she was suddenly aware of a shocking front-page newspaper article staring back at her. The evening newspaper blazed their names in a story about a physician and his paramour refusing to pay child maintenance to a poor single mother and child along with a story to falsely lead readers to believe that Ken and Daisy were milking the system by taking money from several sources all at once.

It was a shock to learn the extent of maliciousness. If she could see this, then so could many thousands of other people. Daisy picked up a heavy pile of newspapers, intending to buy them all but then realized that this was only one store. She could see through the store windows to many shops lining the street. She could not buy all the newspapers on the block, let alone the whole province or stop the papers going onto airplanes, heading to other provinces. Her worst nightmare was to go home and tell Ken.

BLOOD RAN FROM his face. With Daisy at his side, Ken immediately telephoned Marnie Dunnaway at her home. "Have you seen the front page story in the newspaper tonight? ...Why would my loss in court be on the front page of a newspaper?"

Marnie answered. "You were found guilty. It doesn't matter anyway. It's only a game!"

The telephone conversation ended there. Ken hung up the phone. He turned to Daisy in disbelief. "She said 'It's only a game'!"

"I heard her! Your life is wrecked but to lawyers it's only a game! Now I know why Jane did all this under her married name and not the maiden name Anderson she uses in practicing law. Obviously she or Katz called the newspapers. They are doing this to totally ruin your reputation. Why else would a journalist be bothered about child maintenance?"

Ken looked sick with the realization that his reputation was smeared not only in law libraries but also on the streets and in private homes of the general public – to everyone.

Another article clearly telling of an interview with Katz was printed the following morning in the weekend paper with a high readership. As a result of Katz' interview, Ken was made out to be a criminal. The interview had the public assuming the woman was just a penniless mother left alone with a child. The articles failed to mention the poor mother he was talking about was in fact a full-fledged lawyer working in Katz' office and in fact on his letterhead.

"Ken, I wonder if Jane realizes that she is attacking her own son by smearing the name of his father. That is also Andy's name and the name of your other sons, including Stephen. How could she not understand how this will impact her son? And what about the larger family... like your mother? She is obviously only thinking of herself and does not understand that her son is growing up in a hateful environment."

"Such revenge is self serving."

"I think she has lost touch with what kind of man she will raise. He won't always be a child."

"I've heard her say, she expects her son to support her in her old age."

"Oh! Right! I wonder if that's why she had him. He is a support system from his babyhood to his old age."

* * *

STATEMENT in Judge Oliver's Reasons for Judgment:
> ... Wherever the evidence of Dr. Schramm conflicts with that of not only Miss Anderson but of any other witness I accept the evidence of such other witness in preference to that of Dr. Schramm. ...

Regardless of hard evidence, proven in front of Judge Oliver, that Miss Anderson was less than truthful in her testimony about receiving certain money, which in any other case could be viewed as perjury, Judge Oliver brazenly shielded her by writing such a statement in his Reasons for Judgment.

With a pen as his weapon, a little old man in a black robe, abused the power society trusted to him to carry out Justice for all by scribbling statements that completely wiped out the life of a man as it had been lived. In writing his Reasons for Judgment for history, Judge H.A.D. Oliver proceeded to make up his own version of truth, including making up medical advice, to destroy Ken's life in keeping with and carrying out the vengeful agenda of ex-wife and lawyer Jane Anderson, and her lawyer partner, Bruce Katz.

Even though Jane had admitted in court that Ken had high blood pressure when she met him, and she knew that it was uncontrolled by allopathic medication, in his Reasons for Judgment, Oliver wrote about Ken's health:

> ...I find that three and a half years ago Dr. Schramm suffered from elevated blood pressure (as do a great many other people). I find that this is a condition which in the majority of cases can be successfully treated or controlled by medical means and by the use of appropriate medication. ... High blood pressure is a condition which in the majority of cases can be cured or adequately controlled. If medication was required to reduce the respondent's blood pressure, then the failure to take that medication was due to the deliberate act of the respondent. ...

Oliver accused Ken in one paragraph of causing his own illness because of complimentary medicine versus allopathic medicine, and in another he wrote:

> ...I am not satisfied on a balance of probabilities that the respondent was ever disabled from working as a physician either on a full-time or a part-time basis and I am certainly not satisfied of the existence of any such disability at the present time. ...

THE RESULT of the court case was that Judge Oliver did not accept any evidence that Ken had any health concern, nor that he ever did any childcare. Oliver did not acknowledge that Ken ever cared for his ex-wife and child financially. Oliver stated that Jane was only a student when Ken left the marriage, inferring that Ken had left her destitute. Judge Oliver did not acknowledge assets Jane received during separation and divorce, or years of maintenance paid in excess of a court order following divorce. Oliver was determined to ignore everything that Ken gave to Jane and the child of the marriage; instead Oliver painted Ken as a criminal in his Reasons for Judgment.

Oliver went on to accuse Ken of deliberately lying when he filled out forms following Jane's advice, and regardless that Ken's handwriting on student loan forms clearly stated that the matter of child custody and care was before the courts.

Judge H.A.D. Oliver expressed excessive nastiness in writing his Reasons for Judgment. It read like a personal attack.

Ken was ordered to pay all court costs and Jane's legal costs as though she did not work with Katz. Also Ken was ordered to pay back maintenance that conveniently left out thousands of dollars Ken did pay directly to Jane and to daycare, etc. Total damage: Twenty-six thousand and thirteen dollars and six cents. The total had escalated from the $21,700 that Judge Scarth had written. The alternative to paying would possibly be to go to jail as punishment. A sentencing date was set in case Ken did not pay before then. Katz may finally get his wish.

Oliver did reduce future maintenance monthly payments to $350 from $500 and access to Ken's son was further reduced to only three hours two afternoons a week.

Justice and fairness was proven to be a Canadian farce.

When disaster strikes, it sometimes is the small things that provide comedy. In this case it was how six cents got calculated onto such a large sum of money. Jane and Bruce Katz would be able to laugh all the way to the bank with six cents and thirteen dollars along with twenty-six thousand dollars.

Jane and Katz wasted no time. Somehow, with no explanation, they inflated the Judgment figure. A letter to Ken dated December 3, 1990, written by H.A. Massey at Vancouver City Savings Credit Union stated that every last penny had been cleaned out of

Ken's accounts on behalf of a Notice to Garnishee by Plaintiff: Carol Jane Schramm and made out by Bruce Katz. It was another garnish in about a year. Not one penny of a living allowance just before Christmas had been allowed for Ken in the process. The letter stated that on the basis of the Judgment, Katz wanted to garnishee $28,082.45 and the credit union was charging another $50.00 processing fee.

Daisy's family was so shocked and incensed at what happened to Ken and knowing he would go to jail without the exact money ordered in Trial, they arranged for him to have money. On January 11, 1991 he made out a cheque to Katz & Company in Trust for the exact amount of $26,013.06 as Judge Oliver ordered. The garnished moneys simply disappeared again. Through Garnishments more than eight thousand dollars just disappeared.

Through the many court hearings, eventual trial and a progression of Judges, Ken was falsely found guilty of hiding his assets with Daisy even though she was never questioned by any Judge and there was no evidence that she was hiding Ken's assets. At no time was Ken given credit for assets and money he gave to Jane that amounted to many tens of thousands of dollars over and above child maintenance.

THINKING THERE WAS enough that went wrong in this case and clearly without a trusted lawyer to give further legal advice, Ken and Daisy had gone to the legal assistance office with Judge Oliver's Reasons for Judgment to ask for an Appeal. The young man standing at the desk first noted the names involved. He disappeared behind brown doors for about ten seconds and came back flipping his hair with one hand. Then standing firm behind the desk, he declared there had been no error and "No Appeal".

"KEN, I'VE BEEN THINKING." Daisy interrupted Ken's thoughts. They were in the solitude of home, sitting in the living room trying to watch television but really digesting the days just gone by.

"We need to get some perspective on this. Let's put this all together and analyze what has happened to you. Ken, I need you to listen to me all the way through... so that I can get to my point.

I think something has come really clear." Daisy paused... and then started in.

"There are some women who are masters of the masquerade and they expect they can change the man they marry. Men, on the other hand get surprised when the person they thought they married turns into someone they don't recognize. The change the woman wants in her man turns into war when he stays the same. In my opinion, this happened to you. You entered into a marriage with the best of intentions and you believed you could trust the person you took as a partner in life. Very soon, you didn't recognize her and you stayed the same. You believe in a good education so you worked and paid for a high school educated woman to go through university to become a lawyer. You thought you had an understanding with her that once she became a lawyer, you would take your turn and finish the PhD you started back in New England and that you would teach again instead of doing the frontline medicine that supported her education. Well, she became a lawyer and used her legal expertise to destroy you instead of keeping her promise. It's not your fault that she used what you gave her for destruction instead of construction. That was her choice entirely.

"When a man is told to find sex elsewhere, that is destruction of marriage. You were caught in a trap. You separated from her within your own house long before you left the home. You repeatedly tried to reconcile with the help of therapists but she rejected you over and over... and over... and over.

"In separation and divorce, you wanted Jane to have a secure base for herself and your son. Assets and debts of a marriage are usually legally split down the middle. Instead of doing that, you chose to give Jane all the assets... every last penny, and you took all the debts and your part-time medical practice... part-time because you were also looking after her and your child. You were in a shared rental office so your medical practice consisted of nothing but clients and your own training. She couldn't take your practice simply because you spent many years training to be the doctor you are and she is not a doctor. She had a professional career that she didn't have before she married you.

"In law school, unknown to you at the time, but according to what was told to us by a lawyer, she had a reputation of being the rich doctor's wife, showing off in her BMW. She had two close friends from law school. You put out your energy to help all three women in various ways.

"I saw Leslie in action when we delivered Andy to her house. She had a choice about how to treat you; after all, you were doing the women a favor by delivering your child to Leslie regardless that neither you or Andy wanted to go there, but she did not see that. Leslie chose to take the road of brazen attack on you in front of children. You still managed to stay calm and friendly. I saw that and I was appalled but it gave me a first-hand picture of what you had been experiencing with those women.

When I came into the picture after your separation from Jane, I was secure within my own life. I had a job and my own income. I had a family and secure housing. I was doing well enough to be able to support my children and even my daughter in the Winnipeg Ballet School. I certainly did not need anything more. You were simply a bonus for me... a bonus of love. You, the man... is all I wanted.

"Even after leaving the marriage, you continued to pay the mortgage on the house until she sold it years later and you gave her the large profit. What did she net? Thirty thousand or more... all for her? I don't know the exact figure and never cared to know. You even kept the outstanding debt of the money borrowed for the down payment on the house instead of having it paid off out of the thousands she made on the house, and you paid a lawyer's fee to have it sold. You paid a nanny to continue looking after the child and when the nanny was off duty, you took over childcare and helped Jane complete her articling to become a full-fledged lawyer. And not only that, she was allowed to rack up your shared credit cards to the limit long after your separation. In other words, she had almost limitless money to live on while you were paying for it all. On top of that, you paid her extra money in large sums every time she squeaked, was ill or unemployed until you became too ill.

"All you asked for in return was shared parenting of your son and you believed you had that. But, she used your child as a pawn instead of... Oh well, I won't say more about that. Some things are too disgusting to me.

"And the other woman... me. I tried to help. So did my family. You and I thought getting rid of me was her goal but she rejected you so many times that it looked like revenge was the real goal. But for what? That has been the question since she did not want you. I am guessing it was punishment for taking away her right to control you and for losing her status as a doctor's wife, unless meanness is just her true nature.

"You insisted on trusting her because she is the mother of your child... your family, as you said, regardless of divorce. You were completely open with her and she gave you legal advice. You consulted with Jane about all matters and believed that sharing complete information about your life was good for shared parenting.

"When you became ill, you consulted with her about your finances, including bankruptcy and all steps along the way, and student loans. She and her friends advised you about how to do it all.

"Meanwhile, Jane gave up care of Andy to you pretty much full time for years.

"You have many... and I mean many witnesses to all that plus a paper trail about the assets and debts and who got what in the separation and divorce legal papers.

"Then, when bankruptcy ended, she began the vicious trail of harassment by sending weekend Affidavits full of stories that turned all your good deeds upside down by denying that you did any of them. She encouraged you for two whole years to pay for things you believed to be maintenance in good faith and she knew all along that legally this was a garden path to destroy you by then claiming you paid nothing and did no childcare. Regardless of all the witnesses to the contrary, she didn't mind denying the childcare you did and money you gave her. She resorted to calling you names and even denied that you had a health problem. She had her girlfriends believing that she was doing childcare when in fact she wasn't. We know that by the Affidavits they wrote. Oh, I almost forgot, she tried to turn your oldest son against you and had him feeling sorry for her as a financially destitute victim left to be on her own with a child. That was another clue she was playing a game of hide and seek with people by hiding what you were doing.

"Ken, I think it takes a very distorted person to deny all that I have just stated with as many witnesses around as you have and be brazen enough to go to court and tell her version to a Judge and not be afraid of perjury. I believe that is why they needed to change Judges and deny you any witnesses.

"We started with Judge Boyde. For some reason, unknown to us, we found ourselves in Judge Scarth's courtroom. Scarth, in the end, was not one bit sympathetic to you as a father but sided with Jane one hundred percent. He never spoke with you and that seems unconscionable in a child custody case. I thought all child custody cases required a Judge to speak to the parent involved. You had a lawyer who sat on his hands after being threatened. He advised you, and later his boss told you that his advice was completely wrong. He did not defend you. He just sat there and let them run you down.

"You asked for a child custody report because of Jane's distortions and games around your son. You suggested a particular competent and well-experienced psychologist that you knew did good work for children, after which they brought up his name in court and your own lawyer suddenly got some life and jumped up to refuse the custody investigation be done by him. That was about the only time he had some life in court.

"Then, Jane's close neighbor, Mary Murray, another single mother with a son the age of Andy, is suddenly on the case. And Mary is a social worker, working as a counselor for the Correction Branch of government. *Correction?* What on earth does corrections have to do with child custody? She is not a qualified psychologist like the man you wanted to do the custody investigation. At the time I didn't think to ask about her qualifications or where she works. We were duped. In a visit to my house, I watched Mary closely. She saw and heard Andy's extreme excitement about wanting to stay overnight with you and with the grandchildren after being kept away from you for a long time, yet in her report she denied that Andy wanted to see you or us. Mary parroted Jane to the point of also denying what could be easily proven, like the fact that you and I lived as neighbors in False Creek and she knew it. She parroted Jane and wrote that we met when I was your patient. Because of Mary's report, you lost in court with Judge Scarth and your liberal access to your son and almost full time parenting was reduced so drastically that with our bus service, it is hardly more time than a bus ride.

"I am to blame for the disaster of allowing Mary Murray to do the custody report. You asked me about her and I gave the go-ahead. But when she came to the house, I greeted her at the door and I looked into her eyes and saw that she was darkly unemotional and blocked. Her eyes sent a shiver through me. I should have confronted her right then but I didn't. I continued to believe in goodness and honesty but there was none there. I ignored what her soul was telling me through her eyes where she could not hide. And because I was so positive, we didn't even think to question her credentials or how she got the job. When you did, you found out that Mary had been locked into the case regardless of her early promises to you. I am so sorry.

"But... here's the crunch. At least Judge Scarth wrote that he couldn't make a decision about some things because of the conflicting Affidavit information. He ordered an open court trial be held in front of him because he wanted to hear from witnesses for both sides. That at least gave us hope of some fairness. In hindsight, the question is whether or not Scarth would have been fair or was a Trial an excuse to punish you more harshly than he already had done on behalf of fellow officers of the courts, Jane and Katz.

"Instead of Judge Scarth, suddenly, the case is in front of Judge Oliver who has a personal connection to Jane and her close friends. Leslie Baker has involved herself in this case and Leslie articled in Oliver's office when he was a lawyer. He only became a Judge about three or four years ago. It looks very suspicious about how he got this case. He covers his ass by writing that Judge Scarth had not seized the contempt proceedings, which means he could grab it.

"He sided with Jane regardless of her lying in court right in front of him about the eighteen hundred dollars you gave her for child maintenance. When confronted with the cheque that she had cashed, she claimed to have forgotten receiving it. There's no way she could have forgotten. She had been reminded of it a few times in Affidavits you wrote; yet she denied ever receiving it. Judge Oliver deliberately ignored that and regardless of hard evidence, wrote that he would only believe Jane in conflicts with you.

"When you brought in calendars logging your long hours and days of caring for Andy, Katz disputed them even though he had no first hand knowledge.

"Jane signed the paper about the hours you did do childcare and in fact you did more than the paper stated, but in court she claimed she, who is a lawyer, signed a false paper under duress. What duress? You were doing the childcare and paying her lots of money. She had no trouble denying the truth even though there were many witnesses to the hours Andy was in your care. Oliver ignored the calendars and the signed paper and your childcare.

"Your lawyer did not allow you any witnesses for anything except for one, a homeopathic physician. Marnie ruined your only witness's testimony in the hallway in front of people by telling him what to say on the stand. Informed about this breach of conduct right away, Judge Oliver discredited your doctor's testimony. The fact that Marnie made this very basic legal mistake makes me believe that it was done deliberately. Or was she just that stupid? Also, Oliver is ignorant of Homeopathic examining criteria.

"In his Reasons for Judgment, Oliver used the name of a doctor from 1973, someone you had seen 16 years ago, and Oliver stated that there was no medical information from him. As a Judge, he should know that the obligation to keep medical records is limited to seven years. Then in his Reasons for Judgment, Oliver conveniently left out any mention of the more recent doctor that provided Katz and the court with a false medical file. I wonder why. I witnessed this same doctor taking your blood pressure in 1981. At that time, I saw this doctor get agitated, expressing concern about your health and extremely high blood pressure, then writing about it in a thick file. But he sent a false file to court that eliminated any mention of high blood pressure or health concerns. I believe Oliver was concerned that maybe it could be proven as an error so he simply left that doctor's file out of his written judgment.

"Oliver decided he knew more about your health than you or any doctor and without any true knowledge, he threw out any claim to ill health. Oliver who is a lawyer/judge, not a physician, claims to know how to treat high blood pressure and he gives written medical advice on how to treat it without recognizing any other health issues or side effects. That alone, is unconscionable.

"Oliver says that Jane was only a student when you left her, inferring that she was a destitute victim struggling on her own to finish school. I bet back in those years while her friend Leslie was working in Oliver's office, that is exactly what Jane and Leslie were telling him. Oliver refused to acknowledge your generous care of Jane and Andy over the years before or after divorce. Instead, Oliver accuses you of having transferred your assets to me, regardless of the hard copies of legal papers outlining that all your assets went to Jane just seven years prior... actually only five or six years when the house was sold... while you had taken all the debts and acquired no new assets since then. Oh yes, the car that you gave me. Oliver writes about a car. Jane continues to bellyache about a ten-year old car that has gone to car heaven, and was given to me *seven years ago* when you quit driving because of high blood pressure and fear of a stroke behind the wheel, and as pay for a lot of volunteer work I did with you for no pay. *Jane had your BMW and didn't need the much cheaper car.* Oliver actually writes about that car as if it is a present day asset hidden with me. And even though you had been under extreme financial scrutiny by several different professional authorities, he decided you were hiding money with me with absolutely no evidence.

"Regardless of the intense financial scrutiny you were under, Jane and Katz went to great lengths to distort your financial picture, giving the picture that you had played all sources of income at the same time instead of being spread out over years and were completely separate from each other. And according to them, while under this intense scrutiny, you were supposedly hiding money and assets with me. They accused you of deliberately lying when you filled out forms regarding parenting even though Jane had advised you every step of the way. Absolutely no credit is given for the things you paid for each month with her concurrence. You were not given credit for the physical care of your son. They just denied you ever did anything.

"Also... and this is an important flaw your lawyers should have helped you with but did not... Jane and Katz showed your divorce papers in court. It was the Separation Agreement that had the details about Jane receiving all the assets of the marriage, which were substantial, while you kept only and all the debts. The Separation Agreement should have been produced in court to counter claims that you left her destitute and then hid assets.

"Oliver mentions accepting Mary Murray's statement and Jane's other neighbor, housekeeper Marie Brooks. Conveniently, lawyers Leslie and Gail, the friends involved in the case suddenly don't exist, so I suspect there was a deliberate covered up of Oliver's personal connection to Jane and her girlfriends.

"You thought you were going to court about the care of your child and trusted Oliver to be concerned about your child. It appears it was only a ruse to get revenge and Oliver had to be in on it. Judge Scarth had already designated money and custody of the child, so all that was left for trial was revenge. In hopes that justice would be honest and fair and your honest belief that there is some good seed somewhere inside every person, you forgot the fact that the agenda was to make you look like a criminal. As a seasoned criminal defense lawyer, Oliver knows exactly what to do to make someone look like a criminal from the bench of a Judge. You lost this court case before you started."

Ken looked sick as he listened.

"Thanks for listening to all this; here's the crux of what I'm getting to. Judge Scarth was replace by Judge Oliver. I think that Jane and her friends got nervous about you being able to call in witnesses. I think in view of that, they found a Judge who would side with Jane no matter what she did and not question her about perjury... a Judge where there would not be a middle ground or weighing of facts. Oliver was so one sided that he stated that he would not accept any truth from you; he would accept their statements as the only truth regardless of papers that proved otherwise.

"Oliver might be believable if he had at least taken a little from each side and tried to look unbiased. He didn't do that. He's supposed to be a man of justice. Your biggest worry, the wellbeing of your son, was ignored while they took revenge on the child's father. You were surprised to find yourself in front of Judge Oliver who you knew had a personal relationship with the three women. In the end, Oliver called you a few awful names but there are names for people like them. I'll refrain.

"A pathetic old man sacrificed the oath he had taken to uphold justice and instead used his pen as a weapon to rewrite the truth of your life. He made up his own version of your life to satisfy a sick agenda of your ex-wife and her pal Katz. They all think they got away with it."

Ken was still and silent, deep in thought. Sadness was overwhelming. His heart hurt.

"I need to go on," Daisy interrupted the silence in the room. "I have a story to tell you." She waited for silence to give permission to continue. "When I went to live on the Buddhist meditation centre, it was new. There was another couple, also founding members; they had a twelve-year old daughter who was used to her parents doting on her as an only child, but now they had found something else to involve much of their time in. The daughter arrived early on a Saturday morning with her parents and decided to take her resentment out on our teacher, so she found a piece of charcoal and went around the fields writing insults about him on several large rocks. Then she came back to our main cabin and found an old bicycle. She rode it down the country dirt road and about a half mile away there was a downward hill; her bike sped up. She had no brakes. She missed a bend in the road and was thrown through the air into the ditch beside bushes. Her wrist hit a rock. The very same wrist that only an hour before had written on rocks, was broken.

"I have seen Karma work and this is one time it happened fast for us all to see. Mostly, it takes time and we who have wondered about it, never see the outcome. Karma... no matter how or where, comes back to the thrower like a boomerang... and it will... I don't even have to wish it... and we don't even have to guess... it is the owners to own.

"Ken, when a baby is born and dies young, it really has no time to chalk up bad karma in the brief lifetime. Sometimes, the soul has come to teach the parents a lesson. Sometimes, in their grief they are forced into a reality check. They become aware of a higher power... where there is more to life than material goods and greed.

"What has this all got to do with you? Here's how I experience you. You were born as a miracle, recovering from what might have been a devastatingly crippled life. The physician who operated on you had nothing but an anatomy book to go by, yet his hands managed to make you whole as though a higher power guided him. You lived your whole life as a healer and a teacher. You lived with an open heart to everyone else's pain and sorrows. You gave of yourself completely to caring for others. I have never seen you waver in that... ever! Watching you for all these years, I believe you have been born so that others might work out their worst selves and somehow learn about themselves. You are a teacher of souls. You have sacrificed yourself completely. You have always been kind and caring and taught that, regardless of the cruelty and lies and greed you have met. And you live extremely frugally, giving everything away, never keeping for yourself material goods other than books. And even books, you keep giving away to those in need.

"Jane and Andy were beneficiaries of your unwavering generosity. It is not your fault that she did not know what to do with all you gave her. A desperate little boy wants to believe his own mother. It's not your fault she suffers greed, a common fault of the human race. It's not your fault your ex-wife acts like a bully with a gang of followers who waste their lives by bullying one kid on the school playground. Many people got on her bandwagon and helped her act out the way she did.

"You dared to be different and stand by your ethics... and not give up or give in when meeting adversity. What is so sad from my point of view is that I have watched you trying to do good work for humanity. But I have watched this woman act like a vulture to eat you up. She consumed your energy every way she could, leaving not enough left over for your work. I saw your health deteriorate. You got sick."

Ken remained silent, needing a few minutes to reflect on the perspective he just heard.

"I have a little more to say." Daisy waited until Ken seemed to be ready. His eyes were sad as his gaze moved from looking upward into space and back to her.

"I can't help remembering your brother telling you that Jane will outsmart you. The way I see this story is that Jane has used her intelligence to plot a real life kind of murder mystery. You have been the intended victim. The way I see it, she knew about your heart condition and you were meant to mysteriously die or disappear under her relentless war and her intentions would never be found out. Along the way, her lawyer announced intentions to get rid of you one way or another, so we know there was a definite plot. Over many years she mastered the art of drawing you in and pushing you away and drawing you in and pushing you away. Each time she drew you in, she tightened the noose a little tighter as you relaxed into thinking you were building a relationship with her for the sake of your son.

"The cast of characters is interesting to say the least. Jane was the lead player. It all started with her and the play was about her. She arranged the actors to be her helpers. Friends were used to drive you away. Your oldest son was used to hurt you emotionally. Your youngest son was used as a pawn to continually draw you back in and to control you. She used herself as the mother of your son, to act as your advisor about what to do and how to fill out papers. Because she is the mother of your son, you wanted to trust her. When she knew she finally had you trapped in a snare that she had secretly set up, she went for the kill by using the legal system that appears to be easily manipulated and that she knows something about. And by using people working the legal system who were puppets whether they knew it or not... old friends dressed in black that included a made for TV kind of Judge, a neighbor still looking like she should be in a van with Peace written all over it but that belies who she really is, and a work partner that I can't even imagine any woman wanting to be near but she manages to be close to and flaunts to her son... all puppets on strings doing her dirty work for her. I have watched her sit back in court and almost laugh as others worked her dirt.

"However, I think the ending of the story is not exactly what she intended because you are still alive! You are not in jail because my family won't let that happen to you. And because of your determination to stay with your children, you have not fled the country. I believe that she did not count on my determination to stand by you no matter what. I think that is why over her birthday dinner she questioned you about the endurance of our relationship regardless of the difficulties.

"I remember when you gave her the eighteen hundred dollars for child maintenance and she was so cold... not saying anything. I believe that you surprised her with something that was outside of her plan and that is why, even though she wanted the money, she wanted no one to know and thought she could deny you gave it to her; then she was surprised when you had proof. I believe you foiled her ending of the story!

"Ken I'm really sorry but this is how I see things... and have for a long time. It's quite a story. Someone should make it into a movie!"

After a long pause in a silent room noisy with thoughts, Daisy continued, "Look at what you did in court. After five days of them beating you up, in fact pulverizing you, you turned the other cheek and you publicly apologized to Jane for any hurts you may have caused her. Over the years I have known you... you have had many people treat you badly, cheat you out of money, and just plain use you. Yet I have only seen you retaliate once when you threw that midwifery school administrator out of your office because she had treated me badly. You are a man of peace and no matter how bad or greedy people are, you give back forgiveness and understanding, and you continue to be helpful when they ask.

"Apologizing to Jane in court after the years of her cruel treatment of you truly amazes me. I would not have done it. I have had to ask myself why you have so much insight into people, yet you sometimes fail to recognize the bad apples that come your way. On the other hand, I know that you are seeing the child within the bad apple exterior... the needy child looking for help. It's almost like you are a lightening rod or a goal post that attracts them and they can't wait to ram you when they find out you are your own person and not a conventional unthinking dope for them to manipulate.

"You are better than all of them. You are a true man of love and peace... I am not so good as you. I feel like I am in the company of someone too good for this world. I only hope that someday your sons will truly understand who you are."

Ken had no words. His fingers pressed on his chest, a motion all too familiar as he tried to stop the pain in his heart.

THE PLAYERS GOING FORWARD:

In 1997, seven years after hearing this case, Herbert Arnold Dimitri Oliver, better known as Judge H.A.D. Oliver will be appointed British Columbia Conflict of Interest Commissioner and will hold that appointment for about ten years.

Leslie Baker, lawyer, who had articled with H.A.D. Oliver, will teach family law in a College setting.

Gail Davidson, lawyer, will continue her work in International Human Rights. (Ken will continue, as he had in the past, to respect her work and for that reason Ken will continue to be helpful in her work when and if asked.)

Marnie Dunnaway will continue her law practice and a few years later will play another 'game' with Daisy's family.

Jane Anderson and Bruce Katz will continue their law practices.

Mary Murray and Jane Anderson will continue to live a few feet apart as close neighbours in the same housing co-op for more than twenty years and grow old together.

The ill-fitting musician/lawyer will move to the opposite side of the world and teach music in a completely different culture.

38

Fallout

"GUESS WHAT'S HAPPENED here, Ken. In marriage, there is an ability to tell a spouse to 'stuff it' when one person refuses to negotiate or endangers the other. In divorce, with lawyers and judges hired for the kill and determining the law as they interpret it, an ex-spouse can become a captive. I mean to say men are made captives. In divorce, Jane has made you her prisoner, something she could not do effectively in marriage."

They were on their way to do a simple food shopping. Walking along the dusky street, Ken was silent for a moment, and then he nodded and spoke. "You have a way of saying things so clearly."

"I am so sympathetic to men who just disappear to escape women's wrath."

"Something I could not do to my children," he answered.

"Something I could not do to men I knew," she answered.

THE FOOD CO-OPERATIVE store in Kitsilano was small. Ken did not like shopping in supermarkets. He felt comfortable in this store where he had regular relaxed conversations with the manager about the business of healthy food. The patrons were usually local, mostly recognizing each other.

The newspaper articles had appeared only a day ago. Ken had gone across the street for a minute and was not in the store. While paying for the groceries Daisy was accosted verbally by a booming voice behind her. "What a rotten thing Ken has done to you in not paying maintenance!"

Turning her head in shock, Daisy saw Shanti, one of the two women Ken had worked with briefly at the bookstore. Shanti had leaned far out of the middle of the long queue, aggressively setting herself apart with only one foot holding her place in line and spoke so loudly that everyone in the store was involved whether they wanted to be or not. Familiar faces stared at the target – Daisy. She realized in a flash that Shanti had made a mistaken identity, thinking she was talking to Jane, the single mother described in the newspaper.

What Daisy could not figure out in a split second of thought was why anyone would not talk to her quietly instead of yelling in public, no matter what the opinions. Daisy had seen Shanti many times in the bookstore and had always experienced her as an aggressive person with a strange smirk on her face that was supposed to represent a peaceful smile. Daisy had always avoided her, believing Shanti was a pretender in the setting of a spiritual bookstore. This particular woman had been writing articles on spirituality and getting them published in a local magazine where she described herself as a pure thinker with something to teach everyone. Daisy had always suspected she was no more spiritually evolved than a chunk of coal and occasionally read her articles simply out of curiosity about the person's delusion.

Daisy caught the eyes of a married couple at the tail end of the line. Ken and Daisy knew the couple through working as volunteers for the food bank. There had always been friendly conversations on meeting. Now they stared out of blank, frozen faces at Daisy as Shanti continued ranting.

Daisy was in silent shock, no longer hearing what was being said as she gathered up her bags of groceries and left the store – a move she regretted as soon as she got outside.

She stood outside wondering why she just left quietly and reasoned to herself that after the many years of working with Ken and turning the other cheek when clients misbehaved, this was a carry-over reaction to a misbehaving person with problems; or, she questioned herself, is it merely a swift and peaceful way to end a confrontation as she had been taught in her years of study and meditation. But then confrontation was something she had hated all her life. She wondered and was disappointed in herself for not defending Ken on the spot right in public.

Meeting Ken on the street near the store, Daisy was in the middle of explaining what just happened as Shanti came out of the store and was clearly surprised to see Daisy talking to Ken. Shanti's face registered panic. She turned on her heels and ran down the street, disappearing quickly into the evening shadows.

Ken's face showed hurt as he watched the woman run away but he said nothing.

A COUPLE OF DAYS LATER, Ken and Daisy were in a larger grocery store and took their place in a line at a checkout stand with a couple of items. The tall, slender woman in front of them turned around. Jane's friend Gail Davidson greeted Ken as though nothing had ever happened. Ken was completely cordial to her, speaking with her as though nothing had happened. Then Gail turned to Daisy, "Hi, I'm Gail."

"I know who you are," Daisy muttered frostily.

Gail was not fazed and turned back to Ken, continuing to cheerfully talk with him as though they were long lost friends.

Out on the street, Daisy questioned him about being so friendly to Gail and he responded, "Life goes on and my life is not built on resentments or grudges. Besides, Gail does some good work."

Daisy finished the conversation by, "Games! To me it just smacks of lawyers playing games with no consequences except that they do what is required of them to either win or help a friend win. And we are all supposed to carry on as though nothing happened."

KEN AND DAISY walked the beaches following the court case.

"Ken, how can you even think about getting a medical office again with no money?"

"House calls. I've already spoken with Medical Services. They have advised me on how I'm to do the billings for house calls. They have told me that I should bill under the same code as for visits to hospital, home, or institution. I can continue using code 309 for Adjustment Reaction for all diagnosis. So there is no need to change the diagnosis code or explain further." Ken paused to reflect and then continued, "Getting doctors to refer their patients to me when my name has been smeared publicly is the difficulty."

"To do safe house calls, you need a chaperone. I'll work with you part-time and then when the practice gets busy, I'll quit my job at the clinic and work solely with you again."

Ken looked at Daisy's face for a long moment. "I am sorry for what this has done to you. You know she doesn't want me but she doesn't want you to have me."

"I know that."

Ken's voice was pained, "All she had to do was ask me for money and I would have found a way to give it to her. I always gave her extra money in the past when she asked me."

"I know. She just used money as a way to discredit you and me. I'm asking you again not to socialize with her anymore, not even regarding Andy. She is not to be trusted!" Daisy paused, waiting for fallout.

Ken was silent.

"I mean, please don't go to her house even on Christmas and drink the alcohol beverage she offers because she then gets you into what seems like a normal conversation but really she is pumping you for information about us and what you do. She just wants to use anything against you as best she can. She is not to be trusted!"

"I've learned." With that statement, Ken picked up a stone from the sand and threw it, sending it through the air as far as it would go before plopping through the waves into the ocean. "There, I've just thrown away my attachment to her. I thought it was better for Andy to see that his parents could parent together regardless of divorce. I thought spending Christmas morning with them in her home was good for Andy."

Daisy was not finished. "They produced the divorce papers in court to prove Jane has custody of Andy. I was there when Jane dropped off the original papers in your office for you to sign. She was a little surprised to see me but she handed them to me. I read them even before you did. I thought the papers stated you had equivalent of joint guardianship and joint custody. That was the only thing you asked for at that time and she could have everything of monetary value if you could have that. I don't remember anything stating it was only your son's estate."

"I did think I was signing papers that gave me joint guardianship and joint custody of Andy or at least the equivalent – not of his estate. We need to see the lawyer who checked the papers."

THE FOLLOWING DAY found Daisy and Ken sitting with the lawyer. A large brown desk was between them and the lawyer, who looked like every woman's tall and handsome dreamboat. On a corner of the desk was the largest stopwatch Daisy had ever seen. The clock stood at a slight angle so that she can see the hands move, knowing it's job was to measure money by the second and for every word uttered in the room. In her usual flitting thoughts, Daisy could not help thinking how different lawyers have it from physicians because lawyers can charge by the second for phone calls, paper work and any extras when the client is not even in the room and maybe not even in the same country, while physicians need to have the patient present in order to charge and there is no such thing as charging for telephone conversations. As Daisy's mind wandered, she noted that behind the lawyer were rows of impressive looking law books behind glass doors, giving the impression that this man knows the law or can at least look it up in a moment's notice.

Ken outlined the reason for their visit while the lawyer noticeably remained professionally calm and cool, showing no change in expression.

Hoping for some sign of expression, Daisy felt the urge to emphasize her concerns. "I believe a line may have been changed regarding custody after Ken signed the papers. The papers as they are now, don't match my memory of what was handed to me before signing."

In a soft tone that suggested Ken was confident this problem could be worked out, he said, "All I am asking is to see the original papers."

"This is more than seven years ago," replied the lawyer, "I don't have the files."

Surprised, Ken asked, "Where are they?"

"I don't know. I don't remember the details of the papers. I don't have the papers."

"Can you look for them?" Daisy asked, thinking legal files are like medical files that have to be guarded and saved for at least seven years in some lockup. "It's important! The originals have to be somewhere!"

"I have no idea where they are, I just know I don't have them."

Staring at the stop-clock timing this visit with large black hands, Daisy thought about timing, wondering how or if he was going to charge for this visit.

Ken thought... Outsmarted again. I'll never know the truth. Was there ever a moment of honest marriage with that woman?

As they left the office, the lawyer's hand reached over to clamp down on the timer, stopping time in his world.

THROUGH THE YEARS of 1988 and 1989, Ken had been working toward a degree in the Planning department at UBC, hoping in the long run to make a difference in sustainable community planning. His marks had been consistently A's and B's in six Planning courses. Over years, he had also been a volunteer in community planning.

[ks notebook] "...My interest in community development for self help housing and home health care grew out of college experiences in housing construction work; in my philosophy classes with Eugen Rosenstock-Huessy; with Alinsky style community development in Syracuse; learning dairy farming in Vermont; working at the Matador Co-op Farm with mixed farming; house building in Argenta, B.C.; building of an island community at the Coast Range Ranch... my study of self help housing with Charles Haynes; living in, and consulting with housing cooperatives; work in my own Family Health Centre preparing families for childbirth, home schooling, self employment, and the care of their sick and dying members; and most recently my efforts to plan home health care for my parents..."

IMMEDIATELY FOLLOWING THE court case and the bad publicity, Ken was told he was unwelcome to continue studying in the Planning Department at UBC. In being ousted, he was told that the department was looking for grant moneys and he had become a detriment to the department. He was told that there was an active campaign underway by an ex-wife and her lawyer to have Ken removed from UBC altogether.

This was followed by a notification from the University Office of Awards and Financial Aid that there had been an "anonymous complaint".

February 3, 1990 Ken wrote a response:

Byron Hender, Director
Office of Awards and Financial Aid
University of British Columbia
Dear Mr. Hender,
I am writing to request an appeal for special consideration of a decision reducing my student loans and bursaries. I had met the criteria for single parent status on GAIN prior to my application for student loans and bursaries in 1987. I did not meet your criteria of having custody of my son, Andy Alexander Kehnroth Anderson-Schramm. Until January 1989 when my ex-wife, a lawyer, garnished my student loan account for payment of maintenance, I believed I had never relinquished guardianship responsibilities for Andy and continued to have all the responsibilities of a single parent. My belief was based on the Separation Agreement of 1982 which I discussed with my lawyer, Wayne Powell, and I believed to be still in effect. Since separating from his mother, I provided care myself and paid for a nanny especially during his mother's illnesses and his illnesses. In 1985, I enrolled Andy in K-1 at Bayview School and provided daycare. When Bayview School discontinued Grade 1-2 classes, I enrolled him in '86 at U-Hill Elementary where he still does well today. I enrolled him also in University Hill After School Care (Kids Club), participating in and paying for his care from Spring-Summer of 1987 until Fall 1988 when his mother decided to pay her neighbor to provide day care. Then I paid $150 monthly from student loans to her until she garnished my student loan account in January 1989. On the basis of conversations and signed

agreement about our joint care of Andy, I believed I was a single parent providing a second home for Andy with a flexible schedule of access to fit his needs. I discussed my situation fully with social workers when I was going through bankruptcy due to illness and received support as a single parent so when I applied for student loans I believed I was a single parent. I used my student loans and bursaries to provide a home for Andy and for my studies. Enclosed are relevant documents. Your support of my appeal will enable me to continue to provide a home for my son while completing my career change. If you require any financial information, please contact my accountant...

Yours truly,

Ken Schramm

KEN VISITED DOCTORS' offices daily to say he is back at work, in hopes of referrals to rebuild his practice. It proved to be a big emotional as well as physical challenge because he knew that many doctors had read the damning newspaper articles even though they did not speak about it with Ken but instead, made private judgments. Ken needed the referrals because as a specialist, he could not practice his specialty of psychiatry without them. If he had no referrals, he would not get paid. If he did not get paid, the circle of going back to court would start again.

As usual, Ken rose to the challenge. A few doctors began to refer patients, but not the many who did so in the past. The doctor who had referred patients to Ken in the past but had also sent a false medical file into court on Jane and Bruce Katz' behalf, never again made a referral to Ken and Ken never did ask him for one. In a climate where psychiatrists have months-long waiting lists, it seemed odd that referrals were hard to come by for Ken.

He visited the medical clinic while Daisy was on shift and she watched him leave, walking down the street, his back to her. She wondered again how it came to be that lawyers and Judges, without knowing medicine, have such power to decide the health status and medical treatment of people. She believed – no, she knew there was a serious flaw in the Canadian judicial system.

It was with a heavy heart that she watched Ken comply with a court order that sent a man out to work in frontline medicine while he was in danger of an exploding heart. As she watched him walk away, his aloneness wrenched on her heart.

Daisy made an effort to have doctors at the clinic make a couple of referrals to Ken. The newest doctor hired to work at the clinic, called Daisy and Ken into an after-closing hour meeting when all other doctors were gone for the day. Ken entered the meeting unaware of the doctor's agenda. The doctor was brazenly aggressive to Ken and threatened to have Daisy fired because of the referrals; he made it clear he wanted to be the clinic's therapist even though he was a General Practitioner and there was already a psychiatrist working in the clinic. He was a two-faced man. When no other doctor was around, he occasionally had a bad temper with some patients. He nastily, verbally assaulted a young man who came in one evening with a work injury. Daisy was the only witness and the young man ran out so fast, she could not intervene.

When more referrals came from doctors at the clinic, Ken quietly refused to take them.

In trying to be helpful to Ken, Daisy accompanied him on some house calls to see the female patients before her hours at the clinic.

IT SEEMED STRANGE that after years of not seeing each other, paths were frequently crossing between Daisy and the lawyer who had been married to Daisy's musician friend. Daisy discovered that the woman did remember her very well and they had a few friendly conversations. Then one day they found themselves side by side picking out vegetables in a local store and they talked again. They just happened to leave the store at the same time. Outside, in front of the store, Daisy decided to tackle what she really wanted to know. After all, the one-time sweet woman had eaten at her table and now the woman looked sick, had lost a lot of weight, and Daisy was honestly concerned for her.

Daisy dared ask, "Are you okay?"

The woman responded, "Why do you ask?"

"Because you do not look well."

At that the woman shot back, "I've always been thin." She broke away and ran across 4th Avenue in Kitsilano, packed with cars. Rather than go to the corner with lights, only a few feet away, she jogged on her high heels between cars to the other side of the street. She had escaped Daisy.

Daisy was amazed that another woman had taken to running away. But her concern stayed with her, the one time friend was not doing well in her new life. As a health care worker, Daisy felt sorry and wished she could help.

IT HAD BEEN twenty-one years since their 1969 meeting in Regina; fourteen years since living as neighbors; nine years since getting together as partners in love and life in 1981. In the world of numbers, nine is the jumping off point where evaluation of the past culminates and it becomes the point of starting over. At this nine-year juncture in May, Ken and Daisy hit the evaluation point. They were tired.

Ken looked at Daisy and felt sorry he had damaged her life with his problems.

Daisy was sorry for the troubles Ken was having because of her. She wondered what life might be like without Jane and Andy as a ball and chain in her life. She wondered if Ken's troubles were only because of her or if in fact he would have died by now, as he feared, if he had continued living with Jane.

Believing he was doing Daisy a favor, Ken set her free. She went along with it. Each believed they had caused each other enough pain.

As a parting gift, Daisy hoped to fill the empty space in Ken's life with an understanding son. She wrote and delivered a long letter to Ken's son Stephen in hopes that he would finally get a perspective on what had happened to his father. In the letter, she pointed out that the name of Schramm also belonged to all of Ken's sons and to the rest of the proud 'Schrammily' but now that Jane had publicly dragged the name into the mud, it was most important that Ken's sons know that their father was not guilty of any wrongdoing; that it had only been a matter of sly maneuvers on the part of other people that made him seem so.

What a mother would do to her own son weighed heavily on Daisy. She wondered how a mother could be so short sighted as to be raising a son in an atmosphere of hatred and shaming of her son's father. Daisy spent long hours worrying that Andy could not possibly grow up to be a whole human being with a mother who did not understand the necessary connection between a man, his son, and the larger family name.

LYING ON THE LIVING ROOM SOFA, Daisy was having a rare afternoon rest while listening to the radio program of classical music. Sad and lonely now that Ken had rented another apartment, her mind drifted. She wondered what it took for people to crack and go off the deep end.

She remembered a conversation years before with an older woman, who late in life became a Buddhist nun. They were studying with the same teacher, the Venerable Ananda Bodhi, later named Namgyal Rinpoche, a Tibetan Llama. After arriving from England, the woman had been sent to live for a while in Daisy's home. Though Daisy was taking care of her physically, the older woman was in turn drawing on her long experience and had become a teacher to Daisy. A delightful union was struck between the woman with snowy white hair, sparkling blue eyes, a German accent crossed with an English accent, and the dark haired twenty-eight year old Daisy, who had just given birth to her fourth child and was fresh from the prairies, yearning to know more... *more* knowledge. Their conversations were always enlightening, opening up vistas of thought.

For no apparent reason, the nun told this story one afternoon: "I was walking along a cliff in Scotland, overlooking the ocean. I looked down to the beach and saw a younger woman walking with my teacher. I became so jealous that I picked up a boulder and was standing there above them, ready to drop it on his head. I was thinking of killing him. Of course, I came to my senses and didn't drop the boulder. Instead, the other woman has been my traveling companion and here we are, all three of us together in Canada. When threatened, the instinct to fight or take flight is in all human beings. The difference is how that instinct is acted upon."

The nun's teaching of that day was done. Her way of telling a story with a teaching at her own expense, stayed with Daisy. She never forgot the teaching or the story.

That was then; this was now. Then Daisy remembered how she had to run away from her first husband. One night as the wind howled around the house and she waited for a drunken husband to arrive home, she knew her breaking point had come. She realized she was on the verge of serious protection of her children and herself. The instinct was strong not to hurt him if he came home and hit anyone. It was necessary to take flight permanently.

Daisy had been worn down by the endless viciousness of Jane and Katz hurting Ken, bringing out a strong instinct to protect him regardless of any risk of hurting herself. The only reason she had stayed in the background for so long was because she knew a more aggressive approach would have brought him even more trouble.

Ken was a non-violent person. He had lived in fear of his ex-wife. Seeing how viciously his ex-wife and her friends attacked him in Affidavits, in court appearances and personally, it was easy to understand why he needed to leave her home and the marriage. Ken reached a breaking point, but he had become extremely ill, internalizing his breaking point rather than retaliate. In keeping with moral conduct and in truthfulness to his Hippocratic Oath to do no harm, he had to leave his marriage to save his life.

Daisy questioned God, the Creator. She could not condone a good, gentle, caring person like Ken being made to suffer so much, to the point of getting ill as a consequence of trusting another human being enough to marry her and have a child with her, when meanwhile the bad, dishonest, selfish people seemed to thrive. She railed at God in her mind about certain people not deserving to have such beautiful babies when so many good people cannot have babies at all, or they have babies born suffering deformities and health issues.

In examination of these thoughts, she recognized that we do all have the fight or flight instinct; it was the age-old self-protection embedded in our survival instinct. Daisy wanted to protect Ken with her life, to the depth of her own soul.

That memory of the old conversation with the nun brought new insight into what can happen to people internally; it also brought a kind of peace into present day problems.

Daisy hung onto the old nun's words, "The difference is how that instinct is acted upon."

Daisy thought about how thought can affect someone across time and space.

In light of those revelations, Daisy would now have to tame demons and control her mind. If nothing else, her own health would be saved.

Instead, she would try to be vigilant to outguess the opponents' next moves. All she had to do was to think up the worst scenario and then be on their wavelength.

Oh, oh, back to that! she thought.

Then where does positive thinking have room? It will take a lot of work to control her anger and allow positive thinking to take over, and to use the power of peace. Daisy knew she had been given the tools, the wisdom on which to base her life. She decided that the power of positive thinking would be a better way to go; the best thing to do for Ken would be to love him unconditionally and counteract negative forces with a shield of love.

The storm gave way to calm, turning her attention to the music coming from the radio. The long piano cadenzas up and down in Beethoven's Emperor Concerto relaxed Daisy into a mellow acceptance that love is all that matters.

KEN HAD BEEN heading toward the university. Feeling a strong urge to see Daisy, he turned on his heels to follow the magnetic pull.

He found her lying in the living room listening to music. Silently taking a chair a small distance from her bare feet, he waited for a reaction from her. She was wearing short shorts and her bare thighs faced him, causing him to smile with memories.

She was pleased to have him home. Her first instinct was to get up but she relaxed into awareness of his contentment to see her… as is.

In that afternoon, they found a bubble free of trouble. The calmness in the room and contentment of being together nourished the missing spaces in their lives. They spoke softly with each other as time stood still.

39

Ken Wrote:

Writing One's Life 1990

"In 1982 when I read that Dr. Innes Pearse at [age] 80 planned a new version of the Peckham Experiment in Edinburgh, I wrote to Pioneer Health Center Ltd. in London to tell them of my plan to begin a Pioneer Health Centre in Vancouver. After six months of work, I failed to convince my partners to put our business plan in writing and I left to try again. My blood pressure became dangerously high despite medication and I made changes in my diet, exercise, and life style. I went bankrupt due to my illness and discovered homeopathy; it helped me to live.

"I joined Society Promoting Environment Conservation to link family health and environmental issues by forming a Family Health Cooperative. I arranged for the Canadian Council on Social Development to invite the Pioneer Health Centre U.K., founders of the first Family Health Centre, to their 1985 Ottawa Conference on Community Based Health and Social Services. They discussed their concepts of family health care with Jake Epp, then Minister of Health and Welfare, and with a group of 300 health professionals.

"In 1986 we founded Pioneer Health Centre Canada and the U.K. group visited the Single Parents' Program of Vancouver Food Bank at the Unitarian Church, with Finn-Est Institute which advocated principles of Mondragon Workers' Cooperative for housing homeless people, and at Kitsilano Neighborhood House.

"As a volunteer with the Unitarian Church Food Bank, I studied poverty from the perspective of Liberation Theology in the work of Bernard Lonergan, S.J. on conversion through the insights of understanding. His method is based on maxims which question the biases of common sense: Be Attentive! Be Intelligent! Be Reasonable! Be Responsible! Be Loving!

"When I failed to find families to charter a Family Health Cooperative, I returned to full-time graduate study to use the work of Mumford, Rosenstock-Heussy, Page Smith, Innes Pearse, and Lonergan to support our own efforts to build a Food Bank for student families at U.B.C. I needed to learn how to read, write, speak, and live again.

"In 1988 when the proposed Student Food Bank was buried in bureaucracy, I decided to return to my roots in community development and study how people were learning to develop communities. After an intense fortnight of study in conferences organized by my brother Dick on Management and Community Development and Women and Economic Development, I met [name] and decided to study with him at U.B.C. School of Community and Regional Planning. I continued my graduate studies of "How Planners Think" through Local Area Planning in Kitsilano until 1990 when I could not continue because of illness.

"I have lived my life on the boundary where the world of family meets the world of work and school. I come from Pilgrims who built Harvard and Dartmouth Colleges to educate their children and the Indians together in the wilderness. When I was young, there was no extra money or lack of work where I lived. I expected to work my whole life to care for family members, to learn to do all I could do to provide for education of my children and myself. Life, 'The College of Hard Knocks' my father calls it, has been his and my Teacher in the School Without Walls. My first work, interviewing Uncle Bob about the secrets of The Atomic Bomb, taught me not to trust leaders who threaten to destroy all life on earth while lying to their employees about the health risks of what they are really making in their work.

Work and Mistakes

"The work I found at age 12 and continued ever since, the job of healing the splitting of the human race into atoms is too big for me or anyone to do alone. Healing, making us whole again, requires constant rebuilding of communities as safe places for growing fully human beings who can make our living and dying into sacred play so that our grandchildren will have a future. Hidden in the stories of my failures to build any institutional monument is my part in the lives of individuals who rebuild communities and families destroyed by our governments in war, waste, greed, and stupidity, mine as well as theirs.

"I have made wise and stupid decisions and mistakes in my life. To recognize my mistakes, I need to be a member of a family and a community who learn from our mistakes. The only community I know who learn from our mistakes is a community of independent writers. Men like Rosenstock-Huessy and Lewis Mumford teach by writing our mistakes as our own poetry, converting death into life, grief into chance, love into family, war into peace, knowing that the feast of life will soon be over but it is still better than utopia.

"When I began the adventure that became my life, I believed that the world was at war because intelligent caring people devoted all their lives to making money to pay the mortgages (then 6%) which provided homes for their families. They had neglected their poorly paid public duty to discover causes of disease, health, war and peace; and to govern by sharing knowledge with the world's children who might then be able to live in peace with their own children. Because I came to medicine and pediatrics from philosophy and religion, I practiced medicine as philosophy, healing and learning with words, in the Feast of Life as freedom to know the truth by our own efforts and divine grace. I have never doubted that man's duty and destiny is to become divinely human, a loving father, capable of sharing and giving his life if needed for a loved one, especially a woman and a child who represent my future. There have always been Indians as well as children, but few adults, in my story because I grew to atomic fission in a town with an Indian name, a forest full of arrow heads, beaver ponds, fish, turtles, foxes, frogs, birches, and a train that took fathers and mothers away to New York City on week days. This was a world of Franklin Roosevelt, Lewis Mumford, John Dewey, Margaret Mead, Paul Radin, Charles and Mary Beard I learned about in school and at home. It was the world of Teddy Roosevelt, and Winston Churchill I learned with my grandfather and with Eugen Rosenstock-Huessy.

"What have I learned in the years since 1945 of working with families to be healthy and at peace with ourselves and each other? The continuity I experience between my working life as a physician and a student of health appears to be invisible for those with whom I want to share my questions. Others do not share my ultimate concern for the politics and poetics of living, writing, and thinking. Where I see a duty to discuss what we need as fully human beings, others see an imposition on their right to do a job they say they hate to get money so they can do something else they want to do. I'm surprised that people will not do what they are called to do, but will follow orders to do a job that is harmful and to stop others from doing something helpful they would do if they could. I enjoy farmers and others who do what needs to be done so we can brag about what we did by complaining how hard it was to do it. How good food and sweat taste in the salty mouth of the one who brags his complaints!

"I will never build a Family Health Centre in the way that Innes Pearse and Scott Williamson found a patron to support their research. Family home care will continue as the work of bringing families together to plan our homes; a better birth for the next child; convalescent care for members who suffered accidents, surgery, drug effects of chemotherapy; and help with members who are recovering or dying at home. There will be chances for people to find life after illness or disability, unemployment, divorce, death in the family, and to rebuild homes out of a housing crisis. Working with our children learning at home will become practical when we build houses as homes to encourage family living, gardening, and learning. When asked: What do you want to be when you grow up? I say: Alive, I want to be alive when I die!"

Ken Schramm 1990

40

After Fallout

KEN WAS AT the university, having changed direction of study, determined not to give up or give in to his ex and her lawyer. Daisy watched over grandchildren from a grassy knoll beside the outdoor swimming pool at Kitsilano beach. She had not seen Jane and Andy coming her way from behind until she was startled to be looking up from her sitting position at Jane standing over her.

Jane spoke first. "Daisy, will you look after Andy at the pool? I have to be somewhere."

Daisy wracked her brain for a split second to get some perspective and answered politely, "No. Sorry, but no." She could not believe the gall of this woman.

Watching Jane and Andy walk away, leaving the beach, Daisy was conflicted, wondering why she had not taken this opportunity to really tell Jane off. She decided that because Andy was present, better judgment took over. And besides, she reasoned, that is not her way anyway. Then, thinking she was letting Ken down for not grabbing the opportunity to take care of Andy for Andy's sake, she felt bad. She mulled over the surprise of being faced so soon with this scenario by the same woman who had discredited Daisy in court and had Judge Scarth pronounce her unfit to be around. She always knew Jane would one day do this, but now that it happened, because of Andy it somehow was not satisfying to have thrown it back in Jane's face. Circling the pros and cons, Daisy respected herself for not being another of Jane's puppets.

CROSSING 4th AVENUE on the walk home after leaving the beach with her grandchildren, Daisy was surprised and yet not at all surprised to see Jane without her child, meandering along the street, window-shopping. As Daisy watched, Jane disappeared into the women's clothing shop that Daisy had only gone into once and ran out because of the high prices. Andy was nowhere in sight. Obviously, he had been dropped off with someone else. Daisy felt terrible for Andy.

The incident left a horrible feeling of being damned if she did or damned if she didn't. But in the end, it was Andy that was the greater concern than a squabble between two women.

ONCE AGAIN THERE was disturbing news to give Ken. At home, after relaying the story to Ken, they discussed the dilemma Daisy had been faced with. Ken was not judgmental of Daisy. He told her it was not her problem. He expressed his sadness that his son had been used as a pawn in his ex-wife's revenge.

CARRYING BAGGAGE OF intense parental alienation, Andy was back for Ken to care for. Andy no longer went to Ken's home even though Ken rented his own apartment for his sons. Andy had nothing to do with Daisy or her family. Establishing a renewed father/son relationship had to be in Jane's house where Ken continued to have to see the photo on the fridge of Jane on Katz's lap when entering by the main door, or Ken met his son at school.

Andy called regularly when his mother was not home because he wanted food delivered to his house. Ken always responded no matter what the work schedule was. He would travel by bus, buy food, make the delivery and stay for a visit.

Andy called Ken when he was sick which seemed often and Ken spent hours with him, bringing food and any medicine needed. The boy was a victim of damaging brainwashing, resentful in his belief that his own father was a loser who would not and never did pay for his care and gave all his money to Daisy,

Daisy was convinced that the picture on the fridge depicting Jane's intimate admiration of the slayer of the Andy's father and that the boy could not ignore on a daily basis every time he went for food, was a deliberate brainwashing. And... if Ken was to see it, rubbing salt in a wound was accomplished.

Ken insisted that all children and grandchildren always got an immediate response to crisis no matter the obstacles.

WORKING IN MEDICINE had grabbed Daisy and would not let go. A year ago, before the last court case, on a long walk with Ken one afternoon after being fired from the church job, she had discussed her future. "Ken, I'm seriously considering applying to nursing school. I've just been offered a job in a large community health centre. I think nursing school is a better idea."

"Daisy, do you really think you could follow rules without question? You are constantly questioning rules and regulations and challenging the hierarchy. You are always trying to fix something."

"Oh boy! I've been doing that all my life. I've always believed rules are to be broken if they don't make sense or are harmful. After all, mere humans have made the rules and they can be flawed. I can't change. When I was in High School, I got expelled twice for playing hooky. I hate being lied to. I knew the teachers were telling us lies about Canadian History. In those days, even the history books were full of lies about the Indians. I couldn't change it so my way out was to fall asleep in class or get out. My poor mother! The hurt she endured because of my behavior!"

"You don't run away now. You have a way of standing up for what you believe. You are quiet just until you see something that should be fixed."

"I especially get riled and challenging when I see bad medicine."

"It's your decision but do you think you could spend your life in those challenging circumstances?"

The conversation had been a wake-up call. Instead of going to nursing school Daisy had accepted the job in the Community Health Centre where she learned about the extremely competitive world of medical office assistants. Of the many doctors working there, Daisy decided a few were good doctors but over time she disliked and distrusted several because of their medical mistakes or rough treatment of patients.

Ken had told her the joke about himself and other medical students wanting to tape signs on their foreheads to keep certain doctors away from their bodies in case of emergency. Daisy wanted to paste a sign across her own forehead saying: In case of emergency, do not let doctor so-and-so near me.

Then something somehow had gotten into Daisy's eye very suddenly while on the job. Seeing her discomfort, a female doctor that Daisy had taken a dislike to, came toward her with a scrawny hand outstretched, wanting to help as though sticking a finger in her eye would help. Backing up against the desk with a look of horror on her face, Daisy nearly fell backward while trying to get away. The gesture was so clear to the doctor that she backed off.

On what started out to be an ordinary afternoon after Daisy had worked there for nearly a year, a person in a wheelchair was struggling to open the heavy entrance door a few feet away from the front desk. Through the heavy glass window of the door, Daisy could see the woman struggle. Doing what seemed absolutely normal, Daisy responded by opening the door to help the person enter.

The other MOA on duty suddenly left the front desk and went down the stairs to administration offices in the basement. The administrator called Daisy into his office. A tiny man in a small brown suit, with medical knowledge of patient-care only by administration of paper, told Daisy, "You are not here to be a Good Samaritan!"

She could hardly believe her ears. "This is a medical clinic! I helped a handicapped person in a wheelchair through the door!"

The MOA's always left their desks to deliver files to doctors. From day one of her employment in the clinic, Daisy had been acutely aware of what seemed like an encompassing black cloud hanging over the place, affecting the employees. Out of financial need, she had unwittingly entered a portal to a group of people where she clearly did not belong. The place had the facade of being a community health centre but internally it had severe problems and functioned like any other clinic – nothing special about it. It had been a project founded by the same old doctor who had invited Ken to speak at UBC about the Peckham Experiment.

For a celebration of the years open, the old doctor had shown up and while on the job, Daisy had a second chance to evaluate him. She understood the similarity between the old doctor and Ken. Both men had a vision and a desire to provide a place for better health care – to build what was lacking in the community, but because of what lacked in other people and lack of money, they both had trouble making their vision happen. No wonder he had shown interest in Ken's ideas and the Peckham Experiment!

By now Daisy had developed painful bursitis of the left shoulder from dealing with loads of medical files each day. She was aware that the condition could become chronic unless she made a change. Being told she was not here to be a Good Samaritan was the last straw.

She walked out, leaving the tattle-tail MOA to cover the evening shift when Daisy knew very well the woman wanted to go home for the evening. She glanced back over her shoulder with satisfaction to see shock on the hungry woman's face because she was stuck for the next four evening hours, but Daisy also knew the woman had been making trouble because she wanted her daughter to have a job at the clinic and needed someone to leave. Daisy knew the woman's daughter would fill her position by the next day.

Walking away, Daisy analyzed the realization that she had been working in 'medicine' while some of the people she just left behind worked in a 'business office'. What a difference! She acknowledged that Ken had trained her well and he would be proud of her for not stooping to the level of the people she just walked out on. The words, *'If you can't change them, leave them'* ran through her head like a song.

She reveled in the thought that she had given a freebee to a single parent who needed a form filled out for her child to go to summer camp; the form was supposed to cost forty dollars for a scribble. Daisy had been admonished her for that. She knew the woman had absolutely no money and was relying on a non-profit association to send her child to camp. Daisy reasoned the clinic was stealing from the poorest of the poor because they also charged her medical plan for the office visit and a check-up.

She thought out loud, "Ken would never, ever charge a client for signing a form." Glancing around to see who might be listening, she remembered Ken walking the same walk. She had watched his back from the window of the clinic. She was following in his footsteps.

It had been a tough year. It was while Daisy had been working at the clinic that the trial with Judge Oliver happened, followed by the published newspaper articles and the story had even been picked up by a national physicians' rag that each doctor in the clinic had received in their mailboxes. The day after the first newspaper articles came out, Daisy needed to take a private moment in the room filled with files and just rest her head against a shelf until she could emerge pretending all was well. Daisy had no idea whether or not her troubles at the clinic had anything to do with Ken and her being made out to be criminals. She had been wishing someone would talk so that she could explain but no one spoke to her about it.

As she waited for a bus at the bus stop, the same doctor who earlier had threatened to have her fired, arrived a couple of minutes later and asked Daisy for bus fare. She was surprised to see him and even more at his request for money. She wondered if he knew she was leaving for good, but gave him the fare without confiding in him... and never looked back.

Her thoughts were with Ken on the long bus ride home. She could hardly wait to get home where she could telephone him and talk. Just the thought of his soft, soothing voice was comforting.

41

Safe Havens

Living my life backwards from death

In the event of my death,
my critical obituary will read as follows.
It must be critical
or I will not be alive when I die.
The Life and Death (The Living and
Dying) Opinions of Tristam Schrammy.

The significant event of my life I wish to discuss with you is the event of my death which gives all of my life, whatever significance it has or will ever have. My death transforms my life into a poem which dances me to death and back to life. Each family, each person I meet in my daily practice of medicine dances their own story of being alive when I die. For most people in the world, death is an accident that must be explained as an individual occurrence by what deliberate act did this person cause his own death and who else participated in his self destruction by witchcraft, malice, or poison? These questions are asked and answered within the world.

My critical obituary anticipated the denial, blaming, bargaining, negotiating, and acceptances by reviewing all my little dyings, disappointments, failures, crisis, wrong turns, and bypaths. I have died while living my own and other peoples' lives. I am a wannabee someone else myself. My work encourages me to live and die with others and to be others. I have been living my life backwards from the death of others in myself: dead cows, chickens, pigs, carrots, peas, potatoes, beans, grains, and what have you or more importantly who are you having for dinner?

William Carlos Williams speaks/writes. I hear him speaking of the speaking of others that the message becomes the same poem. He does not say what it is I believe it is – will this illness be the last one or will I make it one more time? The doctor asks have you had this before? If the patient answers yes, the doctor says: well you've got it again. If the patient says no, the doctor says: well it's going around. The doctor wisely avoids the ultimate questions which ask and answer themselves. But the patient suffers them actively – he makes my living, he dies my living, I live his dying and die my living. My epitaph: he died his living and lived his dying.

I have been in continuous midlife crisis since I was twelve years' old when Harry Truman decided to kill 100,000 Japanese with one atomic bomb. With that kind of wise leadership, I never expected to live until I was twenty-five. I lived every day as if it were my last like Chicken Little faithfully reporting that if the sky hasn't fallen yet, bombs will soon be falling, unless we learned to grow up and play fair. I presumed my mortality. Now that I am well past fifty, I presume on my immortality and live each day as if it were the first in a long cycle of months and years in which I will be growing older and more childlike forever, however long that is.

I look forward to the progress of stupidity, to discovering the jokes we play on ourselves in the name of progress. When Man thinks, God laughs. Tell us the jokes you played on yourself and unsuspecting. We filled the washroom with paper to greet our roommate returning from his date. So what goes with this obituary? This is a shaggy dog story that goes everywhere but onward and upward, more backward than forward. Smarten up. Give us some more famous last words. **[ks notebook]**

A COMMONALITY BETWEEN Ken and Daisy was the love of learning. As soon as Ken was out of a sick bed and could walk, he had trekked back to the university environment where in his early years he had found people to talk with, exchanging ideas – a place of great comfort. His desire to be in good health took him back to the place where he had always felt his best. Regardless of the behind the scenes active campaign to wreck Ken's studies, the end of Planning spawned a new beginning. He was taken under the protective wing of Sheralyn Calliou, an aboriginal woman, who introduced him into the UBC House of Learning Long House, and welcomed him into the Department of Education where he began the journey of Curriculum Development.

[ks notebook[I am here today because the Creator saved my life when I was ten days old so I could live on the boundary (Chappaqua) of this world and the spirit world, the world of living dying grieving delight... I witnessed traditional healers singing healing songs in Bella Bella 1972. I met Harry Daniels in 1968 who taught me about the medicine bundle. I met Angie Todd Dennis who introduced me to Lou Demerais in 1990 who taught me about aboriginal health and politics; and to George Manual. I met Sharilyn Calliou and Seopeetza who welcomed me into healing stories of the past 500 years – Encouraging me to heal as a wounded father and healer – Helping me face my fears of schooling and failures as a human being.

IN THE DEPARTMENT OF EDUCATION and Curriculum Development, Ken found professors and students who were supportive of each other and people he could talk with and feel safe. Competitiveness was left to other departments.

Ken entered a safe haven in the House of Learning. The aboriginal people accepted him for who he was and they were not influenced by what others said. Ken could feel peace for as many hours as he was in the aura of these people and under their roof. Here he found elder John O'Leary and a place in the men's group to talk and listen, where he knew nothing would be carried out of the room beyond the once a week meetings; confidentiality was understood and respected. He now began his journey to becoming a fire keeper, a respected elder, and participating in ceremonies as an elder sometimes called on to lead prayer at large gatherings.

On a sunny afternoon, Daisy arrived to pick Ken up after he had tended the fire in the morning, enjoyed a potluck lunch with friends, and was now finishing up in a workshop to make his drum. Daisy paused at a distance to watch Ken and John as they put the finishing touches to Ken's drum. Ken smiled as he finished the lacing under John's watchful eye. Daisy was grateful to see Ken here. She had never seen him so at peace; there was transcendence here in the aura of an unseen shield of protection.

Ken looked up as he is finished and saw her. His smile broadens to include her. She approached.

"Hi." He showed off his finely crafted drum. "Will you help me make a drum stick, Daisy?"

"Yes."

ALL DAISY'S ADULT life, she had been in constant schooling by way of night schools and weekend workshops, mostly in the arts or eastern religion and philosophy before she had started to study medicine. Many times her youngest children had accompanied her to adult art classes so that she would not have to leave them at home.

Having left the job at the clinic, she felt a need to cleanse her soul. She woke up the next morning with a yearning to learn how to make bronze sculptures. She had done most every other kind of artwork but never bronze. She went to the library to find out where bronze sculpting was being taught.

Ken was excited when she told him her plan. Even though it was the end of August and enrolment had taken place in early May to fill the classes at Capilano College, she felt a warm blanket of protection in having Ken by her side. They walked the campus with the smell of autumn in the air and the sound of yellow and red leaves shuffling beneath their shoes. Ken supported Daisy by accompanying her with pride as she showed off her portfolio. The magic worked. In Ken's presence, she had more confidence than she would have on her own. The head of an art department took time to explain that he accomplished nothing until he gave up part-time classes and jumped into art full time, encouraging her to do so also. With his advice on how to get into the already full classes, she managed to be accepted in all classes of her choice – art history, sculpting, and painting and drawing. She applied for a student loan and was surprised to be given money, including bursaries to do something she loved.

Life felt like it was starting over. When Daisy worked in the church and the film crew came in, she knew she was in the wrong place as a church mouse and in hindsight it was a blessing to be fired. Then in the most recent health clinic, she felt a deep-seated yearning when an artist off the street was allowed to line the long hall walls with her artwork. The morning of leaving that job, Daisy had stepped out of her front door to go to work and a bird dropped a large wet splotch of several colours on top of her head. She had to re-wash her hair and still get to work on time across town by bus. At the time, she wondered about the myth of good luck if a bird poos on your head; it did not feel lucky. In hindsight, Daisy was now convinced it was a lucky day because she got out of a place where she did not belong and stopped running long enough to recognize the artist inside herself. The yearning gave way to satisfaction and the feeling of belonging.

WITH HAPPY, CREATIVE PEOPLE drawing and painting at easels, sunshine pouring in through large windows over live models posing in their birthday suits, and spending many hours with hands sculpting clay and mixing glazes, and then running off to art history to examine the thinking of other artists, Daisy was sure she had gone to artist's heaven where she could stay in the studios from dawn to midnight with no other concerns, just so long as the buses were still running to get home to shower and sleep and then start over the next day. She was living her passion. She was pleased with the clay on her jeans, a sign of creative fulfillment as she traveled on buses and sea bus across the water with pocket radio buds in her ears playing classical or jazz music.

Always surprised at the newest creation, Ken was always encouraging, wanting to see more of her talents. The happy atmosphere he had always hoped to recreate in his marriages was happening now. He appreciated it all the more because his mother had been an art student and he had loved that about her.

Multiplying grandchildren worked along with Daisy on Sunday mornings after sleepovers. Katie, the small granddaughter who would grow up to excel in the sciences, remarked that "art is really science" as she watched the magic of mixing various mediums to then use to create more magic.

The walls in Daisy's apartment continued to be a museum for children to display their work but now she was adding her own. Long sheets of blank white paper were taped to the hall walls for the toddler grandchildren to draw on and when she forgot to put the paper up, the walls mistakenly become the canvas. No problem! Clean up and start over.

Ken was Daisy's greatest cheerleader. He delighted in seeing the family doing what they loved and found joy walking in on a gallery of new pictures by the children along with Daisy's latest creations. He felt that he was keeping company with a real artist and bragged for her about her, showing off her sculptures to his friends.

Grampa Ken had been with each of the grandchildren through the pregnancy and birth, and was always available to them. In times of illness and whenever someone just needed to talk, Ken was always the concerned and caring Grampa-doctor. No matter what his problems were, the children made him smile. And that's how they knew him... smiling, caring, Grampa Ken.

Meanwhile, he had easily learned how to use a computer, a talent that ran in his side of the family. He discovered that the little finger on his right hand would not type letters separate from his ring finger, a small problem stemming from his birth. Daisy, on the other hand, needed help in making the transition from a typewriter to the computer world. After stubbornly swearing she would never change, Ken took the time to teach her how to write school papers on the computer. In the process, she overcame her fear of new technology and felt liberated by Ken once again.

Daisy had found freedom in art school, a kind of childhood freedom not known since before she had married at eighteen. All her children had become adults and the grandchildren had parents of their own, and midwifery was winding down. In the hours at school, she had no responsibility other than being a moral person, being creative, and pass exams. She was having so much fun being in art school full time that she was less help to Ken. Never the less, he continued to be helpful to her whenever she was in need. And he continued to wait up for her to hear about her latest creation or to talk. Often he fell asleep, waiting.

EXCERPT from draft paper: Remembering the Child, in Education, by Ken Schramm.

...In the Sixties safe places were free schools, rights and peace marches, my rented back porch where I began my private practice with families of students going to jail, a farm school at Goddard College, and a home school on the Matador Co-op Farm. In the Seventies safe places were communities in Argenta, Lasqueti and Calvert Island, my space in a medical building, my living room, and always home visits. In the Eighties, safe places for stories were offices where you can scream and cry and beat up real foam, our midwifery school, my living room and home visits, and Buddhist meditation. Now safe also means a home school for artists of all ages.

What happens in these safe places? Stories and poems and little persons grow safe to let bad demons out good. We are safe places for art, poems, stories, dramas, and families to happen; they do and we live them all again. ...

...When I was studying psychoanalysis, my clients would say whatever came into their mouths three times a week for an hour without losing the invisible thread of their conversation with themselves, their families, and with me. I am surprised by the "natural" order to be found in spontaneous talk and play of dancing, writing, drawing, and painting. All these and more are languages translatable, not reducible into each other. I spent several years of my life translating the languages of videotaped interviews into different systems only to discover that we make meaning with anything and every thing (Percy 1984). ...

People of good will are accountable for their knowing actions with others when we make sense together by being attentive, intelligent, reasonable, responsible, and loving (Lonergan 1973). I believe that childhood is at the root of our crisis as a human family living among families of all life. We have the longest childhood of all animals, needing loving care to live and grow old enough to have children and grandchildren who care for us when we cannot care for ourselves, and who will care for our memory when we die. To remember requires all our abilities as a member of a family without whom we cannot live as human beings.

For more than 1,000 years children of Europeans have been at war with each other and the rest of the world, conquering or destroying whole families of animals, plants, human beings, and all that we call 'inanimate' things, the earth, water, and air on which all life depends. Unless we have a family, we cannot ask who are we, where do we come from, where are we going, how should we remember our ancestors? Educational development of children remembers in story, print, drama, and video media our own childhood of humanity. ...

EVEN DURING THE BLISS of art classes in her safe haven, war crept in. One night, Daisy worked late on a sculpture assignment. She was trying to make a rather large Madonna and child. No matter how she tried to make the clay form the image in her head, the clay kept taking the form of a child wrapped in a burlap cloth looking out into an unsafe world through big brown eyes as she or he crouched on the ground. When finished, it scared Daisy to see what she had done. As it was finished, across the room two pottery wheels started whirling noisily on their own. No one else was around. Startled and now afraid of her own shadow, Daisy turned them off and left the building quickly to take the last bus home. When she put her sculpture in the kiln a few days later, it blew up into hundreds of pieces on the very day the United States started bombing Iraq. Innocent children were being hurt and killed. The sculpture, a Madonna and child, had become a child of poverty, and then became the symbol of children in war. Something demanded that Daisy glue it all together and paint it. It is the *War Child*.

THE COURT CASE that demolished Ken had happened at the beginning of the year. At the end of the same year, Jane extended an unusual invitation that he could not refuse. She invited Ken and all three of his sons to Christmas dinner at her home right on Christmas day. Ken attended – of course! He was happy for Andy, who finally had his mother and father and his two brothers all together.

Ken wondered what that was all about. The event was hardly a safe haven. The only sure thing was that Ken was a man who would always respond kindly and hope for the best no matter what a person had done to him.

42

Starting Over Again

ALL OF KEN'S WORK with families was now in their own homes, on playgrounds, or in schools – wherever the clients needed to be. The separation from Daisy left Ken dangerously vulnerable. He was working alone without the protection of an office or an assistant, and traveling by bus.

Two female clients had been using tricks to entice their bachelor doctor into dangerous situations. Because Daisy was on the periphery, they attempted to get rid of Daisy entirely. Each in her own way directed threats and downright meanness at Daisy when she had, on rare occasions, accompanied Ken in his work. One took to claiming she just plain hated Ukrainians and the other threatened suicide if Daisy did not leave Ken alone with her; then she followed up by harassing Daisy over the telephone. That did it! Because both women were seriously unstable, there was a serious danger to Ken. Daisy launched into action.

Ken's ground-floor apartment and privacy had been invaded by one of the women who merely stepped over the low, stone patio wall and entered through the open glass doors. A secure second floor apartment came available at that time and because Ken had been invited to travel the far north on a teaching tour with an old friend and colleague during the moving time, Daisy and his son Stephen, did the move for him. Knowing that Daisy and Ken had a connection, prompted the manager of the building to offer Daisy the vacant apartment right next door to him. The house they had previously shared had been sold and she was in an unsuitable apartment, so moving next to Ken was a blessing. They were again joined at the hip with side-by-side apartments and with a safety valve. The arrangement allowed Ken to keep a separate place for his sons to live with him or to visit, while at the same time enjoying the company of Daisy and her family easily every day.

Determined to protect Ken, Daisy took her place firmly at his side again and all clients swiftly knew that the doctor was not a bachelor. Problems with female clients stopped. It was simply up to everyone to guess how Daisy fit into his life other than for work, but she was there. The separation had spanned only a few months, but like magnets, Ken and Daisy had been constantly drawn together for conversations, dinners, and emotional support all through those months. They had not been living separate lives. They settled into another new beginning.

HAVING WORKED WITH KEN in an office setting and now on the patients' own territory, Daisy could see why he preferred to work this way. Seeing families in their own homes gave an enhanced insight into relationships, social and financial problems, and needs. It was hard for a family to hide their circumstances when it could be seen first hand and became transparent.

When at home, children were in their comfort zone and acted normally, eating, sleeping, playing, talking, and bringing in friends. They were entirely different than when visiting in an office setting. Children got excited at the opening of a large, blue bag containing art materials that Ken and Daisy now carried into the homes. It never happened that a child would refuse doing artwork. The only problem in some homes was to find a clear table to do artwork on.

On taking over the medical billings again and auditing the past few months, Daisy was astounded at how much free work Ken had been doing while he had been doing his own billings. Even though computer programs had evolved to do medical billings to the BC Medical Services Plan, someone still had to fill out the sheets of information by hand for the computer company to enter and send to MSP. Ken had done so, but never followed through when a billing was rejected. Daisy billed for unbilled work and fixed the billings denied for one reason or another by MSP and resubmitted them. This was proof Ken truly did not work for money and it was completely up to her to make sure he got paid for at least most of his work.

Ken wrote a new information sheet for clients and physicians about the practice:

*   *   *

Ken Schramm, M.D., Psychiatrist
Consultant in Family Home Care
[Ken's 24-hour telephone numbers]
call Daisy, Assistant [number] for appointments

Information sheet for clients

Referrals by physicians only

– prefer Code 309 Adjustment Reaction – 6 months referral

 Home visits only

 Preference to multi-generational families

 Child advocacy

 Children – art, play, plasticine sculpting, painting,
   drawing, storytelling *with parents present*

 Health problems from birth to death

 Orthomolecular medicine (nutrient based,
   removal of toxins & allergens)

 Hypnotherapy, Story-telling and
   Planning – Psychotherapy vs. drugs

 No pharmaceutical/psychiatric drugs prescribed

Informed consent on medical records
(no secret files)

 <u>Problems</u>:

  reducing dependence on drugs

  making decisions about family and health care,
   especially chronic and life-threatening diseases
  (home care)

  inter-generational

  inter-cultural

  chronic pain

  birth and death plans

  lifestyle and career changes

24-hour notice required for cancelled appointments
No forensic work
ICBC & court cases will be referred to medical-legal

*   *   *

STUDYING ART HISTORY for a year and digging through her old photo slides to put together an assignment and being told her photos were like Degas paintings sent Daisy's attention back to previous training in photography. She weighed the pros and cons of enhancing that training by film or television. Either way, she could put previous courses that included screenwriting to new use. In her pink suede shoes with soft soles that made no sound, she was off to night school for the next ten months to get a diploma in the technology of professional television production.

The problem Daisy always encountered in her life was that life had so many interesting things to do, that at any moment she may jump into another venue of learning, much to the excitement and dismay of Ken, who was constantly interested in what she may do next. She felt the same about him. They had an irresistible fascination with each other as they each allowed the other space to explore and then to share what they found.

Daisy had always been entranced by light in colour and had years ago taken classes in making stained glass windows. Because of the danger to her small children, a glass studio never happened. In one of her recent house moves, she had abandoned her box of stained glass and lead, plus other art supplies just before going to art school. (Ken was upset on hearing about that.) Now with a camera, she could carry on enjoying the play of light and colour.

Daisy took to the outdoors often. She experimented with light and shadow, and how colour changed in different hours of the day – how the sun shone on the wings of white seagulls flying over the Kitsilano blue swimming pool water so that the underbelly of the bird took on a blue hue and white light outlined the bird. It was flowers backlit with sun shining through the petals that gave enhanced magic of colour, and the magic hour just before sundown gave a warm golden glow to everything.

One afternoon, Daisy was filming the beach scene where her children had spent many hours. She was telescoping, but not filming yet, for a close-up of a distant scene when a middle-aged homeless woman wheeling a cart emerged from behind a bush and was surprised to see a camera pointed at her. Through the viewfinder Daisy had a clear close-up of the woman's face. She looked right into the woman's eyes and it was as though the woman's soul stood naked. Daisy was shocked and immediately put the camera down. In that split second, Daisy had seen the woman's life. She was clear eyed, not drunk or drugged as our society often imagines street people of being. This woman was living many a woman's nightmare of becoming homeless. She was a woman who had known love and was someone's mother. And she still loved someone, somewhere. She was simply homeless and ashamed. She did not want to be seen. Daisy honoured her wish.

USING VIDEO IN the practice where it proved to be helpful, Ken was adamant that after the clients viewed the tape with him and had a discussion on the same day as taping, that videotapes stay with the clients for their own safe keeping or to be destroyed. No tape was kept by the practice. There was no record kept of sensitive issues where clients let their most intimate secrets be recorded in order to gain clearer insight into themselves and their family relationships.

An exception of keeping a tape happened only once for a family that wanted several copies made because their father had a serious case of cancer and was going into hospital for aggressive treatment. The clients had a small child of a second marriage and teenaged children, who lived in another country with their mother but had come to be with their father. They wanted copies of the dinner they cooked together with their father, then sat and ate together – maybe a last supper – and that is what it was.

THE EFFECTIVENESS OF VIDEO in the practice was played out one week in two different ways with two different families living miles apart. On videotaping one family, the husband and father of small children claimed to be depressed, feeling he was working too hard and could no longer cope. He thought his way out of depression was to leave his family but he was willing to give therapy a try. Daisy held the camcorder by hand and unobtrusively moved around to catch varying viewpoints. During the taping, the husband and his wife slouched in soft chairs, each resting their feet across a coffee table from opposite sides of the room. On viewing the videotape, the husband sat up, entranced. He watched the close-ups of his relaxed face as his feet played with his wife's feet while at the same time he was talking about depression. At the end he exclaimed, "I look downright contented! All I have to do is to work less and spend more time with my family. I don't need therapy. I just need to remember I am really happy!" The family terminated therapy.

The second family had a different outcome. Interacting with each other, the wife let loose an array of loud, angry complaints about seemingly little incidentals. The husband looked increasingly distressed as he moved from sitting upright to cringing in a far corner of the room. Her nagging was relentless. On viewing the tape, he became appalled at what he saw. The wife seemed unaffected, maybe even proud of herself. He had stayed in the marriage for his child, now of college age. He seized this opportunity to ask for a divorce. They were homeowners, so he announced that he would move immediately into their empty basement suite. The announcements made her livid.

Arriving at the home the following week, the door opened and the woman, who was a large bodied person towered over Ken, waving a paper in his face while screaming, "See this! I have the newspaper article about you – you crook! I'm going to report you to your college."

Months after the article had been in the newspaper, the woman had dug it up. It was a concern because she worked in a large hospital among other health-care workers. All the time Ken had been working with this family, she had this secret weapon.

As usual, no matter how ugly a situation was, Ken faced it full on. He made immediate contact with the BC College of Physicians and Surgeons to explain that there was going to be a complaint about him. He never heard another thing about it but that incident served as a reminder that in the background there still lurked the fallout from his ex-wife's wrath.

TO DO HOME VISITS, Ken and Daisy needed to use public transit in all kinds of weather. The weather had become unbearably hot. They were stuck in hot crowded buses, traveling one to two hours just to get to a client for an hour's visit, then on leaving, an hour or two again on a hot bus, sometimes carrying video recording gear and the case of art supplies.

At this time they had several clients that were unreliable. Daisy and Ken traveled half a day in the heat to find no one at home and there had been no telephone call to cancel. This was not billable time, making it a complete waste of half a day. Ken always had a policy of not charging the clients personally for missed appointments as some other physicians were doing. In this case and in most cases, it would be futile anyway to try to bill the client because the clients were poor and collection would never happen.

Daisy complained to Ken, "We are suffering, wasting our time in this heat. I think we should at least have a car to do this job. It is too hard this way. A car is cheaper than a commercial office."

Ken listened. Aware that heart conditions and strokes run in his family, he had given up driving a car eight years ago. He had not wanted to have a stroke or a heart attack behind the wheel and take a chance of hurting someone else. Daisy had loved her bicycle and preferred horses and joked she was born in the wrong century. She would need to add chauffeur to chaperone, guardian and assistant of Ken in determination never to let anyone hurt him again. They leased a car but Daisy needed to learn to drive, something she had never done before.

Andy was still seeing his father on his mother's territory – her home or in a restaurant. The sham was over but the child continued to carry the burden of presuming Ken was holding out on his mother. The car needed for the work in order to comply with the court order became a contentious issue for the boy. He complained to Ken that the car was for Daisy's pleasure only and if it were not for the car, his mother could have that money, too.

AT A TIME when an old friend, a psychologist had taken on a bet with her new husband as to which of them could make the first million dollars at their respective practices and she in fact won the bet, and another rather close acquaintance, a well-known social worker was gaa-gaa over her almost famous and moneyed writer client – Ken was sturdy and true to himself and his morals, always looking out for who he could help without any strings attached.

Daisy's sister Terisa had come on an extended visit to brave Daisy's practice driving before the final driving exam.

"If there ever was a Good Samaritan on this earth, Ken embodies him," Daisy told her sister. "No wonder we belong together! Through thick and thin, for richer or poorer, illness and health, we have a bond."

"Mm-Hmm," Terisa mused from behind her newspaper.

Then on a walk with Ken, Terisa saw for herself what Daisy meant about a Good Samaritan.

They were walking in cold rain of autumn. A lightly dressed homeless man sat on the street by a storefront.

Ken stopped. "Just a minute, Terisa."

Ken walked over to the man, took his own jacket off and gave it to the surprised man, who then put it on with wide eyes looking at Ken in disbelief.

"Thank you, sir. Bless you. Bless you." The man zipped it up, affectionately patting the front of the jacket.

Ken, now only wearing a cotton shirt, nodded and continued to walk.

Stunned, Terisa followed him. "Ken, now you only have a shirt on. It's cold and it's raining."

"Yes. He may get ill in the cold rain. I can't ignore a man less fortunate than myself."

IT WAS KEN'S IDEA to do a video to help Cynthia Hunt in her work to help Tibet's Orphaned Children. Together, Ken, Daisy and Cynthia made a video using the Tibetan children's art, photographs, a dusty filmstrip picked up on the Silk Road, and Cynthia's narration.

While editing the video in one of her 3 a.m. sessions, Daisy was struck with the memory of her Buddhist teacher in 1966. Daisy had been busy cooking at the wood stove on the meditation centre. He had been watching from his chair across the room. Then he got up and before he headed out the door, he turned to Daisy and said, "You will help the orphans." At the time Daisy had no idea of how. Besides, she had her own four children to worry about, so she forgot the comment. Now she remembered with wonder.

The video, "Tibetan Children's Art" played on public television in Ladakh and Dharamsala, and who knows where else. Feedback was that it was a 'smash hit' with the people it was about. Cynthia gave a copy of the video to the Dalai Lama.

43

Ken in Hell Journal 1991/92

EXCERPTS FROM Doctor Ken's Journal named **Ken in Hell**:

December 2, 1991: Today, his teacher Susan and I introduced my son Andy's class to the use of personal journals in learning science.

December 6, 1991: I wrote this for Grade 6-7 science class: **Your Body, Your Life, & Your World in Learning Science:** Here are some ways to use your personal notebook and your public journal in asking and answering questions...

Susan copied the above for each student to have one and I read it aloud for all to hear and ask for questions. ...We spent the hour sharing dreams and discussing their sources and meaning: sleepwalking; two friends dreaming the same dream... dreaming of falling and waking... dreams which seem to foretell the future; dreams as memories... dreams as the result of the work of our brains and our chemistry...

...Susan and I talked about a way to teach math to kids who are having trouble with math; we talked about finger math and learning disabilities...

December 7: Pearl Harbor Day. ...Today I developed swellings of my left hand, right inner arm above elbow, and swollen rings of fluid around my anus. I felt "beaten" after I talked with my ex-wife on the phone about Xmas plans for Andy and asked if she planned to go for more maintenance for next year. ...She said the only private school she is considering for Andy is Vancouver College... run by Christian Brothers. Tuition there would be $3,000, which an increase to $500 would cover. ...I am willing to discuss sharing costs for Andy's education with her. After the past several years of legal hassle just before Xmas, it would be good for Andy and all of us if we had Xmas without a hassle. She passed the phone to Andy who has been sick with sore throat and vomiting.

December 8: Andy is better today but my swellings were worse... I read about dreams in books by Rossi, Tedlock, Coles, Matthews, Piaget...

December 9: ...Today our science students drew pictures with their eyes closed and wrote about their pictures and what they learned. ...Next class we plan to ask what questions have our students put in their notebooks.

I told Doctor... that I do not have the energy to help a woman with cancer who told him the only psychiatrist she could find has a ten year waiting list and who told me today that after months of looking she has an appointment with a psychiatrist on Wednesday. I will talk with her after that.

December 9: I watched William Kennedy-Smith trial on TV and cried, reliving my own experience facing jail a year ago.

December 10: ...I read Denis de Rougemont's "Love in the Western World" ...He analyzes passionate pagan and Christian love in terms of the myth of Tristan and Iseult...

December 11: ...I talked with Andy about Xmas Eve plans for going with Daisy's grandchildren and their parents to Christ Church Cathedral for carol singing. He said he isn't religious. I said everyone deserves a chance at least once in their lives to be in a Cathedral. I asked him to discuss this with his mother before deciding whether he would join us.

I told him I talked with his mother on the phone about sharing the costs of his education at Vancouver College and that we need to discuss it further in person. He says Susan [teacher] is helping him prepare for the entrance exam. ...Later I talked with my eldest son Stephen about this and decided myself that I will talk with Jane, after Andy passes the entrance exam for Vancouver College, about sharing the costs of his education by raising the maintenance retroactively...

I find writing all this helps me feel better. I was/am living Ken in Hell, no thanks to William Carlos Williams. My plan for December is to schedule my work and holiday duties so I can write and research for my courses next year...

December 12: Insights into Daisy's Ukrainian culture ...I told Daisy I am beginning to understand some of the differences between us. I grew up in a Congregational Church with no theology except what the congregation believes... God, who loves you unconditionally, is the only one you can love with your whole heart, mind, soul, and your life. A man and woman marry and raise children to grow in God's love. Love is shared not given because we are born, live, and die in God's love. In my protestant tradition of conscience and conscientious objection to the misuse of power by human beings and the State, icons are associated with the selling of indulgences as a means and a symbol of buying your way into heaven...

December 13: I enrolled in a course at St. Mark's on "Lonergan and Spirituality" and found a book at VST [Vancouver School of Theology] by a Czech historian of Christian doctrine, Jaroslav Pelikan, "The Spirit of Eastern Christendom (600-1700)", to learn about Ukranian Christianity in hopes of better understanding and more closeness with Daisy. Her father is Roman Catholic and her mother Ukrainian Catholic. They married in the Ukrainian Catholic Church and Daisy grew up going to the Anglican Church (a compromise to two Catholic churches with two languages).

Grade 6-7 science students list their questions, group related ones, and discuss them: Susan leads group in guided fantasy just as I have to leave for a family home visit...

I ask them [clients] how they expect change will occur in their therapy... and when they answer through insight and understanding of their past experiences, I talk with them about change is the result of the decisions you make based on your understanding of your experiences and the knowledge you have of your ability to take action, to make promises you can keep.

Friday the thirteenth: no car, no telephone, no good news. G's [church minister client] cancer has grown quickly since September. The good news I found is that the treatment controlled the tumor's growth over the period of intensive treatment with hyperthermia [in a cancer clinic]. The loneliness of protecting each other from our sadness and feeling helpless and hopeless... He finished his first draft of "Dearest Mother" in the tradition of Kafka's "Letter to My Father". He wants me to read it and help him get it ready for ...publication.

December 15: A local Washingtonian composer planned to be an astronomer until at age 12 he heard a song by Schubert in musical appreciation class. He decided that he could begin to write down the tunes he heard in his head. At that time he thought that everyone heard them in their heads. Daisy tells me that when she hears music, that sets off a flow of many images in her head. When she draws, paints, sculpts, or films photos of her family, she feels good. In my world of my body, I find feelings and words with occasional soft images. In dreams my feelings and touches are stronger than my images. Am I a natural protestant? A repressed Catholic? Lonergan's method appeals to me because he emphasizes that knowing is more than seeing. Insights are not simply taking a look inside to see what you see, but to know how you know. I find asking to know is what I do inside and outside. I said to Daisy I'm a good visitor to have around if you want to slow things down; nothing gets done for awhile except a kind of stopping time; what we think or feel or decide or do is experienced and known and evaluated in slow motion. My childhood hero was Ferdinand the bull smelling the flowers, instead of playing war, which I also did.

Daisy and I had a minor war about work before play, money before Xmas gifts. Whenever I'm sick with a cold and feel vulnerable as I do now, I get angry, feeling helpless, worrying I won't be able to continue to bring in money to support people I love and meet my responsibilities. She sees me picking religions she is not interested in. Her religion is art, mine is feeling, thinking, and writing, and Homeopathy where words are remedies, potentized bits of reality, parts that contain wholes.

...Looked for Andy at SUB [at university] video games and realized I would not be so lonely if I could do something with him mornings or at times when Daisy is in the fairies. Divorce makes it even more difficult to be with my sons than their mothers made it when I was married to them. My mother made it difficult to know my father and my wives make it difficult to know my sons. Rougemont writes we make love into passion and passion requires obstacles to keep it alive and to keep us unaware our passion is for death, not for life. I experience images and fantasy as obstacles, competition, distractions which keep people from being in contact with reality and each other. Thank you, Ted Sideras, Greek Catholic, for Sideras Place, our asking, finding, and making place, where I began my work as a family doctor in B.C. [British Columbia]

December 18: In the evening we had a Father and sons reunion of "The Four Musketeers", as Stephen named himself, Peter, Andy and I at [restaurant] for an early Xmas dinner. Stephen and Peter, Christine, Thea, and Morgan Lee will be in Argenta for the holidays with my first ex-wife, Carolyn, and Andy will be with his mother. I really enjoyed being with them after a long struggle to be their father and their friend.

December 19: Met my son Peter for lunch to catch up with him. We talked...

December 27: Woke feeling bloated... terrible with no sense of a future... I spoke with doctor... and he confirmed that I should take [Homeopathic remedy]. I did and felt more alive as I rode the bus and walked through a day of family home visits. I taught focusing to a family seeking life after cancer. He is a poet and she is a social worker. He dreamt that Walt Whitman was throwing shit over the heads of social workers. ...I suggested as a patient he was becoming a participant in his treatment to get the shit out.

December 28: Hurray, I'm awake and alive again!

January 5, 1992: Stephen says the only nourishment he has been getting is our meals together on Wednesday nights. He wants to share with me Morgan's [grandson] growing up. I will do that any way I can...

January 6, 1:30 a.m. I asked my body what these swellings of my body mean and I heard: "I can kill you any time I want. In the meantime I'll just beat you up and cripple you." God/Jane.

Daisy was frightened by the swelling of my hand and arm and worried I would overwork. She arranged an evening meeting to discuss this with [doctor]. I felt quite happy, singing and jazzing with my mouth trumpet and enjoyed my sense of humor. I kidded her that we would each tell [doctor], "I'm fine but my partner is really sick." She didn't laugh nor did doctor... but I did. He spoke with both of us together...

...After Daisy arranged the visit with doctor... I almost ran up the hill, I was so glad to be going back to school...

...I remember Rosenstock-Huessy saying: "Remember, you are always more alive than your most living thought!" Forty years later I know that being alive and knowing that I am alive in my pain and in my joy is my happiness...

January 16: I had dinner with Carolyn, Stephen, and Peter, and then went to the Lonergan seminar for the first time at St. Marks where I enjoyed the company of strangers.

January 23: I missed the Lonergan seminar because of working late, heavy rain, and illness.

January 29: Dinner with my sons. Remembering the sixties in response to Peter's questions...

January 30: ...I found myself speaking to a priest I don't really know... and telling him that I have lived next door to Catholicism but I have married too many times to be a Catholic. I said I believed I had married women with whom I shared a religion only to find later we did not pray to the same god...

I was tired so I did not stay for after class discussion but went to library and home to wait for Daisy to return from her class. Even though I rested at home, by the time she returned I had an itchy swollen right eye and took [Homeopathic remedy] and went to bed without seeing the video Daisy edited for G [client with cancer and his family].

January 31: My right eye closed overnight... I was unable to go to class or work today...

February 2: ...and came alive again. I read "Asphodel" again on the bus and noticed the daisies [in bloom] for the first time.

Read Paul Mariani: William Carlos Williams: A New World Naked...

February 3: I noticed that my hands were wrinkled as if I had soaked them in the bath for a long time and the watery swelling had gone...

February 4: Happy Chinese New Year, I made it through the worst of the winter for me! What story will heal my clients of the hell in being married when their parents divorced?

February 14: I love feeling "A Very Valentine" by Gertrude Stein for Sherwood Anderson. ...I began reading "My Emily Dickinson" and was back to New England again. I remember Emily Dickinson's "I would as soon appear naked in public as read my poems." Yes women are excluded from public writing/reading in a world when progress means killing families, where words are born and grow and live and die. My William Carlos Williams and my very Gertrude Stein give me poetry, spoken conversation, dialogues remembered in bodied imagination.

February 15: ...Whenever I'm freed from work I return to Williams and Stein and the words of speech alive again bodying patients/ce. My journey/journal to hear, write the words being born. Like the Mayans, our task is to bring the world alive again in words which mirror the mirrors of life. Where there are people there are words and things separated and joined, we make art in words which make us and things another world to live in.

February 17: On a morning I hoped to write, I panicked about my heart going from 40 to 80 beats per minute on my beeping do-it-yourself blood pressure machine and after telling myself not to talk with Daisy about the specifics we talk about her fantasy of my funeral where my family, my mother and my brothers and my sisters and my ex-wives and my sons won't acknowledge her and my relationship with Daisy and they all say nice things about dear dead ken and then they go to a restaurant together and after that my second ex-wife and my son's partner, the mother of my only grandson go off shopping together at Holt Renfrew, something they have done together before. I said I think that's exactly what will happen and I want to miss out on my funeral too unless I can ring the bell in my coffin loud enough to scare the hell out of all of them. I said the way they treat Daisy is the way they treat me.

We spoke of the difficulty my mom and dad must have had bonding to me their first child after my birth and seeing my head coming to a point like a dunce cap and my spinal cord showing through the pouch from the hole in my spine at the back of my neck and my dad is holding me in all the photos my mom or granddad took and he is obviously proud of me after I survived the surgery to repair my spine. My mom overwhelmed me with loving kisses and worry I would not be able to make it, and pushed me out the door to meet people and do things I was too shy to do. I was allowed to be angry but not to be anxious and afraid so I learned to overcome or hide my fears and I didn't speak in school until I was 12 and then the grownups blew up my world with their atom bomb. I experienced my life as a gift from God calling me to share what I have with others by being a doctor, a teacher and a physician for families who want to care for their own in a world that seems not to care about their lives except as slaves.

She [Daisy] says she will go to work and take care of me while I write and walk and cook the foods I need to get well and I say I don't want to be a kept man any more than she wants to be a kept woman and she says she understands and I say I appreciate her offer. I think of my mother taking care of my father right into the mental hospital and nursing home...

Later I talked to Doctor... on the phone and then I walked to his office to ask him to take my blood pressure. I wish he would take it away and give me one I could live with better and reassure me I am at least as alive as I feel. On the walk there, I asked myself what do I do when I am anxious and I realized that I ask what it means and I pay attention to the answers and patterns and insights I get, and anxiety changes into something more personal and understandable. I realize I make everything into a religion, even praying, when I use my beeping machine to measure my blood pressure and my life is measured by the numbers and the beeps I get.

I am a shy feeling person who needs to touch and be touched and I make that a religion, too and I allowed myself to bond to my ex-wife in the religious community we shared before I knew we pray to different gods. When I asked my illness to talk to me from all the swellings I was getting on my hands and feet and around my ass and my penis and balls, I got "I can kill you anytime I want" and I asked who are you and I heard "God" and said I don't believe you are god and I heard "Jane" and I believed it was her that wanted to kill me and still may want to and I took that to mean the rest of the world also who want to kill people like me who with Jesus and Socrates and Buddha question the meanings of life and who is truth anyway? I try to say some of this and he [doctor] answers me by taking my blood pressure and doing the lab and ekg requests and we talk of our ex-wives and how we keep hoping for some kind of contact with the Ice Maiden; he calls them the anima and I don't fully understand. He says he wishes more people would understand the other who is represented and present in a couple relationship of man and woman and I hear Walker Percy's triadic relations of man the world maker. I don't talk about that and say I'm shy and overworked and he says be shy and choose who you work with and take as much time for yourself as you need or can.

Our first visit with family grieving over mother's train "suicide". They blame her decision and I blame drugs, doctors, multinational corporations and the voices that told their mother/wife what to do. We are angry and miserable, and we are grieving together, explaining our calamity, in the tradition of witch detection and shamanism.

February 18: Sunny walk to lab for... test. I feel stronger again and ready...

I talk with Daisy about how I began being with her and playing with her when I believed she and I could begin a new life and our love would release my pressure and when I found the pressure increased when nobody, including our children and ourselves wanted us to become a family. Now I feel stuck with having used Daisy for my health and not wanting to use her or anybody else or be used myself. ...I am learning that I do not want to be a priest or a monk either and live a regimented life. I need to write my prayers and remember my Pilgrim family. I want to believe they were more loving than the Puritan George Bush types who took over their homes.

On a home visit I explained that hypnosis is not a bag of tricks but a prayerful knowing of the power of language. The New Hypnosis knows that we do not need to seek a special trance state; we are in and out of dreaming every ninety minutes day and night and recognizing this natural rhythm we can ask permission of our bodies and our partners if it is ok to interrupt our play and our prayer to do or to be something else or not. Asking gives often forced choices in a world of questions and answers. *Being attentive* is having experiences and asking questions. *Being intelligent* with our questions and answers is finding or making patterns in our playful experiences and having insights which are not the same as looking and seeing within or without but rather asking to know the meanings of our experiences which are otherwise invisible and unknown without attending to our own knowing. *Being rational* is evaluating our experiences and insights and questions to judge how we know they are true or false or imagined or meaningless. *Being responsible* is deciding the consequences for others and ourselves of experiences, insights, judgments, and acts of knowing for our own conduct and our chosen actions in relation to the authentically human good. *Being loving* is allowing ourselves to be true to our experiences of being loved by God who is present to us and with us in the world which is his grace and in the desires of our human hearts to ask and to know with whom we are in love in our experiences, understandings, judgments, decisions, and actions. We are healthy when we know we are loved and loving, attentive, intelligent, rational, and responsible human beings. This is how community is made and unmade and made again.

February 19: I went with Andy, my youngest son age 12 to his entrance exam for Point Grey mini school and rediscovered how much I hate Kerrisdale. It is like seeing and feeling him go off to prison in that cold castle. ...With his brother Stephen and I at dinner he [Andy] continues his career as class comic telling jokes... On the phone later he made it clear to me she [Jane] wants him to go to a mini-school and wants him to stay over at my place on Wednesday nights... He really wants to go to Vancouver College... He wants to be a politician when he grows up. I said he would have to be a lawyer first... He said before that he has to be an alcoholic...

44

Journal 1992 - Ken in Hell

AFTER JUDGE OLIVER'S pompous and carelessly flawed medical decision that denied the existence of Ken's illness and stated that in his opinion a little allopathic high blood pressure medicine would solve the problem if by chance there was one and told Ken to get back to work as a physician, Ken continued suffering uncontrolled sky-high blood pressure, a dangerously out of control enlarged heart, and strange swellings that crop up all over his body from head to toe. He would wake up to an eye closed with swelling, or his groin swollen, his hands swelled, or swollen ankles making walking difficult and sometimes impossible. In medicine it is common knowledge that if the external body is suffering, the internal body is also suffering. Ken was not well – just determined to tough it out because now he needed to pay back borrowed money and he wanted a relationship with his sons.

In trying to get well, Ken had many tests done by different doctors. In following a Judge's order to take allopathic high blood pressure medicine and get back to work as a physician, Ken lost the progress to getting well that he had made before going in front of Judge Oliver. Even though he was taking a newer generation of allopathic medicine than he had taken before, it had the effect of making him ill as before with no benefit of lower blood pressure.

Ken continued journal writing of ***Ken in Hell***.

February 20, 1992: I went to see a doctor about my tests: the good news is my blood and urine and thyroid and cholesterol are normal; the bad news is my own doctor who I thought was my friend and whom I paid $100 for talking to me this month left town yesterday for a holiday without even calling me about my electrocardiogram which shows that my heart is still enlarged despite the blood pressure medicine and under the strain my heart is beating irregularly. I told the stand-in doctor who is running from me to the phone and two other patients that my heart is broken. He said if you want it to be and his heart was broken on Valentine's Day and he wasn't going to let it be broken and I shouldn't either. When I said I was overworking because of a court order he said I should forget the court order and go sit on a beach in Mexico. I asked his receptionist where all the people in Mexico are sent? Do they all come here? I've never been in Mexico, don't want to travel, die or leave my body, and have been afraid to exercise or make love for fear of bringing on so many extra beats my heart would race off without me to Mexican heaven or wherever.

Daisy and I worked well together in helping a young couple, both from divorced families, have a practice divorce so that they know what it feels like. On Monday we will see how they are doing their own and their families' lives...

...Before going to the doctor I began making arrangements for my mother to stay at a friend's suite... near her great grandson. I felt pleased at the thought of seeing her as a great grandmom and then my son told me he didn't think we could handle her for more than a week. Reminded me how hard I worked as a child running to catch up to younger brother so I could have a few minutes of play with him and his friends. At that time it often seemed my mom was my best friend. With her eldest son, her three grandsons, and her great grandson here I should think we will find a way to be with her for more than a week if only we can play together.

February 21: I want to know Page Smith in person. His essays have helped keep me alive. He says historians tell what happened.

I spoke with Jane on the telephone. My son is ill. He asked me to visit and bring a movie and some ginger ale. She said I could give him a homeopathic remedy and I agreed to see him between home visits today. We agreed to meet at Vancouver College open house on Tuesday evening and talk about Andy's schooling. I said my mother is coming out in late March and early April to see her great grandson.

I got some bad news about my heart this week. The EKG showed my heart is still enlarged and I am getting extra beats in the ventricles which if they speed up will take me away with them. I hoped after two years of treatment for hypertension that my heart would be less enlarged. [Doctor] told me to stop overworking (remember this is a marathon not a sprint). I worked hard to pay the loan (I took to pay her child maintenance during the time I was ill). I am still willing to discuss sharing the responsibility for Andy's education with her [Jane] on a long-term basis we can both sustain. She told me of her burnout and I said we had done quite a bit over the past year to improve the situation and it would be good for everyone concerned if we could reach a long-term agreement before my mother's visit. She said they were going to see "Macbeth" with a friend and she had seen Gloria Steinem. I said Gloria was asked why she never married and she answered: "I can't mate in captivity." Jane said yes Gloria has had a lot of men. We left it at that.

Second visit with grieving family (over mother's suicide): daughter says if someone is so depressed that they cannot take care of themselves, why does the psychiatrist put them in charge of their medication? I did not give the standard answer and defend psychiatrists.

My client G had a grand mal seizure today while receiving his intravenous cancer treatment. When he woke he could not speak nouns only verbs. When that was reported to him, he found it interesting. He can still write and retains his sense of humor. Tomorrow he will have x-rays to see if there is cancer in the brain, something he had dreaded.

February 22: Sunshine colors through the rainbow drops on the trees outside my windows.

I spoke with Stephen on the phone about Peter and my worry that he was lost and learned... he had rented a room and was doing fine. Neither of us has heard from him despite leaving messages on his answering machine... I said I wanted to talk with Peter about fund raising for Society Promoting Environmental Conservation... I told Stephen more details about my health than I was able to tell him at dinner on Wednesday, especially that my blood cholesterol is normal and my low white blood count is probably viral but may be due to the blood pressure medicine which I think also increases the extra beats of my heart. Stephen gave me his opinion of Jane's response to my telling her of my illness... He thinks my mother's difficulty with accepting Daisy is the same as her problem with accepting my brothers' third wives. I believe she only accepts those that have produced grandchildren. She accepts Jane as Andy's mother but not as my ex-wife who is out to get more money from me.

Lawrence and I are pals. I wish I had this opportunity with my own sons when they were his age. Daisy has given me this gift of sharing her grandchildren. I hope that my mother can see what Daisy and I have shared. I want a blessing for us and our friendship which has brought us and our families so much pain after the joy of new life.

I mediated discussion of starting a new business and learned more gossip about the workings of VanCity [Credit Union] than I wanted to know...

G's wife tells me that he has his speech back but no memory for what happened and no signs of brain tumor. I explained that the loss of memory is due to the seizure and the good sign is that he is recovering his abilities again.

February 23: Fear of being paralyzed by a stroke is paralyzing me. I hope to write myself out of this one. What if it is true that "in the beginning there was the Word and Word was with God" when embryonic heart begins to beat in rhythmic harmony with feeling yes yes yes yes worlds of yes mama papa yes words?

I showed a poem to Daisy and she said she liked it and I asked if she heard the placenta in it and she said I should explain it and I said it is enough that she likes the sound of it...

February 24: Awoke stronger and writing clearer.

February 25:

Raindrops bamboo twigs
twinkling stars
blue green yellow white purple
camera does not what eye can see
Man's reach should exceed his grasp says Robert Browning,
reaching beyond me to worlds of
great grand children

I find it difficult to respect myself for getting $ [dollars] from others' pain. Chinese emphasis on health has drawn me since medical school and I need to follow through with this interest. The block seems to be the lack of context (family) which makes it possible to develop and sustain continuity.

February 29: I survived another Daisy or is it Sadie Hawkins Day without a proposition or even a preposition – Darn it!

March 17: "What do you want to be and what do you want to do with the rest of your life? I have been asking this question while reading the 1992 edition of Richard Bolles' "What Color Is Your Parachute? A Practical Guide to Job Hunting and Career Change." In the Quick Job Hunt exercise he has changed the parts of the parachute to petals of flowers to ask readers to consider where they like flowers to grow best.

 I believe the world and everything in it is alive, especially our thoughts, words, feelings, dreams, and desires. The Creator is present in creation and the world expresses their grace. My response to creation as creature and creator is gratitude when I know I am loved and living in the love of life as their gift to us. When we, you and I, do not know we are loved in life, we react out of emptiness as sick and defensive wounded animals. We are healthy only when we are loved and loving members of a family. In order to do my best, my calling, I need to live and work with others who know that life is love and love is knowing each other in love as the gift of life. I need to be growing and learning, breaking out of the boundaries of myself, my limitations, to know how it is to be someone else, to be converted to know who loves me, with whom I am in love because they made me.

I want to use my skills with people who share the passion of building a more alive democratic world and with whom I feel a sense of ease and understanding and joy and humor without having to be reformed or a reformer, people who live and let live because we have our own lives and don't have to "get a life." I want to make jokes, conversations, stories, books, computer games, dialogues, and other "things" which serve people in building, making, enjoying, and caring for, yes, even protecting our own homes and communities. My central motivation is gratitude for the garden and feast of life I have been given and my desire to share life as love with my children, friends, and relatives in our chosen family of loved ones.

Before I die I want to know that Daisy is happy doing what she wants to do the way she wants to do it and where she wants to do it with whomever she wants to do it. I want to know that I know where I stand, sit, and smell with her. I want to know we are both safe to be and to do whatever we need and enjoy doing. I want to know the same or similar things of my children so that I can share what I know and have with them.

I need to know when my ex-anybodies are going to attack me again for more money or pieces of me, because I want to help my sons to have the education and the work they want while I have the life to share with them.

For and by myself, apart from family, I want to balance my life of love, learning, labor, and leisure so that I can be with other men who are also artists. I want to write stories and dialogues which share what I am learning from living and writing people so that I can keep on learning as long as I live. I want to help build a more responsibly honest, loving and democratic community in Vancouver, in B.C., and New England. I want to join in the planning, design and building of homes on Jericho Lands, especially with native people and our families as partners. I want to make a home with a garden and a studio where I can learn and teach with families who want to take care of their loved ones. I want to live and work at home until I die or move. As Vancouver grows, I want to be ready to either help manage that growth or get far enough away from it to keep on living and working. Before I die, I want to know that I have done all that I can do to help make the world safer and more enjoyable for children, families, and natives. I want my epitaph to say out loud in the hearts of my readers: Ken Schramm was alive all his life and he was alive when he died in the knowledge that he made a home for the family of humankind with all the animals and spirits and dreams of the world as divine grace. He lived his life in gratitude and love and defiance and humor. His body returns to the garden of the earth where his spirit lives and lives his family.

March 30: Ads lie to sell reality. Art lies to tell the truth. The truth of conversation is found and made in questioning the lies of truth, the life in words and individuals as self-making. A clumsy translation of my insight in the opacity of conversation, the hiding of truth in indirection and emptiness challenges me to find and make my truth by misunderstanding others and myself. I have lived inside William Carlos Williams' world for a year of Ken in Hell writing as asking and attending, in a word: prayer. The comparative philosophy of Archie Bahm reads advertising as natural for Americans as salesmen and artificial to Chinese thinkers as cooks and irrelevant to Indians as gurus."

March 31: A Letter to Bill Williams [William Carlos Williams, M.D., deceased] *Dear Bill:*
I have been talking with you inside my life ever since I read your autobiography of your practice as physician and poet when I was a medical student. They called me The Writer on the surgical wards where I was learning to write not cut my cases. All my college, medical school, and internship notes were thrown out by my mother during one of the moves she made in the sixties when my father was too sick to work or help her. I get very upset with Daisy during house moves when she throws away her most precious possessions: her paints and art supplies and her writing. I feel the loss of life and I want to bring it back to life. Since last May when I met Peter Q. [professor] I have been writing and living my life as if I were you writing Kora in Hell every day, only for me it is Ken in Hell living to be reborn as a writer double daring myself and families I see every day to write and live our own stories our own way. It keeps me going knowing you did this before me and did not sell yourself and found your way to live the conversations of your practice as poet physician. Words fail and words heal and fail again and make the world new and naked again.

45

Who is Most Important?

FOR HIS MOTHER'S West Coast holiday, Ken rented the waterfront garden suite on Kitsilano Point in a friend's bed and breakfast home. Only a few feet from the beach, it had a large glass patio door leading into the lush garden that gave privacy behind greenery. There was a view of the city centre to the right and of the bay straight ahead backed by West End, Stanley Park and the North Shore mountains beyond, and an open ocean vista to the left with ships in the harbor that lit up at night like Christmas trees. On a clear day, Vancouver Island could be seen hazily on the ocean's horizon. It was a nice place to rest while at the same time being close to family.

Ken assumed the responsibility of overseeing his mother's care and hoped his family would rally around for more than a week. Because of her strokes, he arranged to pay a salary to his son Peter and his sister's daughter to look after their grandmother around the clock.

The mother of Stephen's small son jumped the queue by inviting the grandmother for dinner right after her plane arrived. That was fine with everyone because of her great grandson.

Immediately on arrival, Ken and Daisy showed his mother her accommodation that appeared to please her. The clock dictated that she must be shuffled out to Christine's house, a block away.

Ken's mother had only time to go to the washroom and do her most important task that was to take a photo of her husband – Ken's father, out of the suitcase. She shared an intimate minute with Daisy as she lovingly showed the black and white framed photo of a handsome young man and explained that this man is the love of her life as she set it out on a side-table to be easily viewed from her bed.

Daisy was moved by the genuine devotion of a woman loving a man for so many years through so much illness and separation by hospitalization.

Ken and Daisy accompanied his mother into Christine's home to find her sitting comfortably as though on a throne at the end of a kitchen table while Stephen, looking frazzled and tired, rushed around preparing dinner. He was lost in bunches of vegetables with lots of large green leaves that he was trying to clean and get ready for cooking or salads. He had just begun preparing the vegetarian dinner after rushing in from work.

Ken and Daisy knew that they were not invited to dinner but had sacrificed precious time with his mother in order to deliver the grandmother to Christine's home on time. Considering Stephen was still at the sink washing vegetables and nothing was cooking yet, it was clear that serving dinner was going to be a while. Since Ken had not seen his mother for several years and had constantly been concerned, actually worried about her, it seemed like an opportunity to have a short visit with his mother and his grandson. They went into the living room. Christine followed on their heels and stated in no uncertain terms that Ken and Daisy were not invited to this private dinner. Regardless of explanations that they knew and were not planning to stay, Christine ordered them to leave her house immediately.

Promptly, without a word, Ken and Daisy walked out. It was clear by the look on Ken's mother's face that Christine's actions surprised and confused her after she had flown clear across the country to see her oldest son as well as others.

Once again, feeling beaten up by a woman whose only power came from having a child, who was Ken's grandchild – Ken took it all quietly, respecting the fact that he had entered Christine's home.

Daisy was angry for Ken's sake. She wondered how that young woman would dare to treat the grandfather of her child in such a manner. She also wondered how Christine could be so insensitive to Ken's mother who had not seen her son for about eight years. Daisy thought back to days when people seemed to have more manners – a time when respect of elders was paramount.

Walking the street at Ken's side, Daisy could feel his hurt. She hated the way these women, mother's of Ken's sons and grandchild, treated Ken. She gave way to sounding off. "Send gifts and money but don't bother me. Doesn't that sound familiar? This is not a good omen for counting on that mother to instill good family values in your growing grandson versus her self-interest, or should I say 'women only' values. Don't these women understand that sons become men? Their self-importance seems all that matters to them."

ATTENDING A REMOTE VIEWING weekend workshop, Daisy encountered another competition about who was most important. The instructor was a Psychologist from the United States. When participants introduced themselves and it was found out that Daisy worked with a Psychiatrist, another student asked, "What is the difference between a psychologist and a psychiatrist?" The Psychologist jumped in with gusto to explain that Psychiatrists simply give medications while Psychologists truly understand people and know how to talk to them. He quickly continued with the workshop.

Daisy was stunned at his self-aggrandizing explanation. She wondered if the so-called learned man really believed himself. Recently, psychologists had been campaigning to be able to give medications without going to medical school. But he left no room for a response to correct him without interrupting the class, so Daisy let it slide.

It was a successful workshop, satisfying a curiosity about Remote Viewing that it was rumored the United States Government had been using in secrecy, but in the end Daisy once again felt a rift between herself and an instructor. She had allowed the guy to keep face. She had allowed the guy to convince a group of people that he was the most important person in a contest between psychologists and psychiatrists. Daisy was disappointed in herself for not standing up for a truth by explaining psychiatry and for not defending Ken in his profession and his way of practicing medicine without giving drugs to people and that he had a myriad of years of training to talk with people. In fact, Daisy knew Ken would never have made himself most important to a group of students.

The alternative in the situation was to challenge the instructor in order to educate the questioner. She left the workshop feeling there was unfinished business. Daisy was too often challenged about when to speak up and take on a challenge. It was one thing to kick-ass and another to have the wisdom to know how or when.

Later, on thinking about it, she decided her own mother had it right when she would never embarrass a person in front of others, no matter what age, but would speak her piece in private with the offending person. Daisy could not count the times her own mother had chastised and educated her in private with a mother's love.

46

The Home Practice

[ks notebook] "I AM A MIXED blood Old American, Scots, Welsh, Danish, French, Irish, German New Englander, father and grandfather, transplanted to British Columbia where I have practiced medicine, using my training in family medicine, pediatrics, psychiatry, and family therapy since 1971. I have visited families in their homes as a family health counselor since my first days of medical school at the University of Vermont in 1954. Since 1990 in Vancouver, I do my consulting in the homes of families who want to care for their pregnant, young, homeless, unemployed, disabled, or sick and dying members at home. Family members are referred to me on Medicare by family physicians for "adjustment reactions" to their health problems. I meet single-parent families in their homes with Daisy Heisler, a single parent and home-schooler of five children and thirteen grand children, who is a lay midwife, family mediator, freelance artist, sculptor, and videographer. We work with families as guests in their homes, assisting them to plan for the care of their members at home: making plans for a birth or death, a career change, home schooling, recreation, life style changes, recovery from abuse or addiction, and finding alternative remedies for health problems labeled fatal, hopeless, or untreatable.

"I listen to family stories, ask questions when I do not understand, tell stories about my life and other people who have survived and even shone despite the odds in similar stories. I introduce families to other people they do not know in my kinship network of friends and family. I keep company with them in hospital emergency rooms where I do not have hospital privileges and help them find alternative remedies when the ones they have don't work. I help with the chores, go for walks with families in labor, and I bring together all the professionals in their lives to meet the family when plans are going wrong, to decide who is doing what, how, and why.

"Families are referred for six months. We spend the first six weeks getting acquainted and making a few changes that all family members agree to work on together. After six weeks of working together, we know each other well enough to decide what we can do together and who else might be of some help. We aim to bring all the generations of a family together, letting them decide who is and who is not family to them, who is welcome in their household and who is not.

"I do not have a waiting list. I speak with family members on the telephone and refer them to others immediately if they are not interested in working as a family in their home with me. I visit families through the cycle of their lives whenever and for as long as we choose to meet.

"We have seen and will see families in their homes and their home communities from Lower Mainland to Vancouver Island, Gulf Islands, Squamish, Bella Bella, Bella Coola, Burns Lake, Quesnel, Dawson Creek, Deese Lake, Atlin, or wherever in B.C. we are invited to visit.

"I give priority to First Nations families and communities because of my friendship with First Nations individuals with whom I am building a support network to improve the health of their families and communities, and those who work with them. We are part of growing networks of families who want to support each other in building homes where we can be born, grow, play, make love, give birth, work, feed and school ourselves, caring for each other when we are sick, healing ourselves in recovery, and knowing ourselves and each other in the safety of our homes, where we can live and die, enjoying our lives in the company of our loved ones."

Kehnroth Schramm, M.D. January 19, 1995

DESPITE BAD PUBLICITY, the practice slowly grew. Once again clients were passing the word among friends and family about the psychiatrist who used alternative methods to drugs. People trusted Ken with their children because he would not give them anything harmful to solve problems. As usual, the promise to keep clients' secrets and a promise not to write anything other than a history and treatment plan was explained before any work began. People trusted Ken when he promised that whatever was going on in their homes would be kept confidential. With trust, he was welcomed into their homes and allowed into the inner sanctums of private lives.

Daisy answered her own question about who is qualified to give advice when on the way to a client's home one day, she said, "At least we have experienced so many problems and pitfalls in our own lives that we can legitimately know what clients are going through. Ken, I think we are more qualified than someone who has had everything go right and only visited problems in books."

Daisy did her best to screen clients about their intentions and as usual, made sure referrals were set up before the first appointment.

Working in clients' homes was advantageous for some people, especially families with children – but it was not for everyone. There seemed to be some other force that brought new clients just as others graduated. In that respect, there was a constant flow of just the right number of clients to work with so that each person had the time necessary for their needs.

Ken's "revolving door", as he called it, offered the security people needed to take breaks and come back when new problems arose, sometime years later.

The practice had evolved. In previous years while working in an office setting, there was a larger number of relationship problems, depressions relating to work, injuries that happened at work, and alcoholism. Though those kinds of problems were still coming Ken's way, the change to his practice in the 1990's was that family crisis more often had additional layers dealing with death by fire, cancer, sex change, psychotropic and street drugs, recent suicides of family members or death by accidents, and the life and death struggles with Aids. The clients taking the challenge of working with Ken were usually people with crisis that could never be resolved by psychotropic drugs but instead needed real problem-solving life skills to either resolve the difficulty or learn to live with it.

The ground rules regarding referrals were the same as when working in an office, but now the risk to Ken by working in homes was too great for Ken to see any woman on her own in the privacy of her home. The rules were clear that there must be another adult present or accept Daisy as chaperone.

At the first visit, Ken continued to tell clients that the "getting to know" period was for six weeks and during that time there would be an evaluation as to whether Ken could offer what the family was looking for or whether there needed to be a referral to other health care or to the legal system because he did not want to mislead clients if he could not help. The clients were informed they were free to leave at any time, especially if they felt no commitment to self-help.

Ken adamantly gave each person the time needed; he never looked at a clock but let the session run its' course. In fact, he had given up wearing even a windup watch. He never walked out on a person in the middle of an emotional upheaval just because a clock said the hour was up. Daisy kept an eye on time, especially when other appointments were booked, but she knew better than to interrupt a client needing extra time. She had heard horror stories over the years about other therapists who ended sessions abruptly. Clients who have had such abrupt endings sometimes found Ken.

A PSYCHIATRIST HAD given a young woman a psychotropic drug that was suppose to help her with grief and depression caused by the unexpected death of her husband still in his twenties. As a widow, she had small children to care for on her own but could barely function because the drug caused her to lose herself. She had been in the middle of an emotional outpouring of tears in the psychiatrist's office when her hour was over. She suddenly found herself out in the street with her emotions. She got into her car and while driving, grief turned to overwhelming anger. Minutes later, she was driving her car on a crowded Vancouver street and realized in a brief moment of sanity that she was using her car as a weapon. Luckily escaping harm, she stopped at an exercise gym where a former client of Ken's suggested she make an appointment with him right away.

Ken responded immediately. The debilitating medication was stopped. The family's healing began as she and the children worked through grief with Ken's help. Over the months, she drew on her talent as a comedian and as a writer. She did comedy routines with Ken as she dealt with her life. Over time, she dealt with an old, severe teenage trauma of being gang raped, and the newest loss in the death of her father that happened while seeing Ken. Through her laughter, tears, and journals, she grew strong. Her husband had died in front of their two-year old child; the child had quit talking. In her strong nurturing, the children grew and thrived. Besides working with the children in their home, when the oldest child started school, Ken and Daisy made school visits to meet with teachers and the principal, and to attend school concerts. The family was able to continue their love for the children's father while getting on with life and forming new relationships without feeling guilty.

VERY OFTEN CLIENTS came to Ken after other methods of medicine had failed. Sometime it was after disaster struck. For that reason, clients were in the process of dealing with major difficulties and they wanted to deal with life-changing catastrophes without being drugged out of their minds.

Sometimes the catastrophe happened because of psychotropic drugs administered by another doctor without proper follow-up, like the family who came to Ken after the woman who was a wife, mother, and grandmother had jumped in front of a fast traveling train while on a psychotropic drug that had a documented side-effect of suicide. To prepare for her suicide one afternoon, the matriarch of the family had carefully emptied her pockets of all items and laid them neatly on the kitchen table; this alone told the family that her following actions were deliberate. Then she walked over to the nearby train station and was caught on surveillance tape, jumping into the path of an oncoming train.

Immediately following the tragedy, the family was referred to Ken. This was clearly a case where Ken and Daisy wished this family had come before the tragedy, and most probably could have avoided the horrific nightmare they were all dealing with.

The dead woman's husband of half a century was elderly, suffering from diabetes and having to undergo dialysis for kidney failure. He and Ken enjoyed each other's company in the home of his daughter and her young family where he lived since his wife's death. Then he went to the hospital for amputations.

Following the amputations and being fed up with the dialysis, he made the decision that he wanted Ken's help in preparing him to die. He was an old soldier who fought for Canada in the front lines of the Second World War.

The days of work were long but after Ken finished his appointments with other clients, he headed for the hospital to be with the old veteran. In the hospital room, Ken sat with him hour after hour, evening after evening, as the man told his stories of a lifetime.

This was one of the few situations where privacy between Ken and the client was desirable. Ken did not need a chaperone. Across the street from the hospital, Daisy waited in the car until Ken came through the late darkness.

One night she asked, "After seeing clients all day and continuing your work on the health committee, you still spend hours with him in the hospital every evening. You must be exhausted."

"I enjoy him. He's a good man. He needs the time to talk out his stories before he lets go."

"A sad story... He wasn't responsible for the drugs a doctor gave his wife. Is he suffering guilt? Blaming himself for his wife's suicide?"

"Not right now. He's gone back in time to tell me his war stories. He needs to talk it out."

"Delayed Post Traumatic Stress Disorder?"

"He had no outlet following the war in order to deal with his experiences. He kept it all buried inside him all these years. I think he is finishing the need to tell stories. He told me tonight that he will be gone in a couple of days... I'll miss him."

"Oh! ...Gosh, I feel sorry." She was actually sorry for Ken now. There was a long sad silence.

On the drive home, Daisy broke the silence, "You know I can't bill the medical plan for all the hours you have spent with him. You have been working for free."

"I don't work for money. You know that by now. I would not stop seeing this man because of money. I am enriched for having known him."

AS CLIENTS, Social Workers were among the most kind-hearted people. At work, they could sometimes be the most difficult people to deal with because of their own system. Too often they were looking over their shoulder to appease a more senior person in the ladder of government employees.

Most professionals Daisy and Ken came across in their work with clients were caring and courteous in wanting to be helpful. Occasionally, they were dealing with someone who had their own interpretation of rules and so often these people came straight out of school with only books as their guide to real life problems of many families.

Ken and Daisy were meeting with a woman and her child born as a result of being raped by a person she met at church. So that the boy would not think of himself as an unwanted child or that he would want to meet his father, she told him that his father had died. Because of her own birth injury that caused cerebral palsy, she needed a wheelchair to get around and social services money to live. They lived in a co-operative housing complex with an internal courtyard and playground placed on top of a manmade hill. Her three-year old child discovered freedom by running out the door to explore on his own. The child never left the hill but the curbs of the sidewalk made it impossible for a wheelchair to run after the small child. The mother needed to negotiate certain paths only. The social workers were adamant that the mother should contain her child and be within arms length at all times.

Ken and Daisy called a group meeting with the social and homecare workers to discuss making a workable plan. On the day of the meeting, the first thing they saw on arrival into the home was a long, black belt placed completely around the refrigerator with a large padlock on it that was big enough to lock a barn door. When Daisy asked the mother what that was about, she was told that the person who had been sent by social workers to teach mothering skills had placed the padlock because the child was going into the fridge to find food when he was hungry.

The situation upset Daisy to the point that she needed to take a walk to get her anger under control before dealing with the padlock. Ken walked with her to calm her.

On re-entering the home, others who had been invited to the planning meeting had arrived and seemed not to be phased about the padlocked refrigerator. Ken and Daisy immediately tackled the subject. The priority was to get the padlock off the fridge and place child friendly food on a lower shelf, and to teach the child about foods he could help himself to. Also, the necessity of a different housekeeper/teacher was discussed because this particular one had been a tyrant in other ways as well. Daisy was relentless on the subject and was determined to follow up. The mother had been frightened into doing things against her better judgment to please the tyrant who wrote reports for the ministry that the mother was not privy to. The mother believed she needed to appease everyone working for social services in order to keep her child – and she was right. Daisy made sure the tyrant was fired and replaced.

In the meeting, Ken determined that the next thing to be done was to get the small patio and private garden area of the home fenced so that the child had a contained outdoor play area. Though everyone thought it a good idea, the BC Ministry and the co-op hierarchy were unwilling to fund the fence. They were instead committed to complaining with no solution.

For the safety of the child, Ken paid three hundred dollars from his own pocket to have the fence built.

It was in situations like this one that office visits could never come close to revealing the real story about what clients actually dealt with in their own homes. No verbal description could relay the total experience of meeting the housekeeper and the social workers in person, or the impact of walking into a home and seeing a belted, padlocked refrigerator. No office visit could expose the reality of the child out of reach on a hill while a mother in a wheelchair panicked because of complaints.

The inevitable day came when a young social worker decided that it was time to take the child from the mother and place him into foster care, given the climate that people with handicaps were given less opportunity to be parents. The social system of the time was known to target people with disabilities and label them as unfit parents. Other parents in the province of British Columbia with cerebral palsy and a woman with deafness had been in the news recently about their fights to keep their babies.

The social worker trumped up a story that this particular mother had beaten her child with a baseball bat and he had bruises on his body. While the social worker prepared the court papers, Ken and Daisy visited the home and videotaped the child in bright sunlight with only his underpants on. There was not even a hint of a mark on the child's body.

Meeting again with the social worker in the home a few days later, the videotape was played for her.

As the tape came to the end, Daisy had a sudden impulse to tell the social worker, "Anyone can become handicapped in an instant by a car accident or any accident."

The embarrassed, young social worker was sitting across the room and facing Daisy, who was determined not to let her get away with lies. Daisy was also mentally critical that the woman never had a strand of hair out of place and always dressed like she had just stepped out of a fashion show in comparison to a mother of an active boy while coping with a wheelchair.

The very next day, the same social worker did get into a car accident that totaled her car. She walked away uninjured but became unsettled to the point that at a conference in days following that Ken and Daisy attended, that particular social worker was seen hiding behind poles so as not to run into Daisy. It was another social worker that pointed the woman out to Daisy, whispering, "I think you make her feel uneasy."

Later, after obtaining the government file through the Freedom of Information Act, they reviewed the file with this mother. Names of reporters had been blacked out, but blaring incorrect information remained on file. The false report that the child was beaten with a baseball bat remained on file as a testament that whoever is in power can write what they wish whether true or not.

Ken's distrust of written files on people and how they could be used against people was proven correct once again.

This family also was an example of how children can use their knowledge of the social system against their parents. The little boy in this family learned fast that he could scare his mother into letting him have his way by threatening to tell a social worker that she abused him.

More than once, Ken and Daisy came into homes where children were wielding power based on their knowledge of a government system designed to protect children – a system that could also ruin families as children acted out unleashed power and scared parents felt they were powerless in the system.

ONE AFTERNOON, Ken and Daisy arrived at the home of twin sisters for a follow-up visit. While waiting for one sister to return from doing laundry, they sat in the living room having a conversation with the twin who had arranged the referrals. She had asked for help for both herself and her sister who had been hospitalized following an overdose of street drugs while in her teens ten years earlier and came out diagnosed as a schizophrenic. The sister was now on psychotropic drugs overseen by a doctor at a clinic specializing in her diagnosis.

The living room was separated from the kitchen by a half wall, enabling people in the living room to a see clearly down the hallway to the back door and through to the kitchen.

The second sister arrived through the back door, exhibiting a fowl mood as she entered the kitchen. She refused to look toward the living room or acknowledge anyone. Walking in with her, attached to her back, was a distinct silhouette of a tall, thin man.

While the twin in the living room was distracted by her sister's entrance, Ken looked at Daisy with astonishment that Daisy mirrored back to him. Under his breath, he asked, "Do you see what I see?"

Daisy nodded. She knew exactly what he was seeing.

After dropping what she had been carrying into the kitchen, the young woman entered the living room. She looked briefly at

Daisy and Ken, and then rolled herself into a grey blanket on the sofa, covering her head.

Several minutes passed in silence. Then from under the blanket she spoke, "I want you to leave."

OUT ON THE STREET, to clarify what they just saw, Daisy asked, "Did you see that male figure attached to her?"

Ken paused in his steps to look at her. "Yes, I did."

"At least we see the same things. I know she fired us because we could 'see' and she... *he* knew it! What can we do?"

"She has a right to fire us. Other doctors are looking after her medications. We are latecomers... ten years late. I have already referred her to Dr. Hoffer in Victoria for his orthomolecular expertise. She is going to spend time with aboriginal elders, so we can step aside. We have a revolving door and we will continue to work with her sister. Working with you verifies other realities because with each other, we can validate what we see."

BETWEEN APPOINTMENTS, while Daisy drove the car, Ken sang to her in his resonant voice. The destination one afternoon was a home high in the mountains.

Making plasticine figures with this family had been helpful. The figures made on previous visits were brought out of the cupboard and placed on the table to play with and change. The sculptures had gotten more elaborate with each visit and now included whole plasticine rooms where the people and animal figures lived.

They had brought a fresh supply of plasticine in the blue bag. While Ken interacted with the small boy and the figure that represented the boy, Daisy helped the little girl finish an extra tall figure with plasticine clothes. After the figure was dressed, the girl surprised everyone by declaring, "This is my teacher. I will turn her back to us," as she placed the teacher in a plasticine room that became a schoolroom.

Her mother, sitting between her children so that she could interact both ways, asked, "She is taller than all the people. Why does she turn her back to us?"

The girl responded with a serious tone, "That's the way she always is!" Picking up a female figure half the size of the teacher figure and placing her in the schoolroom, she said, "This one is you, Mom. You must listen to the teacher because she knows best."

The girl's eyes brightened as though stars lit them. She smiled widely as she picked up a male plasticine figure from a bed in another plasticine room and walked him along with a smaller girl figure. "And this is my Dad in Heaven. He is coming to school with me today!"

AND SO IT WENT... people working out their changes in life.

CHRISTMAS TIME. Ken purchased a gift certificate from the same co-op food store manager who had witnessed the loud criticism following the article in the newspaper. True to Ken's nature, he continued to befriend the man and did not hide.

On arrival to a client's home, Christmas music could be heard in the background along with children noises as they played. Ken handed a gift certificate to the woman who was a single parent of mixed race children.

"A gift certificate," Ken said, "to the health food store for your Christmas dinner. You can buy an organic turkey and all the trimmings with that."

Daisy handed small wrapped gifts to her. "For the children."

The astounded woman took the gifts. Her tired eyes brightened. "A Hundred dollars to feed my kids? My kids wouldn't have a Christmas at all without this."

LATER IN THE AFTERNOON, Ken and Daisy were sitting at a kitchen counter having coffee with a woman while having a private session for the past hour. The timing had been planned to coincide with her daughter arriving home from school.

The child arrived home in a fowl mood. She threw down her bag and kicked her shoes off into the air so that they hit the ceiling.

As though this was normal, her mother asked, "How was school?"

"I don't want to talk." The child's voice spiked, "Cookie!"

She climbed onto a stool to join Ken and Daisy at the counter as the mother handed her a cookie. Two cookies later, the child fell off her stool onto the floor. Getting up, she made a beeline to the living room where she kicked the Christmas tree. Decorations flew in all directions.

Ken had been watching. In his softly comforting voice, he explained what he had seen to the mother. "She looks like she is having low blood sugar after several hours in school. Her out of control behavior increased with sugar cookies that are low in nutrition. We can discuss better snacks for her and not wait until she has low blood sugar. We can discuss food and vitamins."

"Oh! Okay!" the mother responded.

Daisy said, "Food allergies can be from any food and we can help you figure out exactly which foods may be causing problems by a simple chart you can keep without having to go for elaborate needle tests."

Relieved, the mother said, "You know, you are the first people to notice what is going on with her. She has been getting into trouble for mood swings but no one has ever pointed out low blood sugar or possible food allergy. Our GP only offered Ritalin and the school has been complaining about her behavior but not offering any solution other than punishment."

Ken said, "We should see results very quickly and go from there."

Daisy told the mother, "This is why Ken likes to work in the home. He gets to see exactly what people are coping with in their homes. Ken goes to the schools also for the same reasons. So if you want Ken to go to the school, we can do that."

"Yes, I think that is a terrific idea. I'll set up an appointment with her teachers."

IN ALL THE YEARS Daisy had been working with Ken, several families became clients after devastation by house fires. But it was the particularly sad, most recent telephone call that brought a grieving family to Ken after losing two children in a Christmas house fire. In this case, the father chose not to take part; he grieved but thought therapy was for women and children. Ken chose to work with the willing family members and their friends while keeping the door open for the father to join in.

Around the big dining room table, several children and their friends ranging in age from two to seven, found making plasticine family figures fascinating. A few weeks into their therapy, they were more relaxed and a little happier. Ken helped the smallest children make plasticine bodies while Daisy fine-tuned faces with a lot of little fingers helping, and showed the children how to make clothing of their choices for their figures. All the while the children talked about their lost siblings.

In a vivid dream the night before one of the visits with the family, Daisy had seen the sister in a blue dress with yellow and pink ribbons around her waist. In the dream, the little girl told Daisy she is happy that Ken and Daisy are part of her family now.

On the way to the appointment, Ken cautioned Daisy about talking too much but to let the mother take charge of what she is ready for. Daisy found it hard to hold her tongue; instead, she dropped a hint by way of a question when the mother was having her private session.

The mother ignored any hint and told her own story instead. "My children were playing Christmas during this past week. You know... instead of playing house or school, they played Christmas! My daughter suddenly got up and went to look inside a pocket of my coat... a coat I seldom wear, and it was in the back of the clothes closet! Inside the pocket there was a wrapped present... paper earrings that my daughter made for me and hid in my pocket before she died. It is strange how my little girl suddenly went into my pocket in a closet, something she never does! I guess it is even stranger that they were playing Christmas when it is Spring. I wonder..."

While working with the children that day, the older sister had just made her deceased little sister out of plasticine. She and Daisy were dressing her in a blue dress with long ribbons of yellow and pink colours tied around her waist. This was the only time in working with children that Daisy ever steered something. Always the children came up with ideas but today Daisy had suggested the blue dress with ribbons to see if there was any reality to her dream and the message from the girl that came in the dream.

The children's mother came to the table to examine what was going on and looked at the plasticine figure; she told everyone that her daughter did have a favorite dress, "just like this one".

A younger brother leaned over, resting his belly on the table to look at the plasticine figure, and while resting a finger on her, said, "Yep, this is my sister who died in the fire. She tells me not to cry because she is happy."

Meanwhile, the grieving father would come home from work and stay in the kitchen while Ken and Daisy were visiting. He was not listening to his living children. Instead, he traveled to visit a psychic in Edmonton on a lonely search for reassurance that his children do have life after death.

IN A PSYCHIATRIC practice like Ken's, there was a constant flow of people dealing with loss and grief, and since we all die at some point, there was no family that had not been touched by it. Where there is death, there follows question about where loved ones have gone. In allowing room for the dying and the grieving people to express themselves freely in a place where they trusted there would be no label placed on them and no judgment, there was an ever-increasing number of people wanting to talk about their own experiences. The numbers were high in about nine out of ten clients experiencing some form of life beyond this life. Ken's practice of letting people express themselves brought about many surprising unprompted conversions.

A very nice retired social worker asked for help because her only son was dying of Aids. He had received an infusion of tainted blood from the Red Cross before they were aware of the contamination in their blood supplies. She and her son had always been extremely close until he married, but in his wife's zeal to protect him, she protected him away from his own mother. The mother was a devout, church-going Christian believing in a kind of Heaven and Hell. On meeting her, the woman was in so intense grief that she was near death herself. On answering the door to Ken and Daisy's first visit, she could hardly stand up.

She was on so many prescribed medications that she withheld information about them when Ken asked. Ken knew instinctively and telephoned her referring physician, with the woman present and listening, to sort out what she was taking and to work out a plan to eliminate the domino effect. Ken managed to treat her malnutrition, literally feeding her by taking her out to restaurants and buying vitamins and minerals for her out of his own money. He offered Homeopathy for grief. By the time the son died, she was physically strong enough to handle it. She did grieve, as expected.

The young man who had passed away, appeared to Daisy just days later. She was convinced that often spirits make contact with the easiest, most aware person to prove their survival. Because he had been kept away from his mother during his final health crisis, Daisy told him in no uncertain terms, "Go see your mother!"

The next week, Ken and Daisy found the woman transformed from extreme grief to acceptance and contentment. The mother explained that she went to a symphony concert, something she had so often done with her son. She told of how her son sat beside her and held her hand, and when she came home they sat together on her sofa for a long while. She explained how she smelled him and felt him just as though he was in the physical. She was tranquil, talking freely about her knowledge of his survival.

The gift that Ken gave was freedom and trust, enabling people to talk and share experiences no matter how outrageous they may seem in everyday life.

ON A TREE-LINED STREET Ken and Daisy approached their car after leaving another client in an apartment building. Daisy expressed indignation, "That client was telling obvious lies. Did you notice?"

Gently, Ken answered, "We are not here to judge. We are here to listen and understand that this person needs to have her own truth for whatever reason. We start with a patient's own truth and work out from there. This is a beginning, not the end."

OCCASIONALLY Ken encountered a problem about who to refer people to for additional help in a particular area of expertise. Finding the right medical or social help was not easy.

Too often physicians threw up their hands in defeat and instead of a thorough testing, made the common statement, "It is all in the client's head." Following that, the patient might be prescribed a drug for psychotic reasons, or referred to a Psychiatrist where the same thing might happen. A good example was that in British Columbia, proper testing for Celiac Disease was not available in the 1990s and many people went undiagnosed. It was only in the last couple of years that Celiac Disease has been recognized as real. Prior to that, a blood sample could be sent to the United States for more sensitive testing but British Columbia patients were not told that. There were physicians that may treat all the symptoms in separate categories instead of looking for a source of the many problems. The danger in that is that people were actually losing intestines in operations and being drugged with psychotropic drugs.

If a person suffering Celiac Disease consumes gluten, their immune system is attacked and can lead to life threatening illness like lupus, cancer, dementia, and many other disorders that include rheumatoid arthritis. This disease is so serious that to not be diagnosed has been a Canadian disaster. A case in point was when a top specialist in one of the main hospitals, St. Paul's Hospital in Vancouver, looked inside a man who had suffered all his life with symptoms and was even hospitalized as a six-year old child with stomach ailments. The specialist found an ulcer at the top of the intestine and did not bother looking for damage to the intestinal villi, and then dismissed the case, referring the patient to the University of British Columbia where a neurologist, after a few minutes with the man, said it was all in the man's head even though the patient was physically ill, shaking, in extreme pain during the visit, and could not function to go to work.

Daisy had accompanied the man to the UBC appointment and was shocked when the physician came out of his inner sanctums, walking behind his patient and in the waiting room, nonchalantly announced the dismissal of the man to Daisy because it was "all in his head".

Following this circus, the man diagnosed himself after reading an article in a women's magazine and within two weeks of changing his diet to be totally gluten free, he was feeling well and functioning normally. But, one crumb of gluten and symptoms returned.

In Ken's practice, it was often necessary to convince clients to do their own at home testing with a diet change regarding allergies; some were willing and others were not. Diet, for one reason or another plays an important part in changing psychosis. Sometimes it is parents blocking change because they are too busy and they might have to think about something extra, and definitely they do not want the work of keeping a log of any kind. But for those who do make changes, children will often rise from a long-term sick bed and get back to becoming active again and going back to school. In Ken's recent practice there had been children who rose from their beds after a year of illness that kept them bedridden but other doctors could only scratch their heads. During the next ten years, media and public pressure will force the medical community to wake up and take Celiac Disease seriously.

NOURISHMENT AND CHANGES to food patterns were sometimes the most difficult for patients to even think about making. The possibility of gluten intolerance caused some people to fear giving up bread or junk food even though there are alternatives.

A young professional woman had been referred to Ken because she was missing work constantly, suffering undiagnosed abdominal pain and disabling illness. She admitted to Ken that her mother had been diagnosed in Eastern Canada with Celiac Disease. She was an obvious candidate for the home-testing change of diet just in case she had Celiac Disease that can be hereditary. She cringed at the thought and adamantly denied the possibility of Celiac Disease.

At the following appointment, the woman was again home from work with a stomachache. This time, she had prepared a big bowl of white wheat pasta and after Ken and Daisy were seated in her living room, she sat down across the room, facing them with her bowl on her lap. She then proceeded to stuff her face with pasta in deliberately defiant motions. Ken remained his usual calm and waited, while Daisy had to work hard to squelch laughter, thinking that if this person had come to an office visit, this behavior would never be so obvious.

SOMETIMES STRANGE BIASES came to light. On receiving a call late one evening from a potential client who had heard about Ken and wanted an appointment, Daisy explained to the woman that a referral was needed first by a physician. The woman claimed not to have a doctor. In trying to help, Daisy suggested she call a particular female general physician who Daisy and Ken had met through the midwifery connection and had no reason to distrust her because she professed to be so spiritual.

The prospective client phoned back the same evening to say that the doctor "blew her cool and continued to repeat the words, 'I will not refer you to him; he is an Indian lover'!"

After reporting back, the caller was never heard from again.

Daisy had to relay the information to Ken. It came as a complete surprise to him because Ken had referred an aboriginal woman to the physician not long ago. Not only had he referred the woman, but also because the woman was ill, he had walked her to the physician's office and waited for her to make sure she was safe to walk home or to go for further tests. At the time, the doctor never said anything or even hinted to Ken's face that she did not like Indians. This was a reminder to Ken to keep an eye open for physicians who do honor their Hippocratic Oath.

AND SO IT WENT. Multifaceted life was more obvious when visiting so many people in their home environments.

Working in homes was freeing, though not financially the wisest thing to do. Many clients lived in Vancouver but many did not. Traveling daily took Ken and Daisy out of Vancouver to distant places.

The Sea to Sky highway along the seascape and over mountains to the north provided a scenic route to Whistler. Ken would sing to Daisy as she drove the car. Lulled by his singing, she watched the layers of muted colour in the mountains jutting out of the seascape; she thought about Toni Onli's paintings and how he painted these scenes.

The trips through the Fraser Valley were the happiest, bringing Ken and Daisy closest to their love of farms. They drove through areas of tall corn fields and when in season, would stop to buy a feast of fresh corn. Ken sang happily amid the smells of farming as the car purred along the ribbons of curving grey road winding between vast fields of green and gold.

They would go south to White Rock to visit a family in a seaside home. On another day they would head to Richmond to visit families there.

Extra turbulence and drama came with traffic jams that caused delays and occasionally a snowstorm kept them from getting up a mountain to a waiting family. Up the mountains, down the valleys, and across the flats in all kinds of weather – rain, snow, or blazing heat, they traveled to spend time with all kinds of troubles inside their clients' homes.

There were playgrounds, beaches, and schools visited all in a day's work. Sometime one parent played with a child on the playground or built a castle in the beach sand while the other had their private time with Ken; then they would switch. There was the coffee shop that an elderly person enjoyed for a delightful and much needed outing, where Ken treated the client with a coffee and bakery treat of choice and then the trio spent the next hour at a corner table talking. And Ken was known to take clients out for a whole meal and eat with them if they were suffering malnutrition or an eating disorder. His motto was, "Who says therapy must be in an office or even a home? It can be anywhere that is conducive to helping and healing."

The homes differed in many respects. There were the small homes that were obviously housing people with little money and there were the large, rich homes and all sizes and styles in between. Clients were from all over the world and in their home cultural differences were evident. The European, Mediterranean, Icelandic and Northern regions, Indigenous people of North and South America and the Mish-mush mixtures of North American people all showed some evidence of their roots in furnishings, food, and music preferences. The differences would not be so evident in an office setting but in home visits, they provided a daily colourful mosaic.

The homes occasionally held other things, too and presented a danger not only to the clients living in them, but to Ken and Daisy. Walking into a Granville Street hotel that a single man called home and into his tiny room was a good example of what may never be clearly understood by having him come to an office. The drab tiny room was crowded with a narrow bed and one chair, a closet and a few belongings that seem like clutter. On the first visit, the client insisted that Daisy sit on his bed and Ken take a chair. He stood, taking up all the extra space. Daisy hated sitting on the man's bed and would rather do anything else, but he insisted. It was one of the most uncomfortable home visits accompanied by fear of picking up bugs. On leaving, crawling on the hall walls were several giant cockroaches in plain view as other people wandered around seeming not to be bothered. Daisy refused to go back and advised Ken to make his appointments with this man in another location. When the man telephoned for another appointment, Daisy informed him that the meeting must be somewhere other than the hotel. The man argued about having home visits like everyone else. When Daisy stood her ground without insulting his home, he agreed to meet with Ken in the local library within walking distance from his home. The problem had been that he had no money for bus fare.

On the other side of the spectrum, in homes where money and social standing was important, it occasionally took a while to dawn on the client that treating their doctor and his assistant as additional servants was never going to wash because they do not follow orders; nor will they baby-sit small children under the guise of therapy so that the adult can take a break or a nap – as a well-to-do socialite demanded but never got. Ken always insisted that a parent or caretaker had to be in the room with small children.

Homes held people suffering torments of ill health, grief, fear, addictions, trauma of abuse or accident and even life threatening torture with the effects of Post Traumatic Stress Disorder. Commonly, children were suffering loss through broken families; some were sorting out questions of loyalty, life and death, bullying, food and where to sleep.

In dealing with people in their homes, emotions were more apt to run high and be acted out. Daisy was occasionally in line of physical fire. On a first visit, a seven-year old girl spit in her face. The girl was used to having social services come into her home; she was extremely angry about them and thought Daisy was one and the same. It was another case where the supposed helpers had harassed the family and made damning written reports about everything, including the mother's reading material. As a result, the family unit was suffering. Ken was asked to help.

All in a day's work, Daisy felt lucky she wore glasses as shards of china smashed across the floor and flew in her direction. An angry, grieving woman had thrown the cup meant for her husband. The woman was really upset over recent news that in a distant city, her sister committed suicide. With post-partum hormones raging and suffering lack of sleep as a new mom, she had asked for Ken's help.

And then there were the gardens. On many home visits, Ken and Daisy watched the flowers and vegetables being planted and then watched them grow over tea, cookies and conversations about the many troubles and joys that go along with laundry flapping overhead, too much sun, or the chill of evening shade, and children dropping in and out, but mostly dropping in to be a part of a family gathering and to tell their stories. Children looked forward to these visits.

No matter what age the client, it was Ken's devotion to his or her achievement that took Ken and Daisy to churches for weddings and baby christenings, Alcoholics Anonymous cake celebrations, fashion shows, family celebrations of birthdays, school concerts, education milestones, and much more. Ken made time, no matter what he had going on in his personal life, for those who wanted him to share in their special day. He was always grateful for just being asked to participate and he was genuinely happy for all achievements.

ON THE HOME FRONT, Daisy's grandson had been playing on the school playground. He was riding a fast circling carrier when his foot got caught underneath. His leg broke. Rushed to

Emergency at Squamish Hospital, his leg was set and put in a cast. On a visit to Gramma and Grampa Ken a week later, Ken thought something did not look right, as though he could feel or see beneath the thick, white plaster and cheesecloth cast. As usual, Ken dealt with the problem quickly. He got right on the telephone and set up an urgent appointment with the best orthopedic surgeon he knew of at Children's Hospital.

Daisy accompanied her daughter and grandson to the appointment. True to Ken's diagnosis, the bone had been incorrectly set; an error serious enough that it would have caused the child a life-long disability. The bone had to be re-broken and correctly set.

In the recovery room, Daisy was about to learn another lesson. On waking, the boy was in extreme pain. Even though nurses kept pumping more and more painkiller drugs through a vein in his hand, the pain would not subside. As the hours ticked by, the outpatient facility was supposed to close for the night but nursing staff needed to stay on overtime. They could not release the boy because of pain. In looking for clues as to what might be a variable, Daisy realized that the child had been laid on his side by the staff with the cast leg lying across the other leg. She gently changed the position of his legs. To everyone's surprise, there was sudden relief from pain. The problem had simply been a wrong position. They were able to go home and fast healing followed.

Once again, Daisy was extremely thankful for Ken and in awe of him, and wondrous about what seemed like another miraculous healing intervention. Ken had just saved another of her grandchildren from a medical mistake and of a life with a disability.

47

Son Goes To University

IT WAS AN UNEXPECTED surprise to be having breakfast with Ken's brother Richard. He arrived from Vermont on short notice for a Vancouver conference. Richard had grown older, his hair whiter and a few more lines of wisdom in his face, but he had done it gracefully.

As Richard finished his coffee, he set down unfinished toast. "I'd better get going. The conference is about to start."

Ken offered an invitation, "Richard, today is August 9th, Hiroshima Day. Here on the West Coast, we light candles and set them floating in the harbor of the Pacific Ocean in memory of Japanese people. I'd like you to come with me."

"That sounds wonderful!" Richard's face lit up with his usual white smile. "Okay. I'll see you this evening."

Then, in a rush he was gone out the door, heading for a bus.

IN THE EVENING, a crowd had assembled on the dark beach. People were helping each other to light candles in paper lanterns. The small flickering fires threw a yellow-orange glow on the faces of people of Japanese decent and many other cultures. All ages and skin colors had come together for one memory – the people killed by the atom bombs dropped on Hiroshima and Nagasaki.

The bright lanterns of many colours floated out in rows, bobbing up and down on waves as they traveled. Richard and Ken, faces lit by candlelight... were together lighting their lanterns... bending down together in the sand at the edge of the ocean to set them afloat beside each other... standing together to watch them float away... lighting the darkness on their way out to sea.

A Post Card to Hiroshima & Nagasaki
I wanted to send a post card to each one of you
who lived in Hiroshima & Nagasaki more than Fifty years ago.
My uncle Dick would want you to know that he did not know
he was helping to build an Atom Bomb.
He did not even know the chemicals were radioactive
when he put his head down into the centrifuges
to see how they were working.
When he learned the United States Government
had lied to him and to us
about what the Manhattan Project was doing
he quit doing chemical engineering forever.
When I was thirteen he taught me
that good people can do bad things
by following orders full of good words and lies.
There were no secrets about how to make an Atom Bomb
except the secret that you are helping to make one.
We have never seen your pictures or your cities in color,
You are always in black and white
to hide the blood and the burns and the pain.
Only the bombs are exploding in beautiful colors.
My childhood ended with yours Fifty years ago
and I tried to stop the wars
and continue the Childhood of Humanity
and I do not know how to do it without your help
to take back the beautiful colors
from the beautiful bombs
and bring the beauty
and pain of childhood
into all of our lives.
The only way I know
to send this to you
is to burn it
like a candle
with love

8/6/96 ken schramm

"Ken, thank you for this experience. I feel we have come full circle."

"Yes, we are brothers. We have come full circle. Thanks for doing this with me, Richard. It is healing."

Daisy had been standing back, watching with awe... not wanting to intrude on this special moment between two brothers who had come a long way from a bedroom near the eastern seaboard to the west coast beach of another country that shared an ocean with Japan... two small boys in bodies of men finding a kind of peace together... healing old wounds.

DURING RICHARD'S VISIT of only a couple of days, Andy was invited to dinner with his uncle and his father in Daisy's apartment. It was a big surprise when Andy actually showed up to Daisy's apartment because he had not done so since he was about ten years old. Seeming relaxed and enjoying the visit, Andy talked about his intentions to study sciences in university. The conversation turned lightheartedly to the latest styles in expensive jeans that he preferred, causing his uncle to pretend surprise at the prices.

Andy's participation at that dinner had been surprising because he had become increasingly absent. Ken had a hard time making contact and chalked it up to busyness with friends and entering a final high school year.

In order to make contact, Ken resorted to writing letters and did so to discuss Andy's university education which was only a year away, and for the umpteenth time to apologize for problems caused by the divorce. Ken had been getting no response to his offers of financial or other support for Andy to enter university and no response to requests for discussion – just a void.

September 9, 1996

Dear Andy,

I am writing you a longer letter for you to read after we get through this difficult transition in your Senior Year and your application to university. This package of materials for an application to Dartmouth College (a small university) is my way of saying I am sorry for making your life difficult and letting you know I want to help you apply for early admission to Dartmouth College. Applications must be in November 1, 1996 and you will know in December whether or not you are accepted with the necessary financial aid for you to attend. The College must be notified of your intention to seek early admission by October 1st. You can do your part of the application on line at... I have requested the full catalog by e-mail. The Canadian financial aid application must also be requested.

You can read thru' this material and call me when you are ready.

I just want you to know my hopes for you are that you will have as full and as rich an experience of life as I have had because I went to a college in a small town in the wilderness where I spent many happy hours with teachers and students as companions in life. Dartmouth has grown to include women and a native studies program and medical programs which include computers, research and business degrees. The BASIC language was developed at Dartmouth while I was there. My brothers and your brother Peter are teaching, studying and working only a few hours away from Hanover so you would be close to family when you need or want to be close to them. I would be very happy for you to attend Dartmouth in its 1990's incarnation. I believe you would get a good education there that you would enjoy for your whole life. I believe you could also get a good start here in Vancouver at Simon Fraser or UBC but so far I have been unsuccessful in getting a teaching job here.

If you decide you want to be here and make the best education you can for yourself, I will do my best to help. Ultimately it will come down to what you want to do and what you will afford yourself with the support of your mother and me.

Dad

OVER THE YEARS Ken had worked tirelessly to build good relations with all three sons. Since the 1990 court case when Ken was allowed to see Andy again, he had been available to his youngest son at all times, no matter what he had to cancel to be with him for whatever reason, and Ken believed they had a close relationship. The three boys were, each in their own way, making Ken proud. Stephen and Peter had evolved, having lost their teenage attitudes years ago in favor of becoming compassionate men concerned for others in business and in studies. That was all that Ken needed from them. Andy never did go to a private high school, but had been doing well in the public high school he attended. The foursome, or whichever boys were available, had been meeting for a meal together once a week or more often when possible without the intrusion of Daisy or her family. Even though Ken invited her many times, she declined in favor of giving his sons all of him.

SPRING 1997. Ken was delighted to be given a rare invitation to attend the same function as Jane for Andy's grade twelve graduation formal sit-down dinner. It had been many years since Ken had been able to sit at the same dinner table with his ex-wife and his son.

Ken had hoped that one or all of his sons would choose to go to Dartmouth College but Stephen launched a computer business and Peter was studying multi-media in Montreal. Just a few days before the graduation dinner, Andy had informed Ken that for outstanding high grades, he had been offered a Ten Thousand Dollar scholarship for four years to study sciences at the University of British Columbia. Considering that Andy would be able to continue living with either parent and have his Undergraduate Degree entirely paid for, Andy's path to becoming a scientist or a physician seemed auspicious.

It was Ken's hope and dream for himself and his son to share his apartment that was close to the university grounds. He imagined that, with his son studying sciences and possibly pre-med at UBC, the sharing of knowledge would become easier between them.

Usually Ken disliked getting his hair cut because he liked longer hair than he usually ended up with. Once again, he promised to sit calmly and Daisy promised to try to do a desirable cut as she draped him with a white sheet. She combed and clipped, all the while loving to touch him and he loved her touch.

After the hair trim, he dressed carefully. Earlier that week, he had gone to the Salvation Army store and bought a new old, but in very good shape, Harris Tweed jacket. It even had distinguished, English looking, beautifully stitched leather patches on the elbows and braided leather buttons, a fitting look to the professor Ken that he has been. Wanting to please his son by dressing appropriately, he asked Daisy's advice on which tie to wear.

Daisy watched from the window as Ken headed down the street to catch a bus to the dinner. Being environmentally conscious, he always chose not to use a car except for work. It was as though the happy high hopes for the event were visibly tangible around his shoulders and gave a lilt to his steps.

AT DINNER, Ken was taken by complete surprise when Jane and Andy informed him that the scholarship to UBC was being disregarded in favor of Andy going to Queen's University in Ontario.

Queen's had never before been mentioned to Ken. Even though he briefly wondered why disclosure of information had been withheld until now – over dinner, he immediately offered to negotiate paying his share of the expenses to ensure Andy's smooth transition to university.

ARRIVING HOME, Ken expressed to Daisy his shock at being blindsided at the dinner about Andy's plans.

Daisy asked, "Why on earth did they not tell you before the dinner? You've been very clear all along, since he was a baby, that you want to support his university education."

"It seemed to me that Jane was pleased with herself for surprising me in public about Queen's and that they are throwing away thousands of dollars in scholarships."

"And you willingly offered to pay, I'll bet."

"Of course. Andy explained that he would have to qualify each year for a renewal of the scholarship, a stress he doesn't want. I think it is worth spending money to have Andy escape his mother's hold on him. I think it is a good thing for him to be far away from her. I hope Andy will gain some independence and strength of his own. I am happy for this turn of events. In no way would I try to change it. In fact, I am happy to contribute to Andy's new freedom."

"I understand. I keep hoping the boy will grow up and show some independence from her. I've been waiting for some sign of it since the last court case. Maybe finally, it will happen."

AN ONSLAUGHT OF letters and Affidavits from Bruce Katz and Jane Anderson started arriving again. Jane and Katz were turning the event of Andy going to university into reason to go to court for another public fight. They stated that negotiation was not possible.

They were making it clear that if anyone thought they did not mean it the first time, they would do it all over again. They got away with it once and it was clear that Andy's mother had been manipulating the situation again in preparation.

They were demanding that both Ken and Daisy come up with all their personal financial accounting for them. They demanded that no business expenses would be allowed in regard to Ken's income, especially not for paying Daisy. Demands included having both Ken and Daisy cross-examined in Court.

Jane stated that she was determined that her son would not be allowed to work for Ken and be paid for it. The allowance Ken had been paying Andy of One Hundred and Fifty Dollars per month for doing nothing and was over and above the maintenance paid to Jane was conveniently not mentioned, nor did she mention the extra hundreds of dollars Ken paid to Andy.

One Affidavit written by Jane Anderson read as a jealous vomit about Daisy, who was mentioned over and over. There was reference to do **another long court battle** while at the same time she was accusing Ken of being the one who wanted to go to court.

KEN WROTE IN HIS JOURNAL:

"In my family medical and psychiatric practice, I make home visits to families who want to care for their members at home from birth to death. I give priority to homeless, low income, unemployed, aboriginal or immigrant families adjusting to medical illnesses, diagnoses of fatal diseases, or whose members are dying or pregnant, or children with school difficulties. My practice is based on more than forty years of experience and training in family medicine, pediatrics, family psychiatry, family therapy, hypnosis, psychoanalysis, Reichian character analysis and bodywork, aboriginal health, Chinese medicine, and homeopathy.

"In my life I have worked as a construction laborer; carpenter's helper; camp counselor, swimming and water sports instructor; factory worker; postal worker; hospital orderly; medical office receptionist, lab technician, and switchboard operator; house parent in a Children's Home for disturbed children; pediatric interne and assistant resident; Senior psychiatric resident at the Foothills Hospital in Calgary; family physician for a ranch community on Calvert Island and in Bella Bella, B.C.; college health physician at Cornell University and also teacher at Goddard College; university professor of anthropology at McGill University, human ecology at Regina Campus; dairy farmer in Vermont and on the Matador Co-op farm where I also tended pigs, fed cattle, pitched hay bales, and drove a grain truck. During my entire education since age 16, I have worked at odd jobs, as a waiter, babysitter, house cleaner and yards man, book seller, dishwasher, whatever needed to be done.

"In my home visits I use all of my experience and training to help families plan and negotiate for the care of their members at home and in the community or hospital. My services are entirely paid by the Medical Services Plan of B.C. I have no other employer and I am forbidden by law to extra bill for any of these services which are covered under the rubric of 'psychotherapy'. All of the families I visit are adjusting to the stresses, traumas, and abuses, of rapid unplanned change in societies which demand that families adjust to wars and catastrophes of famine, disaster, and genocide in whatever ways they can. I have been

privileged to witness their stories and to share in their family planning for a better and a good life for their children and grandchildren.

"Ever since the Court decided in 1990, despite my bankruptcy due to illness, that I should pay $26,000 in maintenance and court costs, and continuing maintenance for Andy's care, I have made regular monthly payments of $350 to Jane, and for at least two years a monthly allowance of $150 to Andy so that he can learn to manage his own life. Despite numerous invitations to Andy that he work with me in my practice so he could begin to learn what the life of a physician is like, he was not able to accept my invitation until his 18th birthday [Andy said according to his mother] when we began to discuss his designing and maintaining a web page for my practice. I offered a computer to Andy to go along with his $10,000 scholarship to U.B.C. When I was informed at his high school graduation that he was giving up the $10,000 scholarship and would be going to Queen's University, as part of this plan I suggested that I would contribute along with other contributions to a computer notebook for his use at Queens University and in our communicating with each other. I told him I am willing to share fairly and equally the costs of his education with him and his mother. Also I told him that if she insisted on my paying all of his costs as a maintenance payment, I would not be able to pay him anything additional for working with me or buying a computer for him. He was concerned that because we have different views on bioethics, his as a "conservative", mine as a "pinko", I would not want his views presented on the practice web page. I explained that my proposed medical practice web page is to provide my family clients and fellow students information and ideas they could use to make their own decisions and lives, and I need his ideas, thinking, and research to be presented truthfully and fully. We were in the process of discussing Andy's work on the web page for which I paid him $300 in early July to cover this month when I received this application from Jane to vary the maintenance.

"I would not have been able to build and maintain any medical practice and support Andy since the 1990 court decision without the help of my friend and neighbor and colleague, Daisy. Most of my family medical practice is with women and their *children, whom I would not be able to visit without Daisy's full participation. Her experience and training as a Medical Office Assistant, Conflict Resolution Negotiator and Mediator, Midwife, Videographer, Fine and Crafts Artist, Family Counselor, and Grandmother, who has lived and worked with aboriginal families, makes it possible for us to provide insured medical services to families who need them to care for the health problems of their members. We use art and videography to help families plan and provide care for their members through crisis of severe medical illness, death, divorce, disability, unemployment, school problems, career and life change, or pregnancy. Daisy has 15 years experience as a Midwife and Birth counselor; trained to counsel the dying and their families, with 30 years experience; trained as a Mediator, Negotiator, and in Conflict Resolution, with 15 years experience; certified artist and diploma Videographer; 44 years experience in office administration; 16 years experience and certified Medical office Assistant; 16 years training in Psychotherapy, Homeopathy, and caring for patients in crisis (having worked also in an Emergency health clinic)." ks*

IT HAD BECOME CLEAR to Daisy that after all the additional money Ken had thrown at Jane and Andy, his attempts to negotiate Andy's needs were being ignored; Jane and Bruce Katz were waging a war that had nothing to do with money. As before, money was simply an excuse for a hidden agenda that had to be more vengeance with intent to ruin Ken's public reputation all over again, and in the process take Daisy down with him – or worse.

Worried about Ken's health, on July 23, 1997 Daisy wrote to their lawyer, William McLachlan:

...I want you to know how concerned and worried I am that Jane will KILL Ken with the constant pressure and Andy will have NO father.

I see how his health is affected and I am afraid his heart will not withstand the pressure. To my knowledge, he has a damaged, enlarged heart. This is not simply a case of taking blood pressure

medicine and sending the person back to the pressure
cooker. I am concerned that Jane knows this and will
never let up the pressure.

I am concerned that Katz has been hired to do the
dirty work for her and in so doing he will dredge up
a profile of a criminal. Why else would the last court
case be included with the documents for this
maintenance hearing? ...

... I am desperately afraid for Ken's life. ...
(Signed) Daisy

ONCE AGAIN, trying to answer Jane's Affidavits and the contents
of misinformation, Ken registered an **Affidavit No. D141314
Vancouver Registry, dated 24th day of July 1997, stating:**

...I do not agree that the payments are often late... Jane Anderson
Affidavit, the Petitioner is suggesting that I refused a request to
increase child support. On the contrary, the issue of increased
funds for Andy was resolved by my voluntarily paying an
additional $150 per month directly to Andy as an allowance, and
by my assuming payment for Andy's coverage on the Medical
Services Plan at an additional $32 per month. The payment of this
$150 per month directly to Andy was intended to benefit Andy for
incidentals, as well as to assist him in developing some skills in
managing his own money.

...The plan for Andy to attend Queen's University in Kingston,
Ontario was not discussed with me. Andy was accepted as a first
year student at the University of British Columbia and was offered
a scholarship... in the amount of $10,000 payable over the four
undergraduate years. The program... would also have served
Andy's hopes that he proceed on to medical school. ...In any event,
I was not consulted on the decision of choosing Queen's University
over the University of British Columbia.

...I have never been reluctant to assist Andy in attendance at
university. I agree that both the Petitioner and I want our son to

attend university and obtain the best education possible...

As to paragraph 19 of the Jane Anderson Affidavit, I do not agree that the Petitioner made any real attempt to resolve Andy's university costs with me. In approximately mid June, I requested the Petitioner to provide me with a summary of Andy's anticipated expenses. ...

I have tried to speak with the Petitioner about settling the contribution for Andy; however, the Petitioner has refused to discuss the issue with me and has said the matter is in the hands of Mr. Katz, the Petitioner's solicitor.

(a proposal of contribution for Andy's support while attending Queen's University follows, along with Exhibits A to I of financial reports)

...the Petitioner is well aware that payment to me from the Medical Services Commission represent gross payments, which do not reflect any expenses.

(followed by a list of real expenses to run the medical practice)

The Petitioner and her counsel have attempted to characterize my relationship with Daisy Heisler as that of a kept woman. I do not reside with Daisy, and she is not my common-law wife, nor do I pay her expenses, other than the consulting fees that she earns. In fact, I would be unable to earn the level of MSP billings that I presently earn, without the assistance of Daisy Heisler. ...

...As to paragraph 20 of the Jane Anderson Affidavit, I regret that the Petitioner wishes to dwell on past history; however I would say as follows: At the commencement of our relationship, the Petitioner had no university education, and I provided the financial support while the Petitioner went to school. I also paid for the Petitioner's education, including her law school training. After our separation, I looked after Andy while the Petitioner completed her articling year.

In the separation and ensuing divorce, I offered and gave to the Petitioner the assets of the marriage, while I assumed the debts, rather than dividing assets and debts equally. I took this position in order that the Petitioner would have a solid base on which to care for Andy. The family assets included a house on which I continued paying the mortgage until it was sold several years later, whereupon the Petitioner kept all net proceeds.

The debts I assumed during the marriage included all the Petitioner's credit card debts, which the Petitioner had used to the maximum after separation. It was the substantial debts of the marriage that eventually caused me to declare bankruptcy when my health broke down, and I was unable to work. The Petitioner has always doubted the state of my health. In fact, my medical doctor [name] has diagnosed that I have a damaged, enlarged heart and I have dangerously high blood pressure. I am on blood pressure medication to modify my blood pressure; the blood pressure goes out of control with increased stress. I have been advised by my family doctor to minimize any exposure to stress and, in view of my present age of 63 years, my doctor has advised me to retire from the practice of medicine, due to that stress.

After my separation from the Petitioner and after my health deteriorated, I could no longer continue working during the period when I was bankrupt. I received advice from a lawyer that the Petitioner had directed me to, to the effect that I need not pay maintenance during the period of my bankruptcy. In hindsight, the advice was not reasonable advice, although I did not have any money to pay my bills. I provided the Petitioner with transfer of an RRSP (retirement fund) in lieu of some maintenance payments; however, the Petitioner initially denied that she had received it, and when confronted with documents, the Petitioner indicated that she had forgotten transfer of the RRSP. This money was not counted as money toward maintenance for Andy.

Our divorce proceedings also did not recognize the fact that I had been looking after Andy six days a week for years. During the Court case Mr. Katz took the position that I have no proper expenses in my medical practice; however, I do have required expenses, and I could not complete my practice without the help of Daisy Heisler. ...

[Ken and his lawyer, William McLachlan, signed this affidavit.]

A SHOCKING AFFIDAVIT signed by son Andy arrived, in which he stated that even though Ken and Daisy have separate apartments in the same building, he believes they are living common-law because of his "investigation" and found the food was in Daisy's apartment. In his Affidavit, Andy wrote out his continuing complaints about the leased car Ken and Daisy used for work. For those reasons, the Affidavit backed up his mother's reasons to demand Daisy's financial statements.

In the Affidavit, Andy was scathing in his criticism of his father for wanting to pay him for work on a medical website. He complained that he had to pay for his own restaurant meal but failed to mention that Ken had been giving him a monthly allowance to do just that and learn how to get along in the world around him. Andy complained about not receiving enough Christmas presents. Andy ended the last paragraph of his Affidavit with: "I do not understand why my father wishes to provide so generously for Daisy but will not provide money for my support and education. It does not seem fair to me."

KEN ARRIVED in Daisy's apartment looking sad and pale with the paper in his hand. In a soft, sad voice he reluctantly informed her about the contents of Andy's Affidavit.

Her gut response was fury at this ultimate insult to Ken. "How can we ever trust him in the future? I believe his mother coerced him! I can't believe it was his idea to investigate our apartments and pretend to have a good time when his uncle Richard was here. That's so dishonest. He's an adult now. It's time for him to think for himself! I need an apology from him before he comes into my apartment ever again! ...May I read that Affidavit for myself?"

While Daisy was reading, Ken walked to the window to look into the green of the old cedar trees only a few feet away, while reflecting: How can I defend my son? I hope that on his own, my son would not have written such an Affidavit... a public document so warped of truth or understanding... so confused... Daisy is no secret relationship... he was treated like one of her family for years... she is the person who taught him how to wipe his own bum and she wiped his runny nose... It's been almost impossible to have a decent relationship with any of my sons because of their mothers... I have always looked for ways to teach my sons about medicine... to share what I have learned... or just to help them in whatever interests they have... I invited Andy on several occasions to accompany me as a student in my practice... I thought that because Andy expressed interest in studying sciences and probably becoming a medical student, an idea of a medical website that we could work on together would be a source of income for him and that he could be proud for making his own income while learning...

Ken's thoughts took him back over the last few years – Andy's teen years. ...Jane threatened several times to send him to live with me as punishment. I always wanted my son to live with me but having a child thrust into a father's home as punishment does not make a good father-son relationship... Instead of taking advantage of their problems with each other, I did what I would do in my medical practice... Each time they had a flare-up, I would meet with my son and his mother to help resolve their issues... When kids are influenced to be alienated from a parent, it is difficult to overcome... Kids don't want to believe their own mothers tell lies... They don't understand how their own mothers can use them for their own greed and revenge... Andy was alienated from me prior to the last court case and has rarely come to my apartment since... He has never set foot in Daisy's home since then, except for the dinner with Richard, and that appears to have been monetarily motivated by his mother... At Andy's request, we usually meet in Andy's home while Jane is out, and often because he is sick... Many appointments with clients have been changed so that I could look after Andy during his frequent illnesses; I bring food and medicine and just keep Andy company while caring for him...

Ken thought back to the sleepless baby he carried in his arms and cared for round the clock... how he worked around his child's needs in order to support his family financially and be the main caretaker at the same time... how he held his son on his knees and read storybooks to him for hours and years... how they would walk and talk... how his boy with the golden curls had filled his heart with unconditional love... how being forced to live separately from his son has been the greatest heartache in life... causing years of tears... and all else paled in comparison to that loss... second marriage vows down the tube...

Ken's hand went to his forehead as he thought back – How I tried so hard to care for my son... to make up for an incompetent mother... maybe I should not have left the marriage... then I probably would be dead today... but then my son would not have written such an Affidavit... on the other hand, under his mother's influence, even if I had died he may dislike me in a similar way as my other sons did... they have grown up with their mothers' strong influences... I can only hope that someday they will understand me enough to rethink their own lives...

The hurt was strong, affecting his heart – now in severe pain. He kept the pain to himself as the green of the cedar branches came into focus again.

Daisy finished reading and took her place at his side, reaching for his hand. His hand felt warm and she felt comfort by holding on. Ken was always so giving that it was easy to relax and take from him but this time rather than just taking, she wished to comfort him and ease his hurt. She could feel his pain.

She spoke slowly, "The poor kid really doesn't understand you at all, or what you have been doing... for him or for his mother. Even now, at his age, he seems to have no understanding of all the financial support you have given to his mother so that they could have security. This is evidence that he is a victim of brainwashing. He doesn't even understand why you have a leased car, of all things. And Andy thinks he is in competition with *me*! He doesn't seem to know the difference between adult relationships or of a child with his parent. He's obviously mirroring his mother's feelings about us... you... me... and he is taking it out on you the same way *she* has been doing – in a public arena. He's a young man now and..."

"That is my point. He needs to go far away from his mother to find himself. I intend to support him to do that... whatever it takes!"

"Ken, that means he will be far away from you, too."

"I know. I think it is worth the sacrifice to get him away from that woman so that he can grow up and think for himself."

KEN'S WRITTEN AND ORAL requests for information on which to base a common sense offer to support his son continued to be met with silence. Jane refused to answer. Meanwhile Jane continued to accuse Ken of holding things up.

For many days, Ken tried to talk with his son and met with silence, echoing his mother's behavior. Finally, Ken managed a brief, rare talk with Andy and followed it with a note on August 26, 1997:

Dear Andy,

I am writing to clarify what I said to you on the telephone today. I read your affidavit and I am sorry for any hurt that I may have caused you. I fully support your decision to attend Queen's University and I will support you emotionally, financially, and spiritually during your four years of university.

After speaking with you on the telephone, I made an offer to your mother which I believe she discussed with you because I spoke with both of you at your home. The cheques I wrote to you and your mother for your maintenance in June, July, and August, of $650 per month were to communicate concretely the financial support I am willing to give you. Today I told your mother I would continue to pay her $650 per month maintenance tax free to her, and put $5000 into an account to pay my half of your university costs for 1997-1998 [school year]. If she does not want to accept my offer I asked her to tell me what she believes to be fair considering that we will save costs and reduce strain on you by making an agreement now.

I suggest that we review your university cost for 1998-99 next June and decide how we will meet those expenses together. Because you told me today you do not want a laptop computer now and have leased a computer for the academic year at Queen's, we can discuss before Christmas what you want instead of the laptop computer I offered you in June for your birthday and graduation present.

I hope my letter is helpful to you and I look forward to talking with you tomorrow.

with love, your Dad.

KEN HAD MADE numerous offers regarding paying for Andy's education at Queen's. Never the less, a legal notice arrived from Jane and Katz, stating that negotiation is not possible, and again, money already paid to Jane went unaccounted for.

This time Ken's lawyer responded strongly.

No. D141314 VANCOUVER REGISTRY
IN THE SUPREME COURT OF BRITISH COLUMBIA
BETWEEN:
CAROL JANE SCHRAMM   PETITIONER
AND:
KEHNROTH SCHRAMM   RESPONDENT

OUTLINE
PART II

1. Position of the Respondent: The Respondent is not opposed to setting an appropriate level of child support, reflecting university attendance commencing September 1997 for the child, Alexander Kehnroth Schramm, born [birth date].

2. Basis for opposing relief: Although the Respondent is not opposed to setting an appropriate level of child maintenance by negotiation with the Petitioner or by Court Order, the Petitioner is not prepared to discuss the issue with the Respondent, and the parties have been unable to come to terms on an appropriate amount.

3. Material to be relied on: Affidavit of Kehnroth Schramm sworn 24 July 1997, Property & Financial Statement of Ken Schramm sworn 24 July 1997 and the Affidavit Susan Grimshire sworn 25 July 1997.

Dated: July 25, 1997
[Signed by] William McLachlan Respondent's Solicitor
William A. McLachlan, Esq.
McLachlan Brown Anderson
Barristers & Solicitors
File: 40.0074.000

KEN AND DAISY met again with Mr. McLachlan. Prior to the meeting, they had come to an agreement between themselves to make such a generous offer that it could not be refused without the other side looking obviously vengeful to the courts. They had already made the decision that money going to pay for a court hearing and specifically to pay Bruce Katz as happened in the past, rather than the money going to Andy, would make no sense. In the meeting with their lawyer, Ken advised that he wanted to make an offer that would cost him about $60,000 over the next four years.

William McLachlan wrote a letter to Katz & Company:

Re: Carol Jane Schramm (Anderson) v. Kehnroth Schramm:

...Dr. Schramm's first priority is to convey his support for Andy's decision to attend Queen's University. Unfortunately, the Affidavit material has made matters get off track. Dr. Schramm was in the process of preparing response Affidavits to your latest material; however, in view of the prospect of settlement, Dr. Schramm is not proposing to complete response Affidavits, as we would like to focus on getting matters back on track without creating further conflict in the Affidavit material. If it is necessary at some future point, Dr. Schramm will be answering the Affidavit material, and the decision not to file a response at this time should not be taken to be any admission of your material.

Dr. Schramm is prepared...to pay &750 per month...

Dr. Schramm is also prepared to provide your client with a lump sum of $5,000 towards Andy's university costs, ...also pay $5,000 plus 50% of any tuition fee increases over the next three years, covering Andy's four years of under-graduate university. ...

...it is clear to us that Dr. Schramm's payment is well in excess of the Federal Child Support Tables, based on any interpretation of Dr. Schramm's income.

In spite of that, Dr. Schramm wishes to be supportive of Andy. ...

[signed] William A. McLachlan.

A COURT ORDER sealed the matter. Jane Anderson's and Bruce Katz' determination to fight and defame Ken again in a public arena was cut short – *finished!*

The difference between the set up for the court case in 1990 and this time was that Ken now had a strong lawyer, Mr. McLachlan, who really was acting on Ken's behalf.

Daisy wanted to shout from a rooftop but restrained herself and instead told anyone who would listen, "What a different outcome it would have been in the last court case if this clear-headed lawyer had been working for Ken then!"

Damage was indeterminable after all the years of everyone knowing that as far as Ken was concerned, the sun rose and set on his son Andy, and that all Ken ever needed to respond to his son's needs was to be asked. *"Just ask me!"* is... was... and always had been his motto. Informing properly and just asking for what his son needed would have made a difference. Instead, his own son had followed his mother in registering a damning Affidavit in a public courthouse and for law students to get their hands on.

Ken was relieved that his son would now be set free to become an adult.

Daisy ran the visual tape over and over in her head – remembering how happy Ken was to be going to his son's graduation dinner. She hurt for the man who went down the street to unexpectedly be ambushed at dinner – a dinner that was a disguised prelude to another onslaught of nastiness leading into another public fight regardless of Ken's months – actually years, of offers to negotiate the expenses of Andy's upcoming university education and even throwing money at both Jane and Andy to show good faith.

In negotiation and mediation training, Daisy had been taught how to recognize dirty tricks and how to deal with them, but Daisy never ceased to be amazed at the kinds dirty tricks Jane pulled. ...And using her son that way... It boggled Daisy's mind to understand how anyone could be that hateful for so long. ...What wasted energy!

A FEW MONTHS into Andy's first year of university, there came the inevitable phone call to Ken from Queen's. Andy asked Ken to pay him a sum of money monthly so that he could move into a rented house with friends rather than live in student housing.

Ken suspected Andy had no idea about the money he was paying to Jane for his monthly maintenance. This time, Ken did not simply top up the money because if Andy did not know about the money being paid to his mother each month, he should ask her and find out, and use it for his month to month housing because he was not living in his mother's house. Ken told Andy to ask his mother for the Seven Hundred and Fifty Dollars per month that was being paid to her for his maintenance on top of his university expenses.

Would Andy finally wonder if his mother had hidden other maintenance money and assets from him over the years and get that straight once and for all? They could only hope.

THE NEXT FOUR YEARS were full of hope for Andy's independence even though it did not seem to be turning out that way. Andy hardly had time for his father on visits home.

When Andy was at home on holidays, Ken's phone calls were usually met with Jane's voice on the answering machine telling him, "You know the drill!" The rudeness of the message annoyed Ken enough to complain about it to Daisy.

If by rare chance he managed to speak with his son, Andy usually could not see Ken because he had chores to do for his mother and said she would be angry if he did not get them done, or he must have Christmas with his mother's friends instead of having a Christmas or any other holiday visit with Ken. It appeared that Andy's mother continued to control his life. Visits with Ken were kept to a bare minimum and there were trips home when Ken did not see his son at all.

There had been similarities for years with Stephen and Peter. Both mothers had been able to strongly influence the boys by playing games to make sure Ken could not see his sons on Father's Day or his birthday. Carolyn had shown up on Father's day most years or in her place, one of her former boyfriends arrived and the boys spent time with her boyfriend instead of with their own father.

Ken was grateful for whatever time he could get with his sons and it was usually after much waiting to have a lunch with them a week or two before or after an important holiday. Very seldom, in all those years, did he see his sons right on an important day.

48

The Great Spirit Robe

LIFE AND DEATH had been a constant companion in these years. Many clients had been seeking help from Ken to go through the progression of life into death and the grief around it. But personally Ken and Daisy had been losing family members. Ken's father passed away. It had been a long time of trying to help his father by long distance contact with the doctors caring for his father and being grateful when a doctor would listen and follow through with Ken's advice. Loss of his father was accompanied by a concern for his mother who had been fiercely committed to her husband.

Daisy's youngest sister bled to death of a head injury after falling down basement stairs under suspicious circumstances on the ranch in Alberta. Daisy asked the police of the small town to investigate but in the end they said there was not enough provable evidence for any charges even though Daisy was sure there was ample evidence. Shortly after, the rough and tumble cowboy husband (the same man Daisy rode with to round up cattle) rode his horse out of a barn in a rodeo and hit his head on the door jam, dying where he fell. Daisy could not help wondering if he was the victim of his own karma.

Before going to her sister's remembrance gathering in Alberta, Ken and Daisy were doing a course in education at UBC with a professor from California. In discussion, Daisy had talked about a serious bullying situation in her granddaughter's high school. On Daisy's return, they went right back to class. Two teachers from her granddaughter's school, who were taking the course, cornered her in the hallway and told her to "shut up". It had happened twice that she was attacked after a death in her family. Bullying was at the heart of both – adults either bullying or protecting bullying. In no mood to argue on this day, Daisy walked away again.

Daisy's brother Tom and his wife had come from Alberta to visit with Daisy and Ken. As Tom walked away the last morning of the visit, Daisy had a flash of foreknowledge that his imminent death could not be stopped. Soon after, in the middle of the night, her sister-in-law phoned to say that Tom had suddenly passed away. Daisy tried to sound surprised but was not. He rekindled the ongoing question – Do we all have predestined timing of life and death, or can we outsmart death?

Often Daisy would look at Ken, as they were on their way to see more clients, and remark that maybe their own troubles and losses were greater than the clients' problems. Regardless of what was happening in their own lives, they needed to keep working through it all and to focus clearly on each client. It was an art in itself and the reward was in being helpful to someone.

On the other side of living, many grandchildren – fourteen in all had arrived in fast succession. Daisy and Ken had been closely involved. Birthday celebration gatherings grew larger and more often. The favorite gatherings at Szechwan Chinese restaurants got larger, requiring larger tables; babies grew up loving hot and sour soup and spicy garlic chicken that they got their first tastes from in the womb. Ken had a large, busy family that he called his own. He was the children's beloved Grampa. He lived the daily joys and troubles of a large family.

Ken had also been helping his middle son financially while he was a student. Peter had settled in Montreal to study but kept promising Ken that he will soon come back to live with him. Ken continued to hold his apartment for Peter, waiting and expecting him. Before Richard had come to visit, Daisy had given up her one bedroom apartment right beside Ken for a two bedroom down the hall in hopes that they would share the apartment. But months ran into years and Daisy was on hold while Peter just never came.

Over the years, there had been a mellowing of relationships between Ken and his first ex-wife, Carolyn. In son Stephen's home, Carolyn and her mother sat down to dinner at the same table and had a fine social time with Ken and Daisy. Ken had always loved his ex-mother-in-law and Daisy could understand why.

Two elderly neighbors in the apartment building died. In frustration, after years of waiting for Peter and leaving room for elusive Andy, Daisy had enough. "I don't want to be taken out of here feet first with all the neighbors gawking while waiting for your sons."

After six years of living next to Ken, she arranged to buy a home with her family. It came about as a result of her oldest granddaughter wanting a big family home like her friends who were Italian and several generations lived under one roof.

Ken was in the midst of writing his thesis for a Degree of Master of Arts in The Faculty of Graduate Studies, Centre for the Study of Curriculum & Instruction, Faculty of Education at UBC. He pleaded with Daisy to wait until he finished writing and defending his thesis. But when some family moved into her apartment after giving up their home in anticipation of buying a home, she felt pushed into following through quickly.

Meanwhile, Stephen and his children and large dog temporarily moved in with Ken because Stephen's rented home had been sold out from under him. Both apartments overflowed. Ken had to complete his thesis in the midst of this bulging jumble.

In the midst of the chaos Ken did defend his thesis in April 1998 and it was accepted on the same day. He had chosen to do it in his favorite place, the UBC House of Learning Long House, with a celebration lunch following.

In June of that year, he and Daisy became partners as one-third (one-sixth each) owners of a home in North Vancouver. Peter came back at the same time. Regardless of invitations, not one of Ken's sons would look at the home. As a result, Ken again made the decision to keep his apartment where his sons could have unfettered access to him.

After dragging her feet a couple of months, wondering what she had done and wishing to backtrack, it was too late. Daisy reluctantly moved to the new house in the month of August. It was a horrible feeling to leave Ken not only across town, but also across the water.

Ken tried staying overnight at the house and get to UBC in the morning by public transit. The transit system was so inefficient that it took three hours to get from the North Shore to UBC.

He missed the meeting he was supposed to attend. Convincing any sons to join him in North Vancouver was never going to happen. Clearly, keeping the apartment near UBC was a better plan.

Each morning Ken played a tape of Aboriginal music and did his exercises and chanting; he prayed for his loved ones and ended up crying every morning over the loss of Daisy's presence.

Following his morning ritual, his routine was to attend UBC in preparation for his PhD and be ready to see clients in the afternoons and evenings.

AS MUCH AS they liked working with their clients, there were days when on the way to see clients, Ken pleaded, "I'm tired, Daisy. I want to concentrate on my PhD and teach instead of working this hard. My days are numbered if I keep up this pace."

Daisy responded in variations of: "I'm not the one who is making you work. It's Jane and your kids. As soon as Andy is finished school, we can retire. I just wish your kids would respect you and be thankful for your sacrifices... your never-ending support. I wish they would try to understand you instead of being led around by their noses by mothers... I'm sorry. That's not helpful."

It was a dilemma. Ken had been too ill to work once before and got crucified for it. It would be no good to offer to get a different job and support Ken if he was too ill to work and while continuing to work, he needed Daisy to keep him safe. Andy's university and maintenance costs for one year were more than any salary she could make at another job in a whole year and still have a frugal living allowance. Daisy and Ken had no way to change anything right then. Ken's tiredness and ongoing physical pain in his heart were real but they were on a treadmill. Daisy dreamed of the day Andy would graduate.

IT WAS A TIME in Canadian history when men were being beat up in the courts over parenting rights and maintenance. Women had gained the upper hand. New Canadian child maintenance laws were supposed to equal the playing field for parents.

The pendulum had swung but fairness and the long talked about joint custody for the betterment of children's lives was not being utilized. Child maintenance was supposed to be based on actual income but now the payee had a double whammy by also having to pay income tax on money paid out, and some lawyers were not following the rules regarding income schedules.

At the same time, there was no fear of breaking laws because the law protecting children's rights appeared to have no teeth when (usually) mothers ignored court ordered access of the fathers to their children. Mediation was talked about but was hard to come by. Some lawyers were making a good living on the perpetual adversarial route and were reluctant to give it up.

The law ignored parents causing parental alienation even though it had been given a name and was being written about. False allegations could get out of hand in attempts to label fathers unfit to parent and to be called dead-beat dads. The law also got tough and acted out a punishment causing so-called 'dead beat dads' to lose their driving licenses if there was a delay in maintenance payments for any reason regardless of parental alienation. The domino effect was that losing a driver's license meant that some men could not work in order to pay because industrial work was often miles out of town and not on a bus route. Fathers were then jailed. That became a ploy for getting fathers 'out of the way', the intention often sought by mothers who would go to great lengths to do just that.

Games and delays by lawyers in court proceedings were a way of life. Fathers lived their lives with hope of just seeing their children, and crying in their pillows at night. Many fathers were in the news and television documentaries, fighting unsuccessfully to see their children. They hired lawyers who kept the fathers showing up in court but nothing got resolved over and over. The men were drained of large amounts of money that went to support lawyers and courts. Fathers started support groups and did public escapades like climbing poles and hanging signs on bridges just to make statements and have their plight get noticed. All they wanted was to see their children.

During this time of fathers fighting for their parental rights, a young father and relative of Daisy caught his wife in an ongoing affair with another man while he was at work. On being found out when he came across a used condom while fixing her car, she had picked up long pointed scissors and lunged to stab him in a fit of anger; he raised his hand to protect himself and caught the stab in his right palm. He went outside to avoid her rage. She followed, picked up an axe from the woodpile and chased him around the mountaintop where they lived. Though it made an interesting plot for a movie, in real life, he was scared.

Rather than fight on her terms, the young man left the dangerous situation. For two years, father and son then lived together in Vancouver and the mother had weekends and shared holidays with the child. Occasionally, she and her live-in boyfriend would show up stoned and shouted obscenities on the father's doorstep. Then came the Spring holiday after which she did not return the son, but kept him and started him in a local school.

The mother decided to go to court for custody and maintenance. As a single mother she qualified for legal aid but in the background the boyfriend with an income had been living with her for the last two years.

The father had never wanted to ask for financial support and had never collected the automatic child benefit from the government. Instead, he had let the mother collect it. He had never gone for legal custody, not wanting to bother with lawyers.

With the Hearing for her custody case slated on short notice, the father shelled out Four Thousand Dollars to a Chilliwack lawyer who claimed his expertise was in mediation but he wanted the money up front in order to consider taking the case. Desperate to have a lawyer on extremely short notice, the father paid.

At the Hearing, the mother's lawyer asked for an adjournment on the grounds the mother could not be present. In fact, regardless of the Hearing, she had gone to Mexico for a holiday with her boyfriend, leaving the son with an acquaintance from his school instead of the father because of the court case.

Then the games began between the lawyers. Mediation never became part of the game. Several more Hearings held in Chilliwack were rescheduled. The mother did not attend any without saying why but her lawyer kept asking for, and getting, adjournments. Each time the father and his family traveled an hour and a half to Chilliwack for nothing.

Deliberate delays caused weeks to go by. Then the case was moved to New Westminster, home to no one but that was where this female Justice who had allowed all the delays, was working on the new date. This Justice had done nothing on the case except to allow all delays, but for some reason only known to the two lawyers, they were in agreement that they wanted this particular Justice and moved the case in order to follow her to another city.

In New Westminster, the father and his family waited in the benches while another child maintenance case was heard. It was a daunting prelude to what was to come. It was also an example of what happens in Canadian courts with newly renovated maintenance laws that were supposed to protect children, but in fact robbed many children, leaving them even poorer. A young man on the stand tried to explain to the Justice that he had lived only a few months in the home of the woman bringing her child maintenance case to court. He explained that her four children were not his and the mother was already collecting maintenance from the birth father of the children. White faced and scared, he desperately explained that he has a new wife and baby and a low paying job in which he only makes enough money to support one family, his own – and if he has to pay the maintenance requested by this estranged woman for her several children, he is also expected to pay income tax on any money paid out for maintenance, and that would leave nothing for his own family.

Meanwhile the woman who brought the case to court was not required to take the stand. Instead, she and her female friend sat on the bench directly behind Daisy, tittering and snickering all through the Hearing.

The female Justice wasted no time in deciding the young man should pay the woman maintenance as requested for her several children regardless that this was a second monthly maintenance payment she would receive or that the man's new wife and baby would have to starve or fend for themselves. When this decision came down, both women behind Daisy cheered, not caring who heard, "Whoopee! Let's go shopping!" Their legs were running even before their rear ends lifted off from their bench. The clatter of their shoes disappeared as heavy doors slammed behind them.

Then it was Daisy's relative's turn. The mother's lawyer, still in her absence, took this date to make the case that the son had been established in his new school for several weeks, therefore he should not be moved. He also asked that the "poor" single mother needed high maintenance dollars, not at all fitting the father's present salary. The lawyer produced a letter that was not an Affidavit, was not witnessed, and had no verification of signature, from a female counselor supposedly at the son's former General Gordon School in Vancouver that he had grown out of years before and gone on to high school since. The letter stated the boy was better off with the mother. The problem with the letter was that the counselor named the wrong child – the name in the letter was not even close, and she stated an unknown home address in Vancouver as being that of the child; the address was clear across the city on the east side while the father's home was west by the ocean.

The father objected to the letter, pointing out the serious mistakes while his own lawyer remained stony silent. It was as though the Justice was deaf and blind; she ignored the father's objections and accepted the letter as evidence.

During a brief break, Daisy had come out of a washroom. The hall was empty; everyone had gone back into the courtroom except for both lawyers in the hallway discussing their deal. They were visibly startled and bounced on their heels when they realized Daisy was within earshot. As though on a string together, they sheepishly darted into the courtroom to avoid contact with her before a final decision.

Standing straight and steady before the Justice, the father refused to say anything negative about the mother of his child or to allow any witnesses to speak about her bad behavior because he did not want it to affect his son in future. Instead, he spoke only of his own good care and intentions for his son. He kept his high standard of morals intact and lost in court. His lawyer pocketed Four Thousand Dollars for doing absolutely nothing except to show up on assigned dates and deliberately losing.

The female Justice disregarded obvious errors and decided that the child should live with the mother with high maintenance attached for the child on the grounds that the child had been in his new school for weeks and his education must not be interrupted. The mother of the boy never did show her face in court.

ON A WIDER PICTURE at the time, it was reported in the news that a man in B.C.'s north country went out behind a barn and shot himself because a court ordered him to pay more child maintenance than his monthly income could support regardless of newer laws.

With Canadian law gone awry and women seemingly in power, the writing had been on the wall regarding Daisy's friend's case. For Daisy, it was a grim reminder of how Ken was treated in his custody and child maintenance case a few years earlier when Ken had gone to court trying to defend himself against Jane. Daisy could not help wondering about the fallacy that if women were in charge of politics, they would make a more peaceful world. She was not convinced. She had been witness to too much, in both the medical and legal world, to believe women were better than men.

On the other hand, she realized that because of being a midwife to women in their most vulnerable, naked soul moments, an undeniable bond of compassion continues.

ANTONY, DAISY'S SON and his children had come to Vancouver to work for a couple of weeks. He always traveled with his children because he was the main caretaker of the children since birth. He worked with and around his children's schedules and that included cooking their daily meals that his wife came home to. He had been home schooling his children for years and was continuing the home schooling on this trip while at the same time working on some horses in the Lower Mainland that had health issues. He also did some work on his mother's new home, and then the family went back to Quesnel.

On arrival home, he was shocked to see that his wife had cleared his belongings out of his home. His belongings had disappeared. She was out when he returned so he set up a video camera and waited.

As she arrived through the door, she shouted, "Get out!"

Linda, the older woman, who had convinced a guy just out of his teen years to elope with her, now was adamant that she wanted a divorce. Following that, she was on tape running out of the house with boxes of financial statements to hide. It was all caught on tape unknown to her but she then told the children their father wanted the divorce, diverting their anger onto their father. Regardless, Antony never would use the tape. He thought he could keep his relationship with his children without resorting to exposing their mother's bad behavior and lies.

She had waited until the house and country acreage was debt free. She was determined to keep all the assets after eighteen years of marriage and Antony's hard work. He was familiar with her screaming temper and what she did to get her own way. He believed that his wife might roll on the ground to bruise herself and then claim he had beaten her. He made a hasty trip back to Vancouver by himself before she could pull that one or get him involved in a physical or verbal confrontation. It was another case of fight or flight.

On the way back to Vancouver, he remembered how recently he had left the house to work and while driving, within the half hour he had received a phone call from Linda to say his horse Rocky had died. He had gone back immediately. Standing over Rocky's body, Antony was puzzled that he had spoken to his healthy horse less than an hour ago.

Rocky lay within twelve feet of an electrical outlet. It was horrible to be suspicious but when he mentioned it to Daisy, she speculated out loud that his horse had been deliberately electrocuted and there was no way the horse did it to himself.

Rocky always stood out among the Tennessee Walkers being bred and raised by Antony and Linda. This golden-brown horse of no special breed had come to Antony after cruel treatment by a former owner. Daisy had been visiting and had accompanied Antony to pick up hay from a local farmer when they found out that Rocky, who stood watching forlornly, was for sale. Daisy got on his back to test him out and fell in love with the gentle soul. She purchased him as a gift for Antony.

Getting to know each other took time, Rocky would stand and watch Antony while Antony would stand and watch Rocky. Over many days, they would move a little closer until Rocky was nestling against Antony and became his daily companion through the forest and over the hills.

On a visit from Vancouver soon after Rocky's arrival, Loraine and Ron's small son Lawrence was found fast asleep in a pile of hay in the barn with Rocky lying beside him in a guardian position. Rocky, the gentle soul—now gone.

IRONICALLY, Linda hired lawyer Marnie Dunnaway, the same lawyer out of Ken and Daisy's past— the same person who told Ken, "It's only a game."

Games began. In Linda's determination to keep all assets for herself, she pulled many serious tricks in an attempt to get Antony jailed and out of the picture. Out of Marnie's office came false allegations and threats. This all sounded too familiar to Ken and Daisy.

Antony hired William McLachlan, the same lawyer who had recently helped Ken with the second potential court case and managed to out-smart Jane Anderson and her lawyer Bruce Katz so that they had to quit harassing Ken.

McLachlan accompanied Antony when cross-examined by Royal Canadian Mounted Police where Linda's claims were dismissed regardless of an over-zealous female RCMP officer.

Antony's lawyer also called for a report under Section 15 of Family Law to be done by a fully qualified and respected psychologist. This was necessary in order to make an in depth assessment of the whole family before going to court about the allegations made by Linda and her lawyer. The psychologist appointed was the same qualified man that Ken had wanted in his child custody case with Jane, but that his own lawyer had fought against.

Through several days of psychological examinations with the seasoned psychologist, with and without his children, Antony was completely cleared of any and all wrongdoing, and was cleared of even being capable of thinking of wrongdoing. The children, in separate examinations, backed up their father's story of no wrongdoing. The psychologist told Antony that he has a talent for writing children's stories.

For the Supreme Court of British Columbia, the psychologist wrote in his report that in his opinion, Linda is a person who is capable of lying for her own selfish purpose.

In an eight-day court case, Linda's own family produced dishonest financial statements to help her.

Then in what appeared to be a diversion tactic when things were not looking favorable for Linda, Marnie Dunnaway went after Daisy about supposedly causing Linda's infection when she gave birth to her first child in Daisy's home sixteen years earlier. This seemed so far out to left field that at first Daisy was stunned. She was on the stand in a court of law and being forced to speak publicly about confidential patient information.

Daisy explained that at seven days after giving birth, Linda was healthy. She explained that Linda's infection was caused seven days after the birth, when a doctor performed a lancing of Linda's hemorrhoids in his office and the infection following became evident three days after the lancing and ten days after the birth. A hush falls over the courtroom.

In what seemed like another desperate move, Marnie's questions to Daisy were suddenly about another family member who was not in court and had never been involved with this divorce; Marnie questioned why he was out of work. Daisy asked Marnie what the question had to do with this divorce case. She got no answer. In the space of silence where no one intervened, Daisy wondered how Marnie even had that information. She addressed the question by explaining that the former owner of the tiny business had just died of cancer and the business folded only a few days ago.

The diversion tactics to make Antony's family look bad did fail. The strange questioning caused Daisy to read facial expressions of the lawyers instead of watching her step as she stepped out of the witness box. She tripped on a wooden ridge and would have fallen out if Antony's lawyer had not caught her.

Linda's male co-worker confidently took the stand next to testify that he was a witness to Antony causing trouble at Linda's house in Quesnel on a particular evening. Antony's lawyer, Mr. McLachlan, matter-of-factly stated that Antony had gone back to Vancouver on an airplane on that day, sitting right beside him and could not possibly have been at the house that evening.

The box of pornographic magazines that Marnie claimed she had in her office never materialized. Daisy knew that if they had any magazines that belonged to Antony, it was a box full of medical journals that she had given him because of his interest in medicine.

After several days of absurdities and lies, the no-nonsense female Judge gave Linda an hour-long public reprimand.

This astute Judge had seen through all the games and was not being tricked into siding with women.

After an eight-day trial, Antony was one hundred percent exonerated.

The Judge made constructive recommendations about the children and seized the case for the children's sake.

This Judge restored much needed faith in the justice system.

The problem turned out to be that in the children's home, brainwashing continued. The youngest child had express concern to the psychologist, "Our mother would never lie to us."

Oh, yes she would. Linda, as a mother, has done a successful job of parental alienation. She had gotten her way all her life and now she was unafraid. She completely ignored orders by the Judge and everything recommended for the health of the children and their father's right to access. Meanwhile, Linda's co-worker who perjured himself in court was allowed to take the Antony's daughter on weekend jaunts.

Linda had, during eighteen years of marriage relegated the raising of the children, home schooling and cooking of all meals to Antony. Linda had spent much of her home time reading murder mysteries in bed and waiting for her meals to be prepared. Antony had raised the children and worked to make a living around their schedules, in fact taking the children to work on occasion. Now, his children were being withheld from him.

Daisy could not help but think of similarities to Ken's second marriage and caring for Andy. There the similarity ends. The Judges were different in each case. The defending lawyers were different. The child custody investigators were entirely different.

The Judge ordered that Antony be able to pick up his personal belongings and work tools that had been withheld and hidden.

With Linda's henchmen on guard at the country home, Antony was given clothing deliberately torn; irreplaceable family photos ordered by the court to be returned had been crumbled and stuffed into work boots; work tools large and small were deliberately missing parts, damaged and rendered unusable. Linda had complied with a court order that has no teeth regarding quality and was another testament to an ailing legal system.

With sadness, Daisy thought that if Mr. McLachlan had been hired during the first court case that Jane instigated against Ken, the outcome would have been entirely different and Ken's reputation would have been saved.

Through these experiences, it was obvious how valuable the work was that Ken did with clients. Ken was able to help people in divorce to look out for the children first – to be parents first – and accomplish a healthier outcome.

Success seemed to be elusive within their own families. Daisy joked about whether arranged marriages might be better because of the importance of sharing same family values and especially the same ethics, even though she would have been a renegade.

MEANWHILE, Daisy's father had remarried in a small wedding. The woman was a secret alcoholic, only discovered after the wedding when she became a drunken tyrant. On Daisy's visit home for her father's birthday, while talking with her father, the new wife ordered him to stop talking. Daisy watched in horror as her usually exuberant father, the man who taught her about storytelling was damped down. Bewilderment followed by embarrassment was written all over his face. Daisy responded to the woman, "I want to hear my father's stories!" But she knew she would not always be there to defend her father.

They were divorced after a few months but the woman demanded half of all assets that included the home Daisy's father lived in for more than fifty years, and she wanted Daisy's mother pension that was being paid to her father. That sent chills down Daisy's spine because her mother had worked hard for the government over many years for that pension. It became obvious that the woman had married for money. A neighbor, an older man living alone and in frail health had been faithfully cared for by Daisy's father over many years; in appreciation, he gave Daisy's father enough money to buy off the woman legally in the divorce and this gift allowed Daisy's father to keep his home. Because the marriage had lasted only a short time, Daisy's father's pensions were protected.

[Daisy's father did continue his friendship and care of the older neighbor until the man passed away.]

IN NOVEMBER OF 1999, Ken's mother was in crisis and dying. Word came that in an altered state of mind, she was quite sure Ken was at her side in Vermont and once again she was having long talks with her son.

Ken arranged the finances to gather up all three sons from Vancouver and Ontario for quick trips to Vermont. While Ken was in the air, his mother passed away peacefully believing she had been talking with her firstborn.

Ken's loss would also be his gain. Finally, he was able to be at a family reunion of brothers and sisters and their families and his three sons – the first one for scores of years. It would also be the last one.

The few days, while burying his mother beside his father, were laced with sadness but also a gift of the best and longest time Ken had been able to spend with his son, Andy during his college years. During these days, the last photos were taken of Ken with his three sons.

ON HIS RETURN, Ken told Daisy, "I'm an orphan." Ken had lost his father a few years prior and this statement was a bit of a shock as she realized how alone he must feel. He was not only mourning the loss of his mother but he had lost the person he could talk with, his confidante since childhood. No matter what age, a person does become an orphan when parents die.

During the night at his table with pen in hand, Ken wrote to talk with his mother:

Gramma Jean, Mom, I hope you can hear
read my handwriting   drawing
when I think of you being with me, in me, around me,
witnessing me, being me, with you,
living in your our stories, ourstories.

I remember acknowledging Vermont as Abernaki territory, speaking with you at your funeral, reading, performing "a worm's tale", asking Richard, how it went over and he said "right over their heads".

Apparently I was speaking with you in a foreign language like when I came home from Dartmouth College and you told me every time I came home from school, we talked and I had a new religion: another world and another language to live in, I think.

Mom, you were are will be always already, a loyal wife, mother and gramma like your mother remaining within the Congregational Church communities where you met and married Dad and raised us to love life
your five children "diaphragm babies" you called us,
planned and unplanned parenthood, I thought.

When I asked you a few years' ago about my birth,
what was it like for you?
and you said, like all the others, your two brother and two sisters, I couldn't believe you.

I was the first born with a long forehead and pointed head sticking up like a dunce cap, you said, some membrane coverings and nerves of my spinal cord sticking out of the back of my neck.
I thought you and Dad must have been scared of death,

your first born, a monster child, might die at any time from infection or worse, live on completely paralyzed and imbecilic from too much water on the brain, a vegetable human you could not afford after Dad had just taken a $50 cut in pay the week I was born
in the middle of the Depression.
Clean your plates, eat all your food before the Great Depression
The unmourned Morning of my life comes again.

Without your stories of my birth and our schrammily like and unlike all the others
I would not be still living in your our stories:
your father asking his friend, a general surgeon, to fix me, put me back together again

He did with Gray's Anatomy, a lot of luck, and skill,
and Dadad must have paid for it all, I think,
even though he was never a generous man except with his stories,
not wanting to pay for his daughter marrying a poor man, a self
made man, son of a German dirt farmer in New Jersey and a
Danish-Irish-French mother, whose father Dr. Charles Kehnroth,
a physician, homeopath and educator, gave me my name, my
destiny.

Names can always hurt me
being different they always nearly always did
and they made me stronger, too strong for my own good
sometimes.

Then and now there were the stories about your father's relatives
coming over on the Mayflower in 1620 to Cape Cod and
Plymouth Colony,
William Whipple signing the Declaration of Independence in
1775:
Henry Wadsworth Longfellow, poet
Charles Sumner abolitionist

I have lived inside these stories for all my life
until this past year
when mourning your death I almost died an almost healthy
grampa death.
I am writing speaking with you
all your birthdays and mine since I met you
and I want to thank you for living on with me
and ask your help in being the best human being I can be,
learning to live at last always already.

ONE TRANSFORMATION FOLLOWED another along with wonderment of the workings of the universe. Life and death took its turn in the ever changing and evolving lives of people – family and clients.

Going from appointment to appointment, Daisy continued to drive the car while Ken sang beside her. His voice reminded her in tone of a mellow cello resonating inside her chest.

His hair had become whiter. Still the most beautiful hair, she thought, and loved to run her fingers through his curls as he alternated between lengths that brushed over his shoulders to just below his smooth earlobes. Just looking at him made her smile and feel tenderness.

Daisy had turned to colouring to cover grey and was thankful that Ken never made an issue of it. Her 20-20 vision had given way to needing reading glasses.

They looked at each other with appreciation of timeless beauty in the other, even though they were becoming a testament of gravity.

"I love to hear you singing," she told him between songs. "We've now worked together for about twenty years, ten of those doing home visits and you've been entertaining me the whole time with your humor and songs."

"I could not have done any of this without you," he responded.

"Your family has always believed I have been with you for your money but it's been really hard work. So many adults get stupid when they fight over kids and money. I admire how you work with them. You have saved so many kids from disaster and so many parents from being disastrous baggage for their kids. You know, when I took my course in mediation, the teacher – a young woman, swung around the doorway into the room and introduced herself by saying, 'If I can ever negotiate successfully with my own daughter, I'll have it made.' It's kind of like that with us."

"Yes. At lunch on Sunday, my sons told me that instead of leaving them, I should have wrestled the other guy to the ground."

"Really? My God! After all these years! Don't they know you don't fight that way? And their mother would probably have just done what she wanted to do anyway."

"They don't get it."

"Unfortunately, sometimes people only get it by personal experience."

"Daisy, I have to be at the Longhouse early this Sunday to keep the fire."

"Yes. You've been doing that for years now."

"I find peace there. That is where I experience complete acceptance of me no matter what. I wish you would come with me to the sweats."

"I know. I don't like sweating. I'm glad that you have the Longhouse to go to. You have become a respected elder there."

"Will you at least join with me for the feast after the sweat on Sunday?"

When Ken was busy at the Longhouse, Daisy usually used the time to do other things after a week of work. This time she felt the urgency of his request. "Okay. I'll be there. Gee, I still haven't helped you to make your drumming stick."

"I know."

"I hate to make excuses but we are always so busy trying to keep up with working long hours and all the family needs. If I'm not babysitting, you are busy with your sons. I can hardly wait until you can retire and we have time for *us*."

FOR SEVERAL YEARS Ken had been involved with the people at the UBC House of Learning Longhouse. The tall golden-brown wooden walls that housed large guardian totem poles carved to tell stories and held up the roof in the great hall with the circle design in the middle of the floor, had been a place of comfort. Ken's relationship with the people of the Longhouse grew while he became involved with their projects, sitting on a health committee and working on curriculum development, besides being a fire keeper.

When the newly built Longhouse had first opened, Ken and Daisy had brought grandchildren to the opening ceremony. On that first visit, they were aware of peace that was permeated into the building, in the walls with sunlight through the windows casting soft light on the totem poles. Peace came from and was soaked up from the building by the people. And in turn, people gave peace and respect to the building. Long tables laden with cold sandwich makings and cakes were lined up in the great room – a sign of the continuous food sharing to come. The children enjoyed the cakes with fluffy white icing that melted across their tongues.

Following the opening, initially embraced and invited in by an aboriginal woman who for a time became Ken's teacher and advisor, he had now become an integral person to people of the long house.

The Longhouse had become Ken's temple, a place to pray and heal, and meet with people. The Longhouse and its people had accepted Ken's giving back with no questions asked. The Longhouse had been the place that gave him strength to continue to live regardless of his unresolved illness and to get past the humiliations by the people who had done their utmost to ruin him. With prayer and acceptance under the protection of the Longhouse, he had the stamina and resilience to continue working to carry on with his duty to his sons as financier, father and teacher.

As Daisy had watched, she thought over and over that if Ken's sons did not follow in his footsteps and learn from him, the very least they would realize is that he was a man of persistence – a man who did not give in to the illness that nearly killed him several times, nor to the destructive people who tried to get rid of him or kill him... whichever came first. Instead, he was alive for his sons and for the children of his adopted family. Genes ran through his body from the inherited intelligence of the minds of the brave men and women who crossed an ocean on the Mayflower – a family that over many years and much resilience bore descendents that helped to build America.

During the past years, Daisy had been at Ken's side to many of the Long House functions and celebrations. He had chosen the Longhouse in which to defend and gain his Master of Arts Degree in Education. Daisy had been invited to videotape an important health meeting of people from around the province. Many people of the Longhouse had been calling Ken "Grandpa".

In keeping with his promise, Ken would not speak about what went on by the fires, at the sweats, in the lodges, or in confidential meetings among the men. Instead, he would invite people to participate and find out for themselves.

Daisy had watched as gradually Ken had been called on to say prayers as an elder before food was served. He had been honored and thanked several times with blankets and gifts. This was where he found peace of soul regardless of what was going on in his life.

Three days ahead of each sweat, he would prepare by cleansing physically, emotionally, and mentally. At family gatherings, he would refuse even a drop of alcoholic wine with a meal in keeping with the need to be free of anything that was considered a contaminate. It did not matter that no one would know; he would know and as always, Ken was truth.

AS PROMISED, following the sweat on Sunday morning Daisy and Ken sat together among the many people. The potluck brunch was finished and cleared away. A ceremony to show appreciation for several people was underway. Several Pendleton Indian Blankets had been given out and the recipients were wearing them. The last blanket was about to be handed out. The Master of Ceremonies, a scholarly woman who was also the administrator of the Longhouse, called, "Ken."

Ken was surprised. He slowly rose from his chair and walked toward the woman. She held a large flat box. As he approached, she opened it and said, "Ken, this robe is our thanks for all you have given us."

A large, bright, Robin's egg blue wool Pendleton blanket, with many other colors woven into the design, was taken out of the box and draped around Ken's shoulders.

When Ken came back to Daisy, she noticed a tag on one edge. She took it into her hand and read: *GREAT SPIRIT ROBE.*

As Ken took his seat, she whispered, "It's called a Great Spirit Robe. This robe is special... a great honor."

Sunday, April 29th, 2001. Ken wrote in his appointment book: *Sweat – robe; 1st bike trip to Longhouse; Daisy came to potluck!!*

IT WAS A MID-SUMMER afternoon celebration of young boys graduating the summer science class with aboriginal elders. Inside the UBC House of Learning Longhouse several men and young boys circled a drum measuring many feet across. They beat in unison and the sound echoed off the walls, filling the space in an unending circle of sound that lifted the heart to beat along with the waves of sound. Ken and Daisy stood in another circle of people surrounding the drummers.

A young non-aboriginal mother of a twelve-year old half aboriginal drummer-boy stepped toward Ken to touch his hand.

"I want to thank you for all you have done. My son would never have come here and graduated this summer class if you hadn't arranged it. He might have been lost to the streets. I am so grateful."

Ken's gentle smile washed over her in the power of circling sound.

The boys of this family had been told in school they could not possibly exist because all Mayans had been extinct for many years. Here, among these people, they were experiencing total acceptance of who they are. The children had taken their time to get to know and accept Ken's help until they gained complete trust, never missing a session with him.

...And so it was... that Ken and Daisy worked together for almost a quarter of a century, more than ten of those years making house calls... to help families like this one.

LIFE WITH KEN revolved around sharing food. Bringing food to his patients, especially those who were struggling to survive or were in need of sharing teatime with another human being was always important. On the way to many a home, it was necessary to stop and buy something to go along with tea. Ken found pleasure in every excuse to have a food celebration – birthdays, births, Christmas, Easter, graduations and trying to keep Sunday dinners alive with family.

Daisy lost track long ago of how many people rebuilt their lives after meeting with Ken. Some went back to school. Some rebuilt relationships with others and with themselves. Many had changes in their health for the better and some learned to accept changes in life. Children, who had been clients, grew and started their own families and as adults, many remembered Ken. Over the many years, only a handful of clients quit when they hit a bump in the road.

The 'thank you' letters arrived continuously from doctors and grateful clients of all walks of life and were kept in a secret personal file to protect the sender because of confidentiality.

All eight of Ken and Daisy's own children had become adults, giving many grandchildren by now. Five of the fourteen grandchildren were alive and healthy because Ken intervened in their medical care to correct medical mistakes.

Ken could be found on the UBC campus wearing his red jacket and backpack full of books on his back, always ready to be engaged in conversation. He searched out any teacher who would give him the time of day for a conversation. He could be found in the libraries not only in his own quest for knowledge but constantly remembering and searching for what other students, teachers, clients, or family might need in their latest projects. He carried away the load of books and distributed them to whomever. He had no superiority complex. He was totally humble wherever he went.

DAISY WROTE in her journal:

Surrounded by troubles, Ken always keeps his integrity solid. His Hippocratic Oath is his way of life. The people who gave him the 'Great Spirit Robe' are people who recognize Ken for who he truly is.

I am eternally grateful to Ken. He has shown us what it means to be a selfless man of healing… a man with a calling. I feel that I have been in the presence of someone truly too good for this world, someone who had come to heal and to teach. History has not been kind to men who draw attention to themselves by choosing to be different. Throughout history such men have been persecuted.

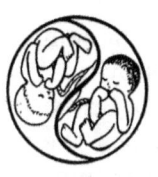

part three

49

Provincial Audit Starts

ON THE WAY to a client's home, a male voice boomed the headline of the noon news over the car radio waves that after a lengthy court case, today a British Columbia physician lost his license to practice medicine in the province of British Columbia because he had been treating thyroid problems with an unconventional medicine. The voice stated that the patients he had been treating were reporting they were being helped and doing very well in situations where the currently approved pharmaceutical drug had previously failed to help. An official spokesman from the British Columbia College of Physicians and Surgeons spoke next. He was a physician turned administrator in one of the top positions at the College, explaining to the public that he did not care about the outcome, he only cared about the method of treatment and the physician who treated his patients with an unapproved method should lose his license.

Daisy was appalled. "If I hadn't heard that stupid man with my own ears, I would not believe it."

Ken was not surprised. "He speaks for the old guard."

"Not to care about the outcome? That's a scandalous attitude for physician."

"Daisy, he *is* the old guard."

The news of a physician losing his license for making his patients well made an indelible impression on Daisy and increased Ken's concern that his time will be coming.

For Daisy, the reality of a system with old men like that College administrator guarding the gates, gave real insight into Ken's complaints about having to be licensed by this system in order to do his work.

What Ken and Daisy did not realize is that this was a prelude to their troubles with the system. It came swiftly.

AFTER FOUR YEARS at Queens University, Ken's youngest son graduated. The news was that Jane attended the graduation.

Andy had little contact with Ken over the four years. It was sad for Daisy to watch. In her critical mind, Ken had helped Andy and Jane gain their university educations and they should have been grateful and thankful. She knew that Ken had to work to pay his way through college and medical school but still found time to be a working volunteer for helping others less fortunate.

Ken was excited with hope that his son, now a full fledged adult in his early twenties, would now give Ken the time of day for the long dreamed of intellectual talks.

Daisy could hardly contain her excitement. Finally the last payment to Jane had been made. Daisy could not imagine what Jane would do with herself because there was no longer any leverage to make more legal trouble for Ken. It was over! **Over!**

After years of trouble and waiting for this moment, Daisy announced with certainty this time, "The worst that can happen now is that you have to attend the same wedding as Jane and perhaps share a grandchild. But she cannot hurt you any more. We are free! Ken, you can retire now!"

IT WAS MIDSUMMER in the year of 2001 – Daisy's birthday. Ken was reluctant to give bad news. He was clearly upset, wanting to protect her feelings by his preamble of asking her to sit down. Stubborn, as usual, she was not in the habit of fainting and refused to sit.

He told her, "I have just received a phone call from the Medical Services Commission. They plan to audit me."

A rush of panic was quickly set aside as Daisy wanted to brush it off and reassure Ken. "That's no big deal. So they audit us! All the billings are correct and in order. They just informed you by phone? Not by letter?"

"Just a phone call. I have not received a letter."

Reassurance was short lived as Daisy complained, "Just when we finished paying for Andy. Darn! I was hoping you could relax and maybe retire now. We go from one problem right into another."

Just then Ken's cell phone rang. Anton Glegg of Medical Services Commission was on the other end of the phone again. "We will be in your office tomorrow morning."

Ken responded, "No you won't. I don't have a walk-in physician's office. I work in clients' homes."

Glegg's voice was loud enough for Daisy to hear. "Then we will send a courier to pick up the records."

"I won't release my patient records to just anyone. My patients have been promised confidentiality."

"If you don't release the records immediately, we will get a court order to search for the records and obtain them by force."

"I will have to consult a lawyer." Ken hung up the phone and clutched his chest. He was having a hard time breathing, his face showing physical pain.

"Ken, are you having a heart attack?"

"I'll be all right. Don't call 911. I don't want their procedures. If you saw what they do..."

Daisy had always understood Ken's adamant request that if it came to life and death, he would choose to die rather than undergo procedures to prolong a crippled life. Most of all, he had been afraid his mind would be dulled by drugs. He had seen too much by being a doctor and would have none of that. She understood that he had no trust that the medical system would treat him with dignity, and these phone calls from the Medical Service Commission seemed to justify Ken's position.

"This puts me in a bind. I want you to live."

"I've been a physician for fifty years, I know what they do. I need to trust you." This was a repeated conversation of long ago.

Ken answered another persistent ring to hear, "This is Anton Glegg. We want all six years of your medical records."

Still in pain but not willing to give in, Ken answered, "This is harassment. I have told you I will consult a lawyer. Send your request in writing. We do not know what you are looking for and we have no understanding of a reason for the audit."

Anton Glegg said, "I will send you a letter."

WAITING FOR SOMETHING in writing about the audit, a couple of days passed but nothing arrived. There was no proof of the caller's identity and no proof of where the medical files would go even if they were released.

Ken and Daisy approached the home of clients and reverently passed by the family cat's new grave in the front yard. Fresh flowers marked the spot under a large cedar tree. As they climbed worn, wooden steps leading to the front door, Ken's cellular phone rang.

Anton Glegg was asserting power again. "We are preparing to search your office for the medical records. What is the address?"

Ken responded, "You have not yet made clear what you are looking for. I am about to see patients in their home."

"We want to browse. Where are the records?"

"I have not yet refused you the records but you will hear from my lawyer first. My patients are entitled to confidentiality. I have not received your letter with your demands as to what you want. This is harassment!"

Clutching his chest, coughing and gasping for breath as the door opened, Ken hung up on Glegg.

The client was a young mother raising children as a single parent. This family had recently had several extremely difficult hurdles to deal with. There was an accident. She had rear-ended a flatbed truck. Her nose had been severed off and hung to the side of her face. Her youngest child, being aged seven was old enough to understand what he was seeing but young enough to be helpless, strapped in the back seat of a car watching his parent bleeding with her nose cut off, leaving a gaping hole where it should have been. He had sat by himself in the waiting room at the hospital while his mother was operated on to sew her nose on. Just days before the accident, the woman's mother had died after months of suffering with cancer, and they were trying to cope with her loss. Also, a close family member suddenly decided he was really a woman and was preparing to have a sex change and was openly dressing as a woman. Physicians condoned the sex change without once consulting with his family. The children had been coping with multiple sudden changes while their mother fought depression over the death of her mother and the scar on her once perfectly symmetrical beautiful face.

Just days ago, this client was forced to travel hundreds of miles to the place of the accident to face a Judge. This single parent was sentenced to many hours of community service to make restitution to society even though no other person had been hurt, nor had the heavy flatbed she hit from behind been damaged. In her sentence, the Judge unwittingly punished the children. As a result, the mother was forced to leave her young children in the care of her teenage daughter several times a week because she had no ability to pay for childcare while she worked for free in the community. Meanwhile, the plan to get off welfare had to be put on hold. Poverty continued.

The mother, wanting to remain clear-headed through the intensity of crisis that was piled one on top of the other, refused psychotropic drugs to help her cope. This refusal stymied several physicians about knowing how to treat her. One physician finally figured out that the family should be referred to Ken because he would be the psychiatrist who would know how to help without the aid of drugs.

[This family will be included in the audit. Ken will be asked to "justify" why he is seeing members of this family even though court records, hospital and medical records for serious matters are already in the British Columbia government system.]

As the door opened, the astute woman immediately saw Ken in distress. "What's wrong?"

Ken answered through fighting for air, "The government auditors want to browse my medical records on patients. They just called me while I was coming up the stairs."

The woman was surprised. "What do they want?"

Daisy answered, "We don't know yet. They haven't answered that question. They just keep insisting that we hand over our patient records. We don't even know who will be looking at them."

Ken assured her, "I won't let them have records containing confidential information."

"Come on in." Once inside, she offered, "I will go to bat for you. I will talk with them."

"I can't let you do that. I promised all my clients confidentiality. I took an oath – the Hippocratic Oath, that I would keep my patients' secrets. I won't let you or any patient defend me by letting yourself be questioned by the government."

Ken's chest pain was scaring Daisy.

Sympathy was written all over this woman. "Well, if you need my help, I will be glad to do anything for you, even talk to the government."

Daisy was amazed that this woman, who already has so much to deal with, was willing to put herself out for Ken.

Ken and Daisy always looked forward to meeting with this family. The family was extremely poor, living in a house so dilapidated that when it rained, water ran through the ceiling and poured down on the children's beds, but they were generous. At each meeting, tea was served. It was not just tea in a teapot; tea was served in the old English manner with fine china collected from years before and some recently inherited from the deceased grandmother. Tea was a ritual, poured with delicate finesse. If the family had any cookies, they were also served. On occasion, there would be a pot of exquisitely seasoned chicken soup on the stove, which they always offered to share. Ken's face always relaxed into a sugarplum, as he tasted the first spoonful.

Ken returned the generosity; often he brought cookies, muffins, or a fruit bread to be served with tea. On birthdays, he brought a box of assorted specialties from the bakery. He delighted in seeing the children's expressions when the box was opened.

When Daisy questioned taking the time to shop for loaves of bread to take to various clients' homes, Ken responded that breaking bread and sharing food with clients was really a ritual of sharing and being thankful, and that it was important.

In the beginning, the children in this family had checked out the visiting doctor and his assistant by roller skating in and out of the house with their friends – running in briefly to say hi, then out again – running in briefly to ask questions, then out. Then they graduated to sitting to have a small talk while having tea. Before long they were asking for help to solve problems at home and at school.

On this visit, the woman set out flowered teacups. Ken relaxed into the warmth of the meeting, feeling much better doing what he did best. With taped classical piano played by her father in the background, the woman discussed her personal concerns before the children arrived home from school.

With Ken's help, she talked about hopes and dreams. She was ready to look forward and make plans. She made the decision to go back to school to study a long time interest. She had never thought she could do it but with Ken's help she saw that she could follow her dream and change the future of her family. Her focus changed from the scar on her face to the excitement of her future.

As children arrived, the quiet of the past hour gave way to activity.

"Hi, Ken. Hi, Daisy." The sweet, lilting voice of the teenaged daughter was heard through the door before the girls actually appeared. She had brought a friend. "This is my friend, Shauna. She wants to meet you. We have decided her parents need counselling."

Following greetings, Daisy explained, "If your parents want to meet with Ken, just tell them that they can call me. All appointments are made by referral from another physician, usually the family physician. I'll explain the referral system to your parents."

Shauna was pleased, "I'll do that."

Both girls twirled to show off their costumes, explaining that they had gotten dressed at Shauna's house because they were going to a teenage dance.

"I love your hats. You both look gorgeous." Daisy complimented them.

The girls explained that they were dressing like Selena, the popular singer.

After dancing around the room, showing all sides of themselves, they settled down to have tea.

Boys arrived from school, dropping their bags on the hallway floor as they kick off shoes and kept on walking in, "Hi, Ken. Hi, Daisy." Somehow they manage to say that in unison.

"Hi." Daisy and Ken also managed unison.

The older boy's face was full of expectation as he asked, "Ken, Daisy, I want you to come here for my birthday on the weekend."

Ken answered, "Yes, of course, we'll come. Thank you."

The younger boy launched into a problem he was having at school and could not handle by himself. After a discussion, Ken suggested an immediate telephone call to the school, before staff left for the day, to set up a meeting that he and Daisy were willing to attend along with the boy and his mother.

The mother called and an appointment to meet with the schoolteacher, school counsellor and principal was set. She was relieved to be able to share the responsibility.

School appointments were a norm in the practice. In this manner, serious matters were discussed, resulting in corrective plans and actions set in motion, relieving students of their anxieties.

LOOKING FOR A LAWYER to handle the audit turned out to be more difficult than expected. The lawyer Ken had known was unable to take on the case because of 'conflict of interest'.

A referral to a couple of lawyers who had already handled audit cases on behalf of physicians brought a new revelation. The game discovered was that these lawyers, who exuded supremacy, were only willing to take on a case if the physician had been keeping their medical practice insurance up to date. Ken had not. He had not been able to afford the high cost of it since he had been ill, bankrupt, and then paying for Andy. For that reason, the insurance he had always carried in previous years had been dropped and not picked up again.

On advice given, Ken called the medical insurance company to find out if his old insurance would cover any of the six years being audited. He spoke with a female physician who was spokesperson for the company. She told him there had been too long an interval by one year; therefore no part of the audit would be covered.

One of the lawyers also contacted the insurance office and reported to Ken that the same woman told him sarcastically, "He thinks his patients love him so much that he does not need insurance." The lawyer assured Ken that the woman had absolutely no sympathy for a physician who does not keep up his medical practice insurance.

There followed the discovery that this particular law firm had worked on other audit cases and had a record of making settlements instead of fighting to actually prove innocence of charges. Because the insurance company would pay regardless of the outcome, the lawyers got paid a sum of money for handling the case – the government got a roll-back of earnings on behalf of the physicians, usually for many years of services – the physicians were allowed to continue practicing medicine for going along with the game while paying the government the roll-back in increments out of future earning. Thus, the circle was completed.

Ken was learning more about the tyranny of these audits.

Ken was so incensed by this information that he did not want the help of the insurance company even if he did qualify for it. He would never agree he did wrong when he believed he did nothing wrong.

Eventually another lawyer in a well-respected firm agreed to talk about the case with Ken. Mr. Wood listened and appeared to be understanding and sympathetic, though cautious about the whole matter. He questioned Daisy every chance he got behind Ken's back as to honesty, trying to find a chink somewhere in the matter, especially in Ken. He mostly wanted to know if there ever was a cheat, even a minor cheat in their medical billings. Ken and Daisy were consistent. Daisy was adamant that the billings always had been correctly done and in fact, they worked many more hours that were not billed for.

She also pointed out that it seemed odd for the government to suddenly want to audit billings for six years when the government had always and continued in present to point out any errors at the time of each billing which was twice a month, and refused to pay until any errors in billings were corrected, or questions about necessity of service were answered, or a missing referral was made. As Daisy explained, there was a long list of computer codes that spit out any questionable billings and no payment was made until all information was corrected, physician referrals received, or a letter of explanation written for additional hours of treatment in one week.

Daisy pointed out that if Ken had done the billings, they would mostly not get done; money had never been Ken's motive for seeing patients and he would rather work for free or on salary.

Though cautious, Henry agreed to take on the case.

NO MATTER WHAT Ken's troubles were, he always was concerned about his fellow man. Walking in the rain in front of a grocery store where Thomas, a young street person sat by the curb, Ken stopped to talk with him as usual, "Hello, Thomas."

Seeing his friend, Thomas's eyes lit up. "Hi. Wish I had a rain jacket like yours."

This was all Ken needed to hear. Instead of shopping for groceries, he and Daisy made a dash across the city to a co-operative outdoor equipment store. After much deliberation, they chose a jacket and headed back to Thomas.

Thomas was sitting where they had left him. Ken handed Thomas a red jacket. "This is for you."

Thomas was thoroughly surprised. He stood up and carefully put the jacket on.

"It even fits! Thanks."

As they walk away, Daisy said, "I hope Thomas appreciates what you have just done."

"He will be warm and dry, that's what matters. I'm not looking for appreciation."

As Daisy rushed past people to get to the grocery store bathroom, she mused, so typical! His own life is in jeopardy. His finances could be wiped out again and he is looking after homeless people. But she loved him the way he was.

OCTOBER 21, 2001. KEN WROTE A LETTER requesting a personal meeting with Bill Edwards, Director of Billing Integrity Program in the British Columbia Government.

"I am requesting an informal meeting with Bill Edwards to negotiate ways I can continue providing family home care services to extended families with multiple health problems, while meeting MSP requirements for accountability in home visit psychotherapy. In my professional opinion, **all** my billings to MSP during the past 25 years since I began my family psychiatric practice in 1976 have been accurate, medically necessary office, hospital, or home visits for psychotherapy, based upon the judgments of the family physicians who referred to me patients who decided how often they needed to meet with me, as well as my own judgments as to my abilities to help them cope with the health problems. Those who did not wish to continue were referred.

"Until I was notified that an audit of my practice would be done in October, 2001, I believed that every insured patient in B.C. is entitled to one hour per day of psychotherapy to help them find healthier ways of living than doing violence to themselves, their friends or family; and by taking harmful prescription or non-prescription drugs. My family psychiatric practice has always been 7 days a week, 24 hours a day, on call for families referred to me. I have needed no holidays and I have taken care of my health in ways that have helped me learn to care for others in less harmful ways than I was taught in my postgraduate medical education.

"When I worked in a hospital, clinic, or other sessional program, I kept the same kind of medical records as my peers, except that I always emphasized the need to recognize and respond to health problems defined by the family, and family physician, rather than by DSM or by their responses to pharmaceuticals. When I assisted Dr. Don Coates at Riverview Hospital Outpatient Clinic in developing the Community Care Teams, I argued with Dr. John Cumming that physicians working in these teams should be family doctors to this psychiatric population. My argument was based upon my experience that my psychiatric patients, who wanted to reduce their dependency on psychoactive drugs, responded well to Dr. Hoffer's recommended orthomolecular regime for hypoglycemia. Blood tests on a dozen of my patients all showed clinical hypoglycemia until Riverview Hospital decided to change their *acceptable levels of blood glucose to exclude those measured in my patients.*

"When I was unable to continue working in community medicine because of cutbacks, I began my private psychiatric practice and continued to work like a family physician to assist family members to take responsibility for the care of families and themselves from birth to death. For the past ten years I have worked with families in their homes or at hospitals when needed. I have not billed for more than one hour per day per person of psychotherapy (The one exception to this was for [client name], whose case was discussed by telephone and letter with MSP, December 3, 1997) despite the fact that I have often attended families for more than one hour per person daily in order to help them care for a sick, pregnant, or dying relative; and prevented hospitalization or drug dependence by helping families make their own support networks of friends and families.

"During these years I have developed a modified problem oriented medical record system based on what I learned working with Dr. Larry Weed, and with Dr. Don Coates whose expertise is the study of stressful life events as predictors and correlates of illness, accident, and hospitalization. My research is summarized in the description of my practice I provide to family physicians and prospective client families which you already have. My MA thesis in education presents my research in the ethics of case making and record keeping as intersubjective violence. In my MA thesis, and my Ph.D. research, I offer an alternative extended family narrative form for doing family work in home visits. The recording of peoples' lives involves issues of confidentiality and accountability based on a personal or professional need to know. I have been able to offer home visit psychotherapy to under-served aboriginal, immigrant, pregnant, and single parent families, as well as lawyers, social workers, health care workers, psychologists, teachers, family and child care workers, only because I could promise them confidentiality. These people would not allow me to attend them in their homes if I did what I have seen and heard other physicians and psychiatrists do: write down everything the person says; use psychiatric, psychological or new age jargon to describe their lives; and insist they take medication prescribed for them without their full knowledge or

consent to accept the side effects of these medications. Because all families I see are referred by family physicians who have already diagnosed and discussed their multiple health problems, and they are willing to take responsibility for the health of their families and themselves, there is no medical need for detailed records about our conversations to help them plan how they will continue to care for family members at home or in hospital. There are no physicians or people who need to see these records because there are no locums or other physicians who cover my practice, nor will my practice ever be sold. Lawyers and others who need access to relevant medical information about these families can get the records or information directly from them. All my home visit psychotherapy is based in conversation leading to making plans to improve their health. No drugs are prescribed which would require documentation.

To continue my practice requires ground rules for accountability to MSP, which we used to negotiate verbally, to be negotiated and written down now."

Sincerely,

[signed] Kehnroth Schramm, M.D.

* * *

THE WRITTEN REQUEST for a meeting with Bill Edwards RECEIVED NO RESPONSE. Ken had believed he was dealing with real people who were willing to negotiate and solve problems in good faith. He was unaware at this time of a hidden agenda.

* * *

The **College of Physicians and Surgeons Spring 2000 Issue 28 College Quarterly** published by the Council of the College of Physicians and Surgeons of British Columbia, printed the following article and distributed it to registered physicians in British Columbia.

"**Maintenance of Confidentiality of Patients' Medical Records**".

Maintenance of confidentiality of patients' medical records has become a topic of increasing concern and discussion. The introduction and increasing use of electronic records, e-mail, faxes, and similar technology, frequently challenge the time

honoured concept that physicians are expected to protect the patient's privacy. Similarly, the introduction of multi-disciplinary practices, community health clinics, salaried or sessional payments to physicians, and a 'team' approach to healthcare, make it more difficult for physicians to assure their patients that their charts and records are in safe custody.

Physicians' ethical responsibilities are best exemplified by Article 22 of the CMA Code of Ethics.

"Respect the patient's right to confidentiality except when this right conflicts with your responsibility to the law, or when the maintenance of confidentiality would result in significant risk of substantial harm to others or to the patient if the patient is incompetent, in such cases, take all reasonable steps to inform the patient that confidentiality will be breached."

The previous CMA Code of Ethics stated more succinctly in Principle IV and Article 6.

- "protect the patient's secrets"
- "Will keep in confidence information derived from a patient or from a colleague regarding a patient, and divulge it only with the permission of the patient except when otherwise required by law."

This ethical principle is also dealt with in significant detail in the CMA Privacy Code, in Freedom of Information & Protection of Privacy Legislation, and in the Privacy Code for physicians' offices in BC.

It is clear from the above that physicians carry the ultimate responsibility for taking any steps necessary to maintain the confidentiality of medical information they possess on their patients.

... It must be emphasized therefore that records created by a physician, about a patient, are confidential and without the patient's explicit written consent are not accessible to anyone except the physician, those to whom he or she has delegated the responsibility, and those physicians co-involved in the patient's care. Patients who provide confidential information to a physician should not be put in the position where other healthcare providers have access to that information without their knowledge or consent. Similarly, governing councils, employers, or health administrators may have the responsibility to provide custody for the health record, but do not have the right to access such information. For example, hospital boards have always assumed the responsibility for establishing medical record departments, which provide regulation and custody of health records. However, a member of such a hospital board has no right to access an individual patient's record. Similarly, the other healthcare providers or physicians who are on hospital staff, would be challenged if they sought or gained access to the record of a patient they had no professional involvement with, unless such access was part of quality improvement or audit requirements.

In a multi-disciplinary practice setting, patients must be provided with the assurance that the confidential material they provide to their physician is protected, and that access to that information by other individuals who happen to occupy the same facility is prohibited, or at least limited to a "need-to-know" basis in special circumstances such as complaints or legal challenges.

While there are many valid arguments for effective communication between healthcare providers, and for sharing of significant information without wasteful duplication, the patient's right to privacy must be recognized and respected.

In summary, physicians have been instructed on many occasions that they have a primary responsibility to protect the patient's health record and medical information, and that they have to assume the role of patient advocate when unwarranted or unauthorized access to that record is sought by other healthcare providers or individuals. This is an ethical requirement in all circumstances. It is especially pertinent in smaller communities where members of the Community Health Councils, hospital employees and other healthcare professionals may have significant social interaction in addition to the provision of professional services and professional interaction.

Cut this out or copy it for your Policy Manual

This bulletin is forwarded to every practitioner registered with the College. Decisions of the College on matters of standards, policies and guidelines are published in this bulletin. The College therefore assumes that each practitioner is aware of these matters.

50

The Audit

KEN WAS ADAMANT that no matter the cost to himself, he would not release any patients' secrets or information of a confidential nature to the government.

In preparation for the audit, Ken and Daisy purged all the files of any information that may be considered secret or confidential by the patient. In purging the files, it was with knowledge that when taking patient medical histories, a lot of information is through second-hand knowledge or interpretations of a person whether young or old; any over-zealous government employee could patch together birth records to pinpoint a parent or a child to a questionable comment mentioned in the history. And since Ken did not prescribe allopathic medicine, it was with deliberateness that no history containing second-hand information about medications should come from Ken's files, but auditors should get that kind of information directly from the prescribing doctor.

The day before the audit was to happen, Ken and Daisy loaded a wheeled cart high with several cardboard filing boxes holding medical records and made their way from the street into an elevator and up into their lawyer's board room in the glass tower. They placed the neatly labeled boxes on top of the giant, glossy, brown table.

In anticipation of the next morning when the auditors would arrive, Mr. Wood was relieved that the files arrived ahead of them. The agreement with him was that he would oversee the audit without the need for Ken or Daisy to be present.

Daisy informed him, "Here are six years of medical records, all the billings to the Medical Services Plan complete for six years and records of payments received for all twenty-five patients that are on the list for audit. All referrals written as they happened are clearly recorded on the front of each patient file folder.

Ken handed his lawyer a large, sealed, brown envelope and explained, "The confidential medical notes have been separated out of the files and are in this envelope. There is no information about what goes on in the privacy of their lives. In other words, no private conversation records are in any of these files or in this envelope. This confidential envelope is to go only to the auditing Psychiatrist, not to the laymen auditors under any circumstances."

Ken asked for reassurance, "Will you be here to oversee the audit?"

"Yes."

Leaving medical files in trusted hands, Ken and Daisy walked into the outside air hoping this would end the problem.

IN THE MORNING auditors arrived, having traveled from Victoria by seaplane that landed within viewing distance from the windows of the destined law office. Dr. Semrau, the psychiatrist who was hired by the government to audit Ken also arrived.

The three laymen auditors shuffled files in the boardroom, then demanded to see complete files on the patients.

When informed that confidential information was in a brown envelope and given to Dr. Semrau, the auditors responded with phone calls to the Attorney General's office in Victoria because they wanted confidential information made available to them.

MID-MORNING, Ken called Mr. Wood, "How is it going?"

Henry informed Ken that the laymen auditors had wanted to see the missing confidential information on all the patients. After two hours of telephone calls back and forth to the Attorney General's office in Victoria, it was finally decided that the laymen auditors were not entitled to confidential information on patients and were now getting on to the audit of what they had.

Ken asked, "Does Dr. Semrau have the brown envelope?"

Ken was assured he did.

THE AUDIT OF THE FILES was followed a few days later by a request by Anton Glegg to interview Daisy. She refused a private interview because she did not trust him after the way he had treated Ken. She feared he would misinterpret her interview unless she had a witness. Mr. Wood arranged the interview to take place in his office over a speakerphone.

Anton was in Victoria. Daisy was in Mr. Wood's boardroom in Vancouver. Mr. Wood was present to witness the complete conversation; he spoke first, "Anton, we have a speaker phone set up here. Go ahead."

Anton said, "Daisy, I understand you work with Dr. Schramm."

"Yes."

"How often are you with his patients?"

"We work in patient's homes. I am with Dr. Schramm all the time while he is working with patients."

"When he sees women, are you there all the time?"

"Yes." Red flags flew in Daisy's head. What a way to start the interview! She was now convinced that she had been right to have a witness; this man is up to no good, trying to come up with something by insinuation.

Anton asked, "He sees a lot of women. What do you do when women cry?"

"Ken is present and he handles the situation. That's a strange question! I act as a chaperone and assistant so that no one can ever accuse Ken of wrongdoing."

Now her shackles were up, believing Glegg was trying to entrap her and Ken. She thought – little does he know I am not the huggy type and the best I do is hand a paper napkin to a crying patient – nor do I take over from Ken when I know he has half a century of experience in handling patients' tears.

Anton continued, "I see. Is there any time that you are not accompanying Dr. Schramm?"

"If a man wants to discuss something with Dr. Schramm without the presence of a woman, I do not participate. That is very rare and I usually drop Ken off and pick him up. Most men accept my presence, not requiring privacy."

"What else do you do in the practice?"

"I do all the paper work, billings and referrals."

"What about the referrals? How are they done? There is one questionable referral."

"One?" Daisy was surprised at hearing a referral was out of order. "Tell me which one and I'll look into it."

"I can't tell you."

Daisy answered, "There shouldn't be any. I make sure all the referrals are made before we see the patients. I do follow-ups by calling directly to the referring doctors offices to be sure all referrals are good. Dr. Schramm is in regular contact with the referring doctors regarding the health of the patients and regarding any medications the doctor may have prescribed."

"How does he do that?" Anton asked, clearly dropping the question of referrals.

"Dr. Schramm talks with the doctors by telephone and he has been known to visit doctors with the patient on occasion when he was particularly concerned. Are there any billings out of order?"

Anton answered, "No, they all match up. Thank you."

The connection was finished.

Daisy was surprised at the whole conversation.

Mr. Wood had been completely quiet while listening intently.

She asked, "How did I do?"

"Good!"

"I think he was trying to make something, anything, of the women Ken sees. Also, he would not tell me which one referral is in question. That's strange since I think he's the head auditor."

Daisy left the office with the sound of Anton's voice ringing in her head. Niggling underneath Anton's voice was an extremely strong intuition that she had just encountered a man looking for an angle to fit his own agenda. That intuition would bear itself out sooner than expected.

DAISY OFTEN STARTED the day with a relaxing cup of coffee while watching a few minutes of morning television before launching into action. One morning soon after the audit, she felt lucky because she clicked into an interview with Stanley Semrau and seemed to have gotten in right at the start. Never having seen Dr. Stanley Semrau, the auditing psychiatrist, all she knew was that he practiced forensic psychiatry. She was surprised that he looked as young as he did regardless of his pure white hair and beard.

Daisy grabbed a pen and paper. Former years of secretarial work came in handy as she was able to keep up and get clear notes of the interview.

Semrau was asked by the interviewer to define his role. In his answer, he referred to himself as a psychiatrist homicide detective. He went on to say, "…I do in most cases read police reports, interview the killers, and understand what was going through their head when they killed somebody. Did they intend to do it? Were they psychotic? Were they doing it because they heard voices?"

The interviewer then said, "So then you act as, can I call you a professional witness? Is that a fair assessment?"

Semrau answered, "Yes."

Interviewer: "You go on the stand and basically deliver what you believe to be true as for the psyche. …"

SEMRAU WAS MAKING the rounds of television stations. On another morning Daisy came across another interview where Semrau bragged about how he gets the goods on people; about being self-taught to do what he does, and how he flies his own private plane to do his job.

Daisy imagined that his income for doing what he does must be extremely high to afford the costs of his private plane. But more than that, she became concerned that Ken would be expected to pay for his plane. She became angry that a man like Semrau had the gall to take money by making trouble for a man like Ken.

IN A BRITISH COLUMBIA **PHYSICIAN'S NEWSLETTER published by the Medical Services Plan for Medical Practitioners** in the **Spring of 1999,** it is written under the heading:

> **Audit, Documentation and Protocols**
> ... **In any case, a medical inspector, who is a practicing physician in the same specialty or area of interest as the audited physician, jointly nominated by the BCMA and the College of Physicians and Surgeons, will be asked to give a professional opinion. ...**

SEMRAU'S DESCRIPTION OF himself gave Daisy a clearer than ever understanding of why Ken was so adamant that Semrau should in no way be an auditor of the kind of work Ken did. Semrau, as a forensic psychiatrist and by his own admission, worked to get the goods on people and then report it. On the completely opposite side of the spectrum, Ken's work was in healing, helping and teaching. Ken was a physician living and remembering his Hippocratic Oath.

After listening to Semrau, Daisy also understood why psychiatrists in general were in extreme danger if they ever found themselves in prison where other prisoners may have had an encounter with a forensic psychiatrist like Semrau. It was clear why Ken had been so fearful of Jane trying to put him in jail.

Daisy told Ken, "It is a mistake that the same spaghetti follows after both your names because there is no way you and Semrau are in the same ballgame. You do different work – as different as night and day or dark and light."

KEN AND DAISY were having a restful couple of hours. They slowed down enough to enjoy each other quietly. Ken was lying on the day bed reading a book just inside the large glass patio doors that were open to the evening scents of the garden. Daisy was painting a picture at the round table by his feet. He occasionally paused reading to watch her and make a comment.

"I like it but I think it needs more red. Daisy, I really do want to marry you soon."

She turned to look at him. His face was soft as he reached for her hand.

She answered, "Yes. It's time for us. You've given more than twenty years over to your sons. It is time for us! Just us."

The privacy of the moment was interrupted as a strange woman made an abrupt and unannounced appearance at the private patio door and shoved a brown envelope at Daisy. The woman had come so quietly that it was as though she had snuck up to the door and then she quickly ran away.

Glancing at the contents of the envelope, Daisy exclaimed, "**It's a letter from Dr. Stanley Semrau Inc., Adult and Forensic Psychiatry, dated November 30th, 2001.** He also sent a copy of this letter to Anton Glegg, MSP Audit Section in Victoria. It has arrived for Christmas. I wonder why these people choose to send Christmas presents like this. **Semrau is asking for psychiatric labels for all your patients for every three months of all the six years audited! He also wants to know which patients *drink alcohol and who uses drugs – any kind of drugs!* He** wants **all the notes on all the visits with patients about what *was said in each and every visit, in detail!* He** wants you to ***justify every minute*** you spent with patients **for all six years!** He even **wants to know about the relatives of your patients!** In other words, he wants you to answer to things about patients even though you would have no way of verifying the information."

Calm and composed, Ken responded, "I will answer him. Psychiatric labels are black and white; there are no grays, no other color. I do not label patients with psychiatric labels. How can a person change if they are labeled? It boxes them in."

Daisy was outraged. "Justifying *every minute* or even every hour is impossible in Psychiatry. They can always say the time wasn't justified when they are looking for excuses. Justifying minutes when working with people about everything from birth to death is impossible! I mean, what if someone needs to twiddle their thumbs for an hour until they find a way to say what they need to say like those teenagers we saw recently. We can't know in advance what a person will say or do or even what their needs will be. Obviously Semrau doesn't understand that."

"That's most likely the truth," Ken said quietly.

Daisy paced in anger, walking in circles, flapping papers, "You have clients that are in high-profile professional positions. They would not like the government to have this kind of information on themselves or their families. They would never have sought help if they thought anyone would give the government this kind of information. I saw Semrau on television a second time where he bragged about being self-trained to... in his words, "get the goods on people". It's guys like him who give psychiatrists a bad name."

Ken said, "We need to challenge them again on confidentiality and the fact that there are no written rules on what are appropriate medical records for psychiatrists doing psychotherapy. I do not write secrets down because once written they can be stolen or subpoenaed to court. What they want is for a psychiatrist to drug patients and send them away for another month. I don't fit the mold. I never have."

This letter encouraged Daisy's outrage that Semrau bragged about himself on television as self-trained to "get the goods on people", and used his credentials as a physician to go after physicians like Ken. She felt outraged that Semrau, on behalf of government, would want to erode the human rights of privacy promised to patients in this country. She felt outraged that Semrau made enough money doing that kind of work to afford his own private plane to fly to and from appointments in order to carry out his work. She felt outraged that Semrau used his medical training status for his own benefit but seemed to have forgotten his Hippocratic Oath to do no harm. She felt complete outrage... and then paused to realize that it would be better to help Ken instead of spreading negative energy because of Semrau.

It was immediately apparent that this stress was already having an effect on Ken. Though he outwardly looked quiet, Daisy could see that the peace of the moment had shifted, disappeared, as they entered yet another debate.

IN PREPARATION OF answering, Ken went over Semrau's written questions.

Semrau wrote:

...To be more specific, I will require the following information for each of the 25 patients:

1. History of the present illness/complaint that gave rise to the referral and need for treatment.

2. Symptoms experienced by the patient, utilizing conventional psychiatric terminology, eg. as utilized in the Glossary of the American Psychiatric Association.

3. Functional deficits experienced by the patient in all important areas of functioning, eg. work, studies, relationships, parenting, recreation, self-care.

4. Childhood and adult personal history including description of family of origin, marital/relationship history, education, employment, etc.

5. Past psychiatric history of the patient, including details of past treatment and response.

6. Substance use/abuse history.

7. History of significant somatic illness and injury.

8. Medications, psychiatric and non-psychiatric.

9. Mental status examination results, utilizing conventional psychiatric terminology, eg. as utilized in the Glossary of the American Psychiatric Association.

10. Diagnosis, utilizing all five axes of the DSM4 classification.

11. Formulation of the biological, psychological and social/circumstantial factors affecting the patient.

12. Detailed treatment plan including biological, psychological and social interventions and in the case of psychotherapy a detailed description of the particular type(s) of psychotherapy to be utilized and required duration and frequency of therapy.

13. An explanation of the medical indication and need for the particular treatment(s) to be employed and their particular choice relative to alternative treatments.

14. Response to therapy including changes in symptoms and level of functioning, including DSM4 axis 5, Global Assessment of Functioning scale.

...The above-listed information will be required as it was current at the time of the Initial assessment phase of therapy. In addition, all of those above-listed types of information which are subject to change over time should be provided as of the date of completion or termination of therapy and where therapy extended longer than 4 months, at 3-month intervals during the course of therapy

... For patients with major mental illnesses such as severe depression or psychosis, do you prescribe psychotropic medication? If not, why not?
... [signed by Stanley Semrau, M.D.]

* * *

KEN RESPONDED to Semrau by letter dated January 18, 2002:

...You then request detailed information about my patients in the language of the American Psychiatric Association, i.e., DSM. In fact, I have provided you with "life stories" [McHugh 1998: Part V] similar to those I share with my patients and their family physicians orally and in writing, allowing each of them freedom to interpret these stories and to ask any questions they want because they need to know what I am thinking and doing with them. I expect that you might ask me about what I do with my patients in home visit psychotherapy because my practices are being audited, not those of my patients. To write about them without their permission is a violation of their right to privacy in their homes and in their personal lives; and a betrayal of the trust and respect they offered in sharing their homes and their life stories with me. Among aboriginal families I know, their life stories belong to specific people and can only be told within the requirements of protocols interpreted by authorized local elders. Acknowledging your authority to audit my practices to determine the medical necessity of the medical services I provided while respecting the cultural and family stories of my patients, I want to answer your inquiries about how I practice home care psychotherapy.

I understand that the primary reason for the audit is that my billing profile of practice differs significantly from the norm of psychiatrists practicing in B.C. Certainly I spend more time with each patient than the average because home visit medical psychotherapy must allow enough time for family members to plan self-care from birth to death at home. All my patients are referred and re-referred to me by physicians who have diagnosed their health problems and decided that they need psychotherapy. My family medical practice began in the fifties when DSM1 and psychiatric medication were introduced into medical practices. I learned to work with patients without and with psychiatric medication. Since I began family medical practice in B.C. thirty years ago, my practice has been devoted to the care of individuals and families who take responsibility for their health and their care of family members at home. I was family physician for eighty people, including a family providing in home palliative care to their mother with breast cancer, who were building the Coast Range Ranch on Lasqueti and Calvert Islands. My practice there challenged me to make full use of all my experiences in family medicine, pediatrics, psychiatry, and anthropology. In 2004 I will have been a family health counselor for fifty years since I was given responsibility as a medical student at the University of Vermont for home, clinic, and hospital care of a pregnant family under supervision of my clinical teachers during my four years of medical school. At that time, we provided home care for the families of Burlington, Vermont in our last two years of clinical work. Along with home and clinic visits, I was also a house parent for preteen children living in the Children's Village of Burlington. Please see my enclosed resume and a description of my home visit psychotherapy practice for a summary of my experiences integrating education and medical practice in my care of under-served aboriginal, immigrant, refugee, and single parent families caring for their members at home; and lawyers, physicians, teachers, social workers, and students who provide services for these families. Just as you are a specialist in Adult and Forensic Psychiatry, I am a specialist in family home care psychotherapy.

My pattern of practice has remained essentially the same since 1991 when I began an exclusively home visit psychotherapy practice with 32 patients in response to a need for home care which was then publicly discussed in the media and at U.B.C. The only change known to me is an increase in the fee for home visit psychotherapy which I believe is a factor in the judgment that my pattern of practice is deviant and expensive. M.S.P. includes home visits in the same fee item as hospital or inpatient psychotherapy which makes it impossible for anyone to analyze only home visit data in order to compare my practice with any other psychiatrist who is billing for home visits. As a Ph.D. candidate in education at U.B.C., I am in the unique position of researching my practice as a way to educate myself and others to make home visits in culturally respectful and sensitive ways. My M.A. thesis encourages writing of one's life as a case in order to understand the ethical practical difficulties involved in writing health records which survive the lives of those who have been recorded.

On the basis of my consultations with the Unified Family Courts of Richmond, Surrey and Delta, I can appreciate that in your specialty as an adult and forensic psychiatrist, you use DSM as your standard for evaluating your clinical records and psychiatrists who practice as you do. I am asking you to consider that those who do home visit psychotherapy exclusively have different practices than you do, perhaps because we were educated in different times and places. Teachers in my generation of medical psychotherapists include my younger colleague from S.U.N.Y. Upstate Medical centre, Peter Breggin, M.D., author of "Your Drug May Be Your Problem: How and Why To Stop Taking Psychiatric Medications" [1999]. Paul R. McHugh, M.D. has described a similar program to that of Upstate Medical Center in the Department of Psychiatry and Behavioral Sciences at Johns Hopkins University School of Medicine with Phillip R. Slavney, M.D., in "The Perspectives of Psychiatry," Johns Hopkins University Press, 1998, portraying the ways psychiatrists think and work. On September 4, 2001, Reuters Health reported: While the current edition of the Diagnostic and Statistical Manual of Mental Disorders (DSM) brought reliability into psychiatric diagnosis, it failed to address validity, according to Dr. Paul R. McHugh, chair of the Department of Psychiatry and Behavioral Sciences at Johns Hopkins University. Dr. McHugh proposes a new conceptual structure for the next edition of the DSM, due to be released in 2007. Rather than diagnose patients based on symptoms, as the DSM is used to do, he suggests that conditions be identified according to four "perspectives": the Disease, Dimensional, Behavior, and Life-Story perspectives. In psychotherapy, the Life-Story perspective includes the others. I agree with Dr. McHugh that DSM is not valid for psychotherapy, and the Life Story perspective is relevant for my family home visit psychotherapy practice. From that perspective I will answer your questions:

Responses to inquiries 1 – 14 on page 2:

...Within the requirements for patient confidentiality and accountability to M.S.P. for my part-time family home care psychotherapy practice described in my information for referring physicians, I believe the information I have provided meets all written requirements for adequacy when read, and then reviewed with me, by a practitioner who does home visit medical psychotherapy. The complexity of defining, teaching, applying, or judging "standards and guidelines for the psychotherapies" is presented in the book by that title edited by Paul Cameron, M.D., Jon Ennis, M.D., and John Deadman, M.D. and published by University of Toronto Press, 1998. In Chapter 2, "General Guidelines for the Practice of Psychotherapy," contributors Ray Freebury, Jon Ennis, Carolyn Rideout, and Martha Wright discuss 'assessment of competence': "It is essential in all instances, that assessors be fully conversant with and trained in the modality of psychotherapy practiced by the clinician who is undergoing evaluation" (page 39). The modalities of psychotherapy I practice have emerged over a lifetime of premedical, medical, and postgraduate medical education in philosophy, family medicine, pediatrics, psychiatry, cultural anthropology, family therapy, hypnotherapy, history of science and medicine, community planning, and education, providing languages other than that of the American Psychiatric Association in the Diagnostic and Statistical Manual of Mental Disorders (DSM). After almost fifty years of home visit medicine, I find patients and physicians understand each other and make needed changes through our conversations when patient confidentiality is respected. At U.B.C., the importance of ownership of our stories for aboriginal health and family practice is recognized. My family home visit psychotherapy practice developed from my family practice in Rivers Inlet and Bella Bella, B.C., influenced by many teachers of aboriginal elders and writers as well as by the philosophical and realistic concerns and writings of Ian R. McWhinney, M.D. about patient-centered medicine in family medical practice as taught at U.B.C.

[In this space of the letter, Ken answered additional questions about recording time, administration and billing procedures. Then he continued as follows.]

...MSP billings are based on the appointment book entries and the hour or half hour for psychotherapy for each person even though I often give more time to family members than is billable in order to mediate conflict within their home.

...When I began my home visit psychotherapy practice, M.S.P. told me that I should bill for 00652 even though it includes hospital and inpatient visits as well as home visit psychotherapy; and that #309 is the correct I.C.D. code for adjustment reaction, which is the only diagnostic category I use for the reasons I provide in my information to referring physicians. M.S.P. has *never told me there was anything wrong with my billing practices. ...My education in family therapy included my residency with Karl Tomm, M.D. at the University of Calgary in the MacMaster Model... and with Drs. Bill Hanley and Lee Pulos in hypnotherapy and self-hypnosis, using story telling as taught by Milton Erickson, M.D. My home visit psychotherapy is conversation for family members to make plans for improving their health, caring for others at home, involving community resources and building their social support networks.*

...The clinical rationale for hourly and half hourly time units is based on the time needed to provide respectful, confidential, culturally sensitive, and appropriate individual psychotherapy for family members coping with serious medical illnesses in their homes. I bill only for the actual times when I am attending my patients.

...My case summaries include similar information and life stories that I provide to family physicians orally or in writing on a need to know basis after six weeks of home visits and after six months of home visit psychotherapy. I have never seen any written requirement from MSP to provide the kind of confidential information you suggest, nor to follow any specific pattern of reporting in psychotherapy.

...I do not prescribe any medications for my patients because their home visit psychotherapy helps them make their own health choices. Patients on medication are referred to me by their family physicians to find other ways to deal with their health problems by making lifestyle changes. I often do psychotherapy with other individuals who are taking psychotropic and other medications under the direction of other physicians, supporting them in making their decisions about medication in consultation with the prescribing physicians. From the beginning of my medical, pediatric, and psychiatric education, I have attended patients who are coping with emergencies with and without psychiatric medications. Peter R. Breggin's book on "how and why to stop taking psychiatric medications" asks readers to think about their ultimate resources in emergencies for which they may be seeking relief by taking medications, and guides them in finding the resources available to them in their families, communities, friends, and beliefs. In a B.C. health system where the greatest increase in cost is from widespread use of pharmaceuticals and

hospitalizations, my home visit practice is needed to provide alternatives to meet the health needs of responsible individuals caring for their relatives at home from birth to death. ...

Sincerely,

[signed] Ken Schramm, M.D.

A SUDDEN FREEZE was put on Ken's income for services billed to MSP. This was accompanied by the Medical Services Commission demands in writing that patient medical files be submitted to Victoria for each and every service before any money could be released.

Ken had informed all clients about the audit. In order to submit daily files to the British Columbia government, Ken informed all clients about the latest government demand before any session began so that they could go along with it or bow out. At each session the client or client's parent jointly wrote with Ken what general information was to be released and carefully left out what should be confidential. At the end of each session, clients and Ken signed the notes together to clarify that they were in agreement. Then the files were couriered weekly to the government for unknown people to read.

In a query to the BC College of Physicians and Surgeons about the files being couriered, Ken was told that this demand by the government was a violation of patient confidentiality.

At the same time Ken was informed that a representative of the BC Medical Services Commission had reported to the BC College of Physicians and Surgeons that he kept no records.

A LETTER FROM ROBERT MUSTO of the Attorney General's office dated July 29, 2002 addressed to Ken's lawyer followed, stating his point of view about the freeze on payments to Ken:

> **...Your letter mentions "as recent absolute refusal by MSP to pay any of Dr. Schramm's accounts". This does not accurately reflect MSP's actions and may leave an uninformed reader with the false**

impression MSP is acting in an arbitrary or high-handed manner. Mr. Edwards' letter of July 2, 2002, and D. Watson's letter of July 23, 2002, both indicate MSP will pay Dr. Schramm's claims once he establishes he has rendered a benefit. ...MSP has a duty to the public, and other practitioners, to insure the Plan only pays for insured benefits. MSP's request for confirmation of an adequate medical record in support of Dr. Schramm's claims is a reasonable and measured response to the audit findings and Dr. Schramm's stated opposition to record keeping.

...I wonder however if Dr. Schramm is under the mistaken impression that College requirements and MSP requirements are the same. MSP of course, will be assessing Dr. Schramm's medical records against Payment Schedule criteria, not College criteria...

[signed by Robert Musto]

* * *

DAISY FOLLOWED THAT by writing a letter to Ken's lawyer:

... I am a witness that Ken actually did all the work claimed for. I was present but not there without Ken. So no other person did the work for him.

It seems to me that if MSP requires Ken to produce more information about his clients, then it has to be in writing for each and every doctor doing psychotherapy in the province. Semrau's opinions on what should be written should be disqualified. That is very dangerous information that Semrau is asking for and no person in this province should have to live with that, especially if not informed <u>before</u> seeing a Psychiatrist that this is the type of information the Government will keep on them.

The other question is in regard to justifying the need of a doctor visit. It is absurd for a physician to be able to know in advance whether there is a need which will justify a billing to MSP. Whether it is a physical complaint or an emotional complaint, the need cannot be justified in advance. ...Imaginary or real problems can arise suddenly. ...In Ken's situation, he relies on the family physicians, who make the referrals, to decide whether it is necessary and justified to see their patients. Referrals to Ken are always for six months and that alone tells me that work with a Psychiatrist is expected to be that long and since they are renewable, that the work can take much longer. ...Since the referrals have been renewed many times for some patients, then the referring physician must make that judgment also. I am sure every Psychiatrist in this province, except the Forensic Psychiatrists, has long-term patients and others that come and go quickly just as Ken does. ...

This is a very crazy situation with the doctors in this province.

Sincerely,
[Signed] *Daisy*

51

Victoria Hearing

a patient's privacy act
whether i am blissed or pissed
is none of your business
                    Kehnroth Schramm, M.D.

AUTUMN, SEPTEMBER 24th, 2002, over a year since the audit began, Ken traveled by ferry in the early morning to attend a mandatory Hearing in a Victoria government building. His lawyer, Mr. Wood met Ken there.

The auditors, including Dr. Stanley Semrau lined up at the table.

Ken looked around the room and made a mental note that he was probably the only one to have taken the Hippocratic Oath, other than Semrau who admittedly "gets the goods on people". Ken assumed the others seated with Semrau were civil servants with their own set of loyalties.

The surprise was that Semrau displayed confusion and seemed unfamiliar with this case as he shuffled papers. Ken suspected none of the laymen auditors had read his written answers to Semrau's request for patients' confidential information, so now it was for their benefit as well as for Semrau that Ken presented his argument.

For those present, Ken verbally repeated much of the information in his letter. He had brought a backpack full of books written by authors that backed up his arguments. He did a show-and-tell with the books and pages mentioned in his letter. He explained again for all to hear that while DMS diagnosis codes may work for a forensic psychiatrist, the system has serious shortcomings in actually working with families who are dealing with life from birth to death. He explained again for all those present that in the scores of years before this auditing event, Medical Services had always communicated immediately about any problem with billings and that MSP allowed an allotted time to fix any problem or lose the income for the billing.

Ken reiterated the fact that he took the Hippocratic Oath and has always lived by his promise to be a healer and to protect his patients' secrets. Ken explained that even in this situation of being confronted by civil servants on behalf of the government, he will not divulge any information that his patients have confided to him while believing that a promise to keep confidentiality will be honored.

Launching into the reasons why this particular auditing team was not qualified to audit a physician doing psychotherapy in the privacy of patients' homes, Ken brought out the back up material. "This is published by the University of Toronto Press, 1998". Ken held up the book, then opened it and read: "In Chapter 2 of 'General Guidelines for the Practice of Psychotherapy', contributors Ray Freebury, Carolyn Rideout and Martha Wright discuss 'assessment of competence'. Here is a quote from page 39: 'It is essential in all instances, that assessors be fully conversant with and trained in the modality of psychotherapy practiced by the clinician who is undergoing evaluation'. End of quote. It is my understanding that no one in this room is trained in my modality of medicine."

People around the table somehow seemed shrunken in their seats, as though deflated.

Turning to Semrau, Ken continued, "Your work and mine are very different. I am a specialist in family home care psychotherapy. I do not do forensic psychiatry. I do not write reports for the courts as a forensic psychiatrist. My work with people depends on confidentiality so that patients can be honest. Accurate diagnosis and realistic treatment plans depend on patients' trust in their physician. Patients cannot trust and be honest if they believe their physicians will betray their promise to keep confidentiality."

Semrau shuffled papers.

Ken looked around the room. Everyone was quiet.

Holding up another book, Ken's voice maintained a quiet confidence as he repeated previous information given to Semrau. "Within the requirements for patient confidentiality and accountability to the Medical Services Plan for my part-time family home care psychotherapy practice described in my written information for referring physicians, I believe the information I have provided meets all written requirements for adequacy when read, and then reviewed with me, by a practitioner who does home visit medical psychotherapy. The complexity of defining, teaching, applying, or judging 'standards and guidelines for the psychotherapies' is presented in this book by that title edited by Paul Cameron, M.D., Jon Ennis, M.D., and John Deadman, M.D. and published by University of Toronto Press, 1998. If anyone would like to look at this book, please do."

No one offered to even touch the book.

Through the silence, except for the sound of confused shuffling of more papers, Semrau asked about a patient by name.

Ken responded, "This patient is not on your list of patients being audited."

Ken was told that he should talk about her anyway.

Assuming this was intended as a trick question, he calmly explained, "I will tell you only what is already in public record. She was in a car accident and suffered a brain injury. She was hospitalized, put on several different psychotropic drugs. The side effects accumulated, jeopardizing her physical ability to function in the basics of daily life. She was having severe flashbacks and hallucinations. She lost her marriage and has since been divorced. She has two children. Her eight-year old daughter is now living with her ex-husband, some distance from the city and visits with her mother only on weekends. Andrea [fictitious name] is now before the courts in a dispute with her own mother over custody of her youngest daughter, aged three. Through consultations with her family doctor, who prescribed her most recent medications, we have been helping Andrea to reduce the drug dependency. We have met her youngest child with the grandmother, and as a threesome with Andrea. Also, we have met Andrea with her social work team. Our main concern is a favorable outcome for the child. We have arranged for Andrea to have in-home domestic help until she is able to function better. Other than that, I will not tell you what she or anyone else has said, in keeping with confidentiality. Do you think I needed more justification for seeing this person or her child?"

The auditors look stunned and remained silent.

Ken explained again that he does not prescribe psychotropic medications and gave his history of being trained to work without the necessity of giving drugs. He also explained why his way of working is cost effective in the long run.

The meeting was suddenly ended.

Ken was not finished. "One more thing, Dr. Semrau. I have written to you and to the government auditors through your legal team, requesting an answer to my questions regarding keeping medical records appropriate to psychotherapy. The present written guidelines of both the Medical Services and the College of Physicians and Surgeons of B.C. are for medical practices that do physical procedures, not for a psychiatrist doing psychotherapy. There are no guidelines for psychiatrists. I have received no answer after several written requests over a time period of more than a year. I need to know in writing what is required to keep practicing medicine in this province and not run into this problem a second time."

There was no answer.

The silent auditors gathered themselves up and were leaving the room.

Disappointed at getting no answer to his question, Ken and his lawyer started to leave.

Semrau caught up to Ken at the doorway. "Dr. Schramm, I admire your integrity! You are the only doctor in this province who has refused us all the patient information we request."

LATE AFTERNOON FOLLOWING the meeting, Ken was on a windswept deck of a large, white ferry heading back to Vancouver. Clutching his chest, having difficulty breathing but hoping the cool air would help, he called Daisy's cell phone. "Daisy, I am sick. I'm having a hard time breathing."

"What do you think you are sick with? Is your lawyer with you?"

"Yes, he is. He says he will drive me to my apartment. My nephew was sick with a flu on Sunday when we had dinner together. It's probably that."

Daisy was traveling with her sister, having visited a person in a Nanaimo hospital. She had gone on the Nanaimo trip believing that Ken would be fine in the company of his lawyer and not need her. "Ironically, I'm also on a ferry just a little north of where you are."

Now she was upset that she left him when he most needed her. They were traveling the same waters just miles apart, having boarded at different terminals and going to land at different terminals. They could not reach their hands across the water to touch each other. They were both upset for the same reason.

FROM HIS APARTMENT, Ken called Daisy. She was upset that he decided to go to his apartment to be sick. She then asked, "How did the meeting go in Victoria?"

"They all had nothing much to say. Semrau seemed unfamiliar with the case. Then he apparently thought he would catch me up by asking about a client who is not on the audit list. I told them only the information that is already public record and not more. Then as I was leaving, he caught up to me at the doorway and told me that he '*admires my integrity*'."

52

September 2002 Collapse

FOLLOWING THE Victoria Hearing, Ken was back at work continuing to see clients, now convinced he had no flu though he was weak and increasingly slower in movement.

It was just a few days after Victoria when following behind Daisy up the stairs to the third floor of an older apartment building without an elevator, Ken took a few more steps and collapsed quietly to the floor in the hallway near the patient's apartment door.

While knocking on the door, Daisy had not heard him slide to the floor but then she heard his soft voice saying quietly, "Daisy, I can't get up."

She looked down where Ken sat on the floor, leaning against the wall with his legs outstretched. He was smiling up at her whimsically to keep a good face on his embarrassment. She recognized that he was in serious trouble; his face and hands had a white pallor, a marked contrast to his red jacket.

The client opened her door.

"Hi," Daisy said, trying to sound calm. "Ken has just collapsed."

Ken, still trying to smile, explained slowly, "Just give me a minute, I'm having trouble breathing."

Daisy expected the client to offer something to help Ken but her response was, "I don't want to catch anything!"

Daisy's attention had been toward Ken but she briefly turned toward the client in disbelief, "You won't catch anything."

The client quickly closed the door, leaving Daisy to help Ken to his feet and hold him as they walked with difficulty down the stairs. They each quietly worried about what it meant, neither wanting to frighten the other.

Nudging at Daisy also was the thought of the client who had just refused to help Ken. The reason they had been seeing her was because a heavy truck had crashed into the young woman's small car and she had been hurt, resulting in loss of lifestyle, job change and separation from her husband. Following the losses and dealing with residual pain, she had been referred to Ken because of his reputation for helping patients without giving drugs. She had since been mending remarkably well. She had been putting her life back together by being able to go back to work and renewing her relationship with her husband even though they were still living separately. The same client started her appointment a week ago by announcing her fear of dying and finding out she was the only person who survived death and was alone in the afterlife.

Daisy had asked, "Why would you be the most important person in the universe? What about the rest of us?"

The woman admitted that maybe she ought to think about that.

Pushing the thought of the client aside, Daisy told Ken, "I'm taking you right home." She meant her home where he could be safe. Mostly, she wanted him to be safe from the world and all the nastiness of some people in it – all those nasty and stupid auditors, selfish clients, and anyone else who had ever hurt Ken.

Safely in the car but before driving away, Daisy said, "I can't believe the woman wouldn't even offer you a glass of water or some tea. I would have asked you in and tried to comfort you."

Ken seemed slightly stronger now and answered, "Not everyone is like you. That's why you are my partner."

"I just think she is so selfish to be worried about herself when you are on the floor. I know I should understand but I'm really ticked off at her after all you've done to help her change her life around."

Ken quietly explained, "She hasn't finished her growth. Don't take it personally."

"That's what is so special about you. You never criticize people. You always look for their positive side; always looking for changes they can make. I know that the difference between you and me is that I still make judgments and you don't. But I hate it when you are treated badly!"

"I'm a physician. I can't take it personally. Daisy, please take me to my apartment."

"Darn that apartment! I want to take you home with me."

"I'll be alright. I just need to rest and I'll call one of my sons to help out. Also, I'm supposed to be at UBC in the morning. The apartment is close and your place is far."

"You have been keeping that apartment for your sons for so many years and most of the time you are alone in it. I think it's time to just give it up and come home with me for good. Your sons are all grown up... years ago."

"I'll think about that tomorrow. Tonight I just need to rest."

Daisy was concerned that as usual, his sons would all be too busy to help their dad, but she could not say that. "I'm taking you there against my best judgment."

"I understand."

While driving the car, Daisy took a hard look at what she had done, realizing that she, too, had treated Ken in a seemingly uncaring way. Casting stones would not make her look any better. She had been so involved in keeping appointments on time that she had been overlooking his deteriorating health. On the other hand, he had done his best to keep it to himself. He had just slowed down until he broke. But now she realized that she should have known.

She thought back to just yesterday. She was running ahead of Ken on the way to see clients, trying to be on time. When seeing clients in the West End of Vancouver, they always felt lucky to find any parking at all. After parking the car, Ken had been so slow walking the block uphill that by the time he caught up to Daisy, she had already rung the doorbell of the apartment building. He was upset and having a hard time catching his breath. The client opened the door at the same time that Ken blurted out loudly at Daisy, "You abandoned me!" His face was red and white with anguish.

The client's wife had been diagnosed with a reoccurrence of lung cancer that was now spreading across her chest, and she was undergoing chemotherapy. He was shocked that the doctor and his assistant appeared to be arguing. They had barely gotten to know these clients but it seemed better to cancel today, explaining that Ken had become ill. Daisy offered to phone later.

In hindsight, Daisy realized that she should have known Ken was in real trouble on that hill because as she glanced behind, she could see that he was walking slower and slower.

Then he had seemed to recover over night and today they continued on to another appointment that had been set a week ago, only to have him collapse to the floor in front of a client.

Daisy could not avoid thinking about the times over many years that she rushed Ken from appointment to appointment. She was used to him slowing her down. He always insisted on staying until the client finished in his or her own way; and if it was important to leave and come back the next day, they would squeeze in an extra appointment to fit the situation. Daisy could not count the times she booked the day so solidly with no breaks until Ken would beg for some food. But what was happening now was a new kind of slowness.

With Ken resting beside her as she drove the car toward his apartment, she thought how the clock had started to rule... Me – I was the kid who lived in a timeless zone, playing on the stunt pole in the playground, preferring to be late for school in favor of timeless bliss of viewing the world upside down and working muscles that hated sitting still in a desk... My family and I had lived in an Inuit village with people who only ten or less years before had been Nomads... Time was kept by the chores that needed to be done to care for people... If a meeting was called in white man's time, the people may show up hours late because family's needs and household chores like getting water came first... It was a timeless zone where there was more sky than anything else except for white man keeping the clocks running regardless of the weather or needs of people... And there was the aurora borealis with the timeless music of the universe that is like listening to eternity...

Daisy mused that self-assessment had a way of leveling out the playing field between people. With Ken ill, she had time to think and regret how she treated him at times. Under her breathe, she said, "Hindsight is sometimes better than foresight. Insight is not always available."

"Yes, and where is that coming from?" Ken asked.

"You have suffered at the hands of a clock and I have been winding the clock. I was just thinking how I treated you by rushing you to keep appointments and walking ahead of you in a hurry to be on time; trying to make up time for when people's needs were more than the clock time. I am so sorry. I am so-o sorry now."

TOWARD EVENING Daisy received a telephone call. "Daisy, please come and get me. I can't take care of myself. I'm too ill."

This was the second time that Ken, normally so independent, had called for help; the first time was when he fell ill and was bedridden in the '80s.

Leaving his apartment on Daisy's arm, neither he or she realized that he would never return to it.

IN DAISY'S HOME, Ken collapsed completely. He struggled to keep breathing and could barely sip anything for thirst. Daisy nursed him throughout the night, staying awake around the clock – watchful as he desperately clung to life. She played Solitaire and Mahjong on the computer all night long by Ken's bedside. Not a game player, it was the only way she could stay awake and alert.

At dawn, Ken informed her, "I'm in heart failure. I thought at first I had the flu. It's heart."

"I know. You should *not* have gone to that meeting in Victoria."

"I thought I could handle it."

"I wish you hadn't gone. Your health is more important."

Ken had been asked to speak the next night at a gathering of physicians determined to fight and support each other about the way audits were being conducted. He regrettably was forced to cancel but sent a hope that he would attend at a later date, perhaps in a couple of weeks. He was still hopeful of a quick recovery and did not realize that weeks of near-death illness would follow.

After the first night Ken had refused to be in a cave of a bedroom. He asked to be moved to the living room where he could look out to the garden and there was an overhead fan for air movement. He had to be upright. He was propped against pillows of many colours and covered with a brightly coloured blanket the aboriginal people had given him. He had many bouts of not being able to breath and slipped off the sofa to crash onto the floor in his struggle to breath. Along with no breath came *fear* – fear of falling – fear of dying. He had lost all sense of balance and was afraid of falling out of bed after falling many times. The larger, overwhelming fear was not of dying so much as he was not ready to leave his family. While clinging onto a thin thread of life, Ken fought smothering and the horrors of it.

Daisy thought smothering to death was horrifying. In imagining death, it was how to get there that was the scary part, not what comes in the afterlife. But the thought of losing Ken was more than horrifying. She was not ready for that either.

Ken's body swelled with water from head to toe until he looked like a dripping balloon. His clothing no longer fit. Heavy legs sprung many holes that wept. Plastic was placed beneath thick towels under his legs and feet to catch the running water. They would become sopping wet and needed to be replaced every couple of hours with dry towels. The washing machine and clothes dryer were running day and night for the towels and sheets in the attempt to keep Ken clean and dry.

Ken continued his struggle to breath with the aid of a humidifier, fan and air conditioner all running at once. He could not lie down and breathe. Instead he remained propped by pillows in an upright position hour after hour, day after day. He could not sleep, afraid that if he fell asleep, he might not wake up. He became sleep deprived.

The holes in his legs grew even larger and regardless of keeping him clean, some open sores at his ankles became infected.

Antony was on call around the clock. He got out of bed in the middle of the night – many nights, no matter what he had to do the next day as a medical student. He set up a massage table and did the Chinese massage and moxa treatments that calmed Ken when he had a crisis of being unable to breath and seriously looked death in the face. The treatments helped.

A physician of Chinese medicine had Ken soak his feet in large pails of medicated water that had to be boiled up fresh twice a day.

After a couple of weeks, Ken was calmer. He wanted grandchildren around him even though he was still too ill to do anything but express love for them and to know that they cared.

To be dressed properly, he needed safe, comfortable clothing, especially for visiting grandchildren. He could not just wear his under-shorts. He needed soft cotton lounging pants for at home and jogging pants for when he would be ready for out of the house medical appointments. His jeans were too stiff for his sore body and no longer fit his waist.

Ken found it difficult to be without Daisy even for a few minutes. Son-in-law Ron agreed to stay with Ken while Daisy and Loraine made a dash to shop for the new clothes. Needing an anchor to life, Ken wanted to hold hands with people near him and Ron was no exception. He asked Ron to hold his hand. Ron was embarrassed, not used to holding hands with a man.

Ken had been telling everyone who came near him that he loved him or her. Ken had no armor and was genuinely in love with everyone and innocently told Ron he loved him. Ron was even more embarrassed.

It was hard for Daisy to leave Ken even for an hour. It was a fast shopping trip. Loraine liked the brightly coloured pajamas with lively designs on them. She thought they looked right for healing.

Bringing back red cotton lounging pants with little cartoon dogs printed on them, and a green pair with Christmas trees, Ken's eyes lit up when he saw them. He loved the humor.

DAISY BECAME severely exhausted as one night had turned into weeks of serious illness. She caught a few hours sleep whenever she could but many nights there was no sleep. She drew pictures and played more computer games to stay awake – watchful. Playing games on the computer was something she never thought she would ever do, considering it a waste of her time before. Watching the food network on television kept her entertained because of an interest in cooking.

Son, Antony was exhausted by long day classes, necessary study time, exams, and on top of that being on call in the night when Ken needed him. He continued to heroically set up a massage table in the middle of the night when Ken was desperate.

Daisy would not entertain the idea of hospitalization. Ken wanted to be at home and she adamantly wanted him at home, going out only for necessary medical appointments.

Ken gained a little strength and started to eat. There was hope that the worst had passed. Daisy tried to keep the world at bay while he recovered.

With the help of Traditional Chinese Medicine and Homeopathy, Ken was slowly on the mend. His body lost the bloating. Water stopped running from his ankles; the many holes, some as big as an inch wide and deep to the bone in his legs and feet were visibly healing.

On the way to the bathroom, on Daisy's arm one evening, Ken paused, turned around and said in his soft voice, "Get lost!"

He told Daisy that a spirit behind him had asked him to "Come home."

He smiled at Daisy, "I told him to get lost. I want to stay with you."

TO BE WITH Ken now was to watch a person look death in the face and come back with absolutely no armor. He had undergone a complete stripping away of all the ways human beings build coping mechanisms and defenses throughout life. Ken loved everyone. Ken was now completely innocent and vulnerable.

Ken lay on the living-room sofa, covered with blankets and from his bed, reached out his hand to hold hands with any and every visitor, proclaiming his love to anyone who came near.

Daisy watched with renewed sense of humor at how people were taken aback. Having built such a distrust of feelings and resistance to open affection, people simply did not know how to respond or what to make of it. At first, the temptation was to recoil and then with embarrassed reluctance, they went along with giving Ken their hand to hold.

The thin veneer Ken had adapted for himself, through a lifetime of problems, just slid away; it vanished. Ken was naked in this world. Ken had become a pure spirit, the embodiment of pure love continuing to inhabit a human body.

Children and animals were not fazed and did flourish in open affection. Jonah, the grey cat lay with Ken day and night, keeping a constant vigil over him. Devoted granddaughters had a lifelong closeness and understanding of Ken's innocence, experiencing him through their own innocence. Maria and Katie, now in their late teenaged years, kept him company by day and night, reading and talking with him. They continued sharing their troubles and concerns. Ken gave them guidance from his bed.

Daisy mused that it was no wonder Ken had always said he got along best with children and animals while having difficulty with adult humans. In the medical practice, children and animals would be all over him with affectionate trust. Looking back, Ken had always been extremely caring and loving with absolutely everyone from the street people who may be sick and dirty to the self-absorbed ball-crunching career woman or a ruthless man, to the sweet and sometimes spitting and kicking children. Ken had always looked deeper into the person, regardless of the outward garb or behavior, to find the child within and to love the child within. Daisy could see more clearly that Ken had always been too good for this world and had functioned with a very thin protective shield that was now gone. She understood the good fortune – the privilege of knowing him. She wondered how she got so lucky.

It was from his bed that Ken reached his hand for Daisy's hand. "Daisy, I want to marry you by Christmas of this year."

"Yes, I want to marry you, Ken. We can do a Christmas wedding."

"I want to do that with you." Ken smiled. "I wonder where we should have the ceremony. I would like it to be right here, at home."

"I think that would be nice."

Daisy watched over him as he napped peacefully now for the first time in weeks.

THERE WAS NO income to pay for two dwellings. The week after Ken had become ill, his son Stephen had helped by moving Ken's belongings to Daisy's home. The separate apartment that had been for his sons, and a barrier to getting on with marriage was finally gone. It had become clear that his sons would not be looking after him. The obligation to keep an apartment and keep a part of himself separate from Daisy and her family for his sons was over – complete.

In a burst of energy, Ken got on the telephone to his family and to Daisy's family, happily announcing his intentions to marry Daisy by Christmas. It was as though he had a new lease on life, something to hurry and get well for. He gained some strength.

Daisy was excited but unsure about marrying Ken while he was ill. She wanted him to be of sound body and mind so that his family could not accuse her of taking advantage of a sick man. Meanwhile, she dreamed of what she would wear to become Ken's bride.

As Ken questioned and dreamed of where the wedding should take place and wondered who would attend to witness the vows, she thought about sewing her dress... a soft cream coloured material because Ken likes soft material, trimmed with a mix of dusty rose, blue and lavender embroidery and beading. In keeping with her mother's Ukrainian heritage, she would for sure wear a wreath of flowers with ribbons crowning her head. And maybe Ken would wear a crown of flowers because Ukrainians do crown the bride and groom in the marriage ceremony. Most of all, she wanted to please Ken.

It was harder to imagine what Ken would wear because of his health. He did not yet fit into uncomfortable pants and shirts. Ken loved humor and a good laugh. It was easier to imagine that he marries Daisy in his comfortable cartoon pajamas and they would be married with humor and comfort.

All Daisy wanted was for him to be well and they could marry in anything, anywhere, and hopefully people present would be supportive.

OCTOBER 2002. CANADIAN THANKSGIVING. Ken was not yet well, but he wanted to join the family for dinner. Leaning heavily on Daisy's arm, he slowly climbed the stairs to sit with the extended family at the dining table on the second floor of the house. He had only enough energy to stay five minutes and could not eat a turkey dinner yet, so with help again, he made his way back down the stairs to his bed.

The family breathed a sigh of relief at how much better he was. Ken had just proved that he was alive!

53

American Thanksgiving

AN ARTICLE WAS PUBLISHED on pages 18-20 in the **College of Physicians & Surgeons of British Columbia 2002 Annual Report.**

... Some demands for medical records leave practitioners vulnerable to ethical and legal transgressions. ...

... In an ideal world, the work of the College and its Ethics Department and of the Committee might be more manageable if physicians and their patients all recognized and acknowledged that:

> **- pain, sickness and death are part of life;**
>
> **- modern medicine can do good, but that good is limited, and carries risk of harm;**
>
> **- all of us are owed dignity and respect;**
>
> **- without trust (truth-telling, promise-keeping), all is lost;**
>
> **- the doctor-patient relationship is a partnership; rights and obligations to autonomy and accountability belong to both. ...**

..."Moral credibility is ours to establish and ours to lose": (quote taken from) Pellegrino, E. The Caring Ethic: The Relation of Physician to Patient. The University of Alabama Press. 1985.

T.P. Seland, MD, FRCPC, Deputy Registrar

R.H. Morton, MD, Chair, Ethical Standards and

Conduct Review Committee

* * *

MEANWHILE, LETTERS AND PHONE CALLS explaining Ken's illness to both the BC Government and the BC College of Physicians and Surgeons had apparently no effect on learned men; some of who were physicians and lawyers. They were revved up to wage warfare on a man who was fighting for his life with heart failure and could only get out of bed for a few minutes at a time.

In their campaign following the audit in Ken's lawyer's office, Government lawyers had complained to the B.C. College of Physicians and Surgeons that Ken kept no medical records.

Even though Ken had received a letter from the B.C. College of Physicians and Surgeons telling him they would wait until he recovered from illness, they hired Miller Thomson, a Limited Liability Partnership, with 'Affiliations Worldwide' and offices in eight major North American cities, and with an intimidating looking letterhead. The intimidating tactic of stern letters written by lawyer David Martin started as early as November 8th. He suggested a two day Hearing. They were deaf to letters from Ken or his lawyer stating that Ken needed time for reasons of illness. They wanted Ken at a Hearing or else.

AMERICAN THANKSGIVING was extremely meaningful to Ken. Days before American Thanksgiving November 28th, 2002 he called his sons to invite them for dinner in his new home with Daisy. All three agreed to come.

In the night, Ken sat at the kitchen table writing out the menu and over several nights he wrote about other concerns.

Nov/02 Menu & Shopping list
Turkey roast(s), legs & thigh
Turkey gravy
Cranberry sauce – 2-3 bags (unblanched from Oregon)
Beets for roasting & beet greens
Roasted pumpkin, onions, garlic
Mashed potatoes
Baked apples

Things for Ken to do re "Thanksgiving"
Will Stephen & Andy come here after 6 p.m.?
Set-up (my) phone, computer & "office"
Hypericum spray for Rt. Ankle
Rest & Sleep & wait for phone person
Chores *Shave & Wash*

PLANS:
(What to do about) car lease
Henry to negotiate a small home visit psychoRx practice to repay him &
MSC & Income tax
Copies of mortgage & letter from Dr. Blackman

Wedding: *options – civil house, garden*
Who would be the marrier merrier marrier?

Income: *teach course @ aboriginal research with E.?*
Writing health records with informed consent & respect for Hippocratic
Oath: do no harm & keep patient secrets

My Next Thirty (Minutes? Years?)

Xmas: Daisy...LOVE...*beyond Xmas dinner & presents for the*
kids/grandkids – what? a heart with new tires (retired?)

Take/make the time for loving, enjoying, living
Cross-country skiing & story making – scrapbooks??

> *Smelling cinnamon*
> *Remembering mother*
> *How do you write the places of times,*
> *the homes of blessed memories?*

KEN PROUDLY SHOWED his lists to Daisy for approval. He took pride that he was beginning to read and write again after weeks of not being able to do so, and even write a small poem again.

This Thanksgiving menu and written wish for his sons to come was a milestone to healing. Daisy prayed to God that his sons would show up but would not believe until she could see them.

Practice writing at the kitchen table in the small hours of the morning and the late hours of the night with a cup of medicinal tea while regaining strength, Ken wrote poetry, food lists, bits of memoirs, and notes to his mother in keeping with their conversations of years ago – and optimistically kept hoping to get back to work and to UBC.

THE YOUNG MEN did arrive for Thanksgiving dinner as promised. Ken was happy. Daisy was relieved. Ken, wearing his red doggie cartoon pants, tried to help in the kitchen to prepare the food. It was the most fun Ken and Daisy had in years. Having dinner with his sons seemed to give Ken a jump on healing power. Success!

AS KEN GAINED a little more strength, he would stand for a few minutes just outside the back door, facing the garden with his hands stretched outward, praying and thanking the Creator. He was completely unguarded... open... thankful... hopeful of healing... hopeful of gaining enough strength to complete his work and be in this world for their children... hopeful that he and Daisy could begin again and finally have their wedding.

Daisy and Ken delighted in small things like Ken being able to eat a light meal while sitting at the table. They were grateful and happy that Ken could simply hold a pen and write again, something he had not been able to do for almost two months. Daisy sat beside Ken as he sipped tea and read the poetry he wrote in the night while he could not sleep. Finally, no ex-wives were trying to beat at them. They did not have to rush around looking after other people, and Ken's sons seemed glad that Ken was being looked after. No family member was making a stink about their relationship. For the first time in twenty-three years, Ken and Daisy were enjoying comfortable togetherness in one home. They only wished for Ken to get well.

IN THIS STATE of Ken having no armor, negative forces were at work in the background with the intention of harming Ken. Along with David Martin's letters, there was the never-ending onslaught from within the darkness of Victoria's public servants, to slay Ken regardless of the fact that they had been informed of Ken's life threatening illness.

An email letter from Robert Musto, of the BC Attorney General's office dated December 4, 2002, with copies to Bill Edwards and Anton Glegg, both of the BC Health Executive, arrived in Ken's lawyer's office. Musto stated that he was sending some figures for consideration re: payback; reasoning that there were a significant number of services rendered where there was no referral or re-referral. He then stated it to be only a framework for discussions and to call to discuss these numbers and the underlying assumptions.

It was clear that the audit had shifted to throwing things against the wall to see what sticks or what could scare Ken enough to simply agree to pay back some amount of money.

DAVID MARTIN was hard at work on behalf of the BC College of Physicians and Surgeons. Even though no Hearing had yet established Ken to be guilty of misconduct, David Martin of Miller Thomson outlined in a letter dated December 18, 2002, that he was instructed by the Preliminary Review Committee **that in view of Dr. Schramm's misconduct... if this matter were to be settled by an Agreement short of an Inquiry Committee hearing, the following is the punishment:**

> **- Erasure from the Register and transfer to the Temporary Register**
> **- A 3 month suspension from practice**
> **- Payment of 1/2 of the College's costs**
> **- A reprimand**
> **- A requirement that Dr. Schramm keep proper medical records and monitoring of his record-keeping to ensure compliance**

* * *

REGARDLESS OF KEN'S fight for life and several requests for time to get better, letters from BC government employees and from lawyers representing the BC College of Physicians and Surgeons swamped Henry's office on their way to Ken, undermining healing.

Irate, Daisy wrote a long letter with pictures of Ken's legs, chastising the whole bunch of stupid, bad boys – physicians and lawyers alike. But she was most angry at the physicians turned administrators at the BC College of Physicians and Surgeons who had taken the Hippocratic Oath and seemed to have forgotten that their duty in taking the oath was to take care of people, especially those who are ill, and not to cause them harm. Ken's lawyer cautioned her about sounding angry. She did not care; she was angry that these bad boys seemed to have no moral fibers in their bodies. In her letter, she wrote about her experience in a clinic that cost society untold amounts of money one Saturday afternoon when a patient on her shift called on the phone to tell her he was about to commit suicide. She was familiar with the disturbed patient and called 911 to go to his house because the clinic doctor was out delivering a baby and the man's psychiatrist who was also the clinic's psychiatrist, was not answering his phone; instead a fire truck with on duty firemen, police and an ambulance all showed up at the man's home. Daisy pointed out that such a shamble of expense would never have happened in Ken's practice because Ken would have been available and quietly taken care of the person. It hardly mattered because they all ignored her letter anyway.

CHRISTMAS CAME. Ken was still struggling to live and again he tried to enjoy Christmas dinner with the family but within a few minutes had to retreat to his bed without eating.

December 2002 wedding plans took a back seat to all the troubles that just kept coming. They hoped for healing in the Spring.

54

Questions

JANUARY 2003. "Who brought up Judge Oliver's Judgment against Ken?" Daisy asked.

IT WAS DURING the third week of January that Ken and Daisy went to Mr. Wood's office. Ken looked weak and as though he had shrunken in size but he was glad to show Henry that he was *Alive*! His ankles were no longer swollen with fluid but they continued to have large open wounds left by the draining holes, some larger than an inch and deep to the bone. Daisy was eager to show Ken's ankles to Henry. She lifted his pant legs and watched Henry's shocked facial expressions. She always looked for compassionate reactions toward Ken in order to sort out who was real and who was phony. Henry was genuine. When Ken had fallen ill, Henry had couriered a large, expensive bouquet of flowers to Ken with a card. Daisy had received the flowers in awe that a *lawyer* could be so caring. But at the time, Ken was struggling so hard to hang onto a thread of life that he refused to have the flowers near him, saying, "I appreciate the thought but please put them in another room. I'm not dead and I don't plan on dying."

Never the less, the lawyer who cared, showed it – several times now.

KEN WAS RESTING on the sofa, covered by a blanket and his protector grey cat lying on his legs.

Daisy had in her hands the answer to her question. "It says here that government lawyer, Robert Musto has looked into your past and found Jane's old Judgment against you, which they say makes credibility an issue and that they would have to investigate the claim of 'impecuniousity'. That's their word. I don't even know what that means except it must mean something awful."

It was evident that the BC government was figuring out how to make use of Judge Oliver's Reasons for Judgment, brought about by an ex-wife's disgruntlement a dozen years earlier, to further ruin Ken's reputation as an intimidation tactic.

Ken took in the news quietly, but looked devastated as though he had just been physically beaten.

"Ken, the good part is that you told your lawyer about the Judgment in your first consultation with him. You have been completely open so he can't be surprised about this. He should only be surprised at the tactics used by a government lawyer."

Daisy did not know how to protect Ken in the continuing attacks. She wished she could take care of it all without telling him the bad news that came almost daily.

"We've been battling the government for about two years," Daisy said wistfully. "They are really working hard at breaking you down. Now they are resorting to attacking your character, not just your work. It's horrible how your ex-wife did so much damage that it is affecting you even now."

Ken remained silent but the color had drained away from his face. He was defeated and ill.

REPEATING KEN'S EARLIER QUESTIONS, Mr. Wood sent another letter dated **January 20, 2003** to Rob Musto:

...In order to decide whether or not he can continue with a home visit psychotherapy practice, he requests responses to the following questions:

1. *How often may he bill (weekly, monthly, yearly) for the same individual receiving office or home visit psychotherapy?*

2. *With whom may he negotiate flexibility in frequency and duration of individual home or office psychotherapy daily or weekly to plan for the complexity of family home care and decision-making?*

3. How many re-referrals may a patient obtain from their family physician to see him?

4. How is he to know that patients are actually referred or re-referred by family physicians? Can he rely upon explanatory codes?

5. Beyond his clinical notations which will address what he did, what treatment is planned, and how it is evaluated, what additional records will be required by MSC (e.g. referral and re-referral letters)?

6. Will the required reimbursement sum be economically viable, allowing for the payment MSC claw-backs, overhead, legal fees, and taxes?

7. What "order of practice" is proposed to be imposed on Dr. Schramm?

8. Would the rules imposed on Dr. Schramm be for him alone, or for all Psychotherapists?

9. How might Dr. Schramm avoid another expensive and stressful audit?

While we realize that a reimbursement to MSP may be imposed on Dr. Schramm as a resolution to this matter, you will already appreciate that the inevitable implication that Dr. Schramm has deliberately abused the system in some manner is **not** true. ...

In that regard, although you refer to a significant number of services rendered for which there was no referral or re-referrals, I do not believe that we have ever been provided with the particulars of that determination. My recollection is that Mr. Glegg had referred to only one instance of a non-referral being unearthed, but, in any event, the MSP explanatory codes appear to contemplate that non-referrals are monitored at the time of billing (e.g. H2). Since confirmations to MSP of referrals and re-referrals by a family physician are also the function of the family physician, is it not reasonable for a specialist to presume that the referrals and re-referrals have been approved unless MSP indicates otherwise? It is difficult, if not impossible, to address these matters effectively years after the event. ...

KEN HAD RECEIVED NO ANSWER to his questions during the Victoria meeting or in previous written queries. Believing in good will and that there must be a mistake because of gaps in written rules, Ken wrote another letter through his lawyer to the BC Ministry of Attorney General, Legal Services Branch.

February 3, 2003 – on behalf of Ken, Mr. Wood asked again for a solution to the unwritten rules that were a glaring omission in the Audit process.

It had been like talking to a blank wall. The questions, asked several times verbally and in writing, were never achnowledged in any form by BC Medical Services Commission or the BC government legal team. Musto and his team had a one-way manipulative talking system.

55

Retirement 2003

February 2. 2003

D.H. Blackman, M.D., Deputy Registrar,
College of Physicians & Surgeons of B.C.
Dear Dr. Blackman,

Thank you for your kind letter of November 22, 2002.

Enclosed please find a letter from my family doctor. I have been seriously ill with congestive heart failure and viral pneumonia after my meeting in Victoria with M.S.C. auditors. In your letter you say that the College will defer taking further action against me until I am recovered.

In the meantime, a letter dated December 18, 2002 was received from David Martin, lawyer for Miller Thomson threatening punishment and payment of half the College's cost (which I assume means his fees also).

I have not practiced medicine since September, 2002. I have no M.S.P. income and no insurance to cover my living expenses. I have no money nor assets with which to pay M.S.C. and the College. Just getting by daily is a problem. I cannot afford a lawyer and I cannot attend any meetings myself. My heart will not stand the stress.

I am seriously considering retiring from the College and my practice of medicine. I would appreciate your help in securing a delay in the proceedings against me until further notice. Thank you for your kindness.

Sincerely,
Kehnroth Schramm, M.D.

March 21, 2003

D.H.Blackman, M.D., Deputy Registrar,
College of Physicians & Surgeons of B.C.
Dear Dr. Blackman,

re: Retirement

Due to serious illness, I find that I cannot return to practicing medicine. I hereby retire from the practice of medicine and from ever billing Medical Services Plan of B.C. again.

My last letter to you, along with a letter from my physician, outlining my illness and possible intent to retire was answered by David Martin, lawyer for the College of Physicians and Surgeons. Mr. Martin warns that he may still pursue me but that possibly the retirement will be accepted and along with that the College will publish that I retired in the face of disiplinary action again me.

I would like to point out to you that this would be publishing a lie since I am retiring soley because of ill health and cannot continue with any hearings or actions at all.

When I met with you in the Autumn of 2002, I fully intended to work along with you and continue practicing medicine. During the latter part of September I became so ill that I was close to death for several weeks. My condition has improved, but not enough to continue working, attend hearings, or battle for my good name.

I would appreciate it very much if the College of Physicians and Surgeons would allow me to quietly retire.

Thankyou.

Sincerely,

Kehnroth Schramm, M.D.

MARCH 21, 2003, Ken's lawyer, Henry Wood, wrote to the law firm of Miller Thomson:

>*Attention: David Martin*

>*I write to confirm that Dr. Schramm feels compelled to retire from medical practice. His health is such that it is neither feasible nor advisable for him to attempt to carry on. However, I write to emphasize that he is retiring because of ill health, not because of the disciplinary process invoked by the College. Any publication that might suggest otherwise, directly or by innuendo, would unfairly besmirch him and the highly principled dedication he has demonstrated throughout his professional life.*

>*Yours very truly,*
>*(Signed by Henry Wood)*

AS A RESULT of being ill for months, there was no money to pay the substantial annual physicians' licensing fee for 2003. As of March 31, 2003 Ken was suspended from practicing medicine in British Columbia for non-payment.

THE SCENARIO NEEDING discussion in Mr. Wood's office was that Medical Services Commission had sent another Agreement they wanted Ken to sign.

Ken looked at the papers and grabbed his chest. He excused himself and left the room.

Daisy was torn about running after him or staying to take over. She decided Ken would be safe for a few minutes with the secretaries. In the interim, she gave Henry a hard time over clauses she was reading.

Coming back into the room, Ken appeared to have recovered enough to participate. "This is the exact same Agreement they asked me to sign two months ago. I have outlined changes needed. I told them then I will not sign a false statement and they have refused to communicate about it. They have not answered any of my questions."

Clutching his chest and gasping for air, Ken explained, "When I first started home visits ten years ago, I consulted with the Medical Services Plan and they told me how to do the billings. I have followed the rules as set out then and in their printed manual. MSP has never told me there was anything wrong with my billing practices. I have to say again that with no clear agreement as to what is an appropriate pattern of practice, there is no way to do a practice if I was well enough to continue."

Daisy jumped in again, "Right. I've been doing billings for over twenty years – twenty-three, in fact. MSP has always audited billings as they happened, twice each month. If there were any questionable billings or referrals, we were always informed immediately and allowed six months to fix the problem; three months is the present time limit. There is a booklet of codes; each rejected billing was given a code for me to refer to so I knew exactly what the problem was. If there was a questionable billing, we just were not paid or if payment was made, it was clawed back within a month until MSP was satisfied. We always knew where we stood from month to month. Regardless of these safeguards, audits are being sprung on physicians for six or seven years with no way to fix any problems that the commission makes claim to regardless of the safeguards we have always worked with. It doesn't add up."

Ken was bewildered. "They also do not answer me on any question I have raised about confidentiality, or on the reasons not to label patients, or on how to do my psychotherapy practice without running into trouble."

This had all been said before to the lawyer. The papers were laid down and chairs pushed back in preparation to leave.

Mr. Wood had worked many hours trying to negotiate and explain his client's position and beliefs. Mr. Wood was up against endless financial resources of government and numerous government employees all paid by taxpayers. The government employees, who held the pot of gold to dip into, refused to budge by sending the same proposed Agreement a second time and at the same time refused to acknowledge or answer any of Ken's questions about procedure for a practice like his. They refused to acknowledge the gaping hole in written information the government provided to all physicians.

Standing beside his chair, Ken stated emphatically, "I would rather be held responsible for paying back all my earnings for six years, than settle for ten percent and be forced to sign a false document. I will stand by my Hippocratic Oath and keep my promise to my patients. I will not save my own hide at the cost to my patients!"

AS THEY MADE their way to the car, Daisy thought out loud. "According to MSC, we have worked six years for absolutely nothing and it cost us money just to work! They are forcing us into bankruptcy. If they beat us to court, which is obviously their next step, we will be indebted forever to them, and so will our children if I interpret that Agreement correctly. ...No! We have to go bankrupt first. It's more honorable for us to go bankrupt than for you to go back on your promise to patients."

APRIL 2003. Ken could barely walk on the day of the trip to the Trustee of bankruptcy. Even though the car was parked within ten feet of the door, on entering the office, Ken needed to sit on the first chair by the door and rest before he could go farther. Ken's illness was shocking to the Trustee. He paused and waited for Ken to revive even a little. One look at Ken and everyone in the office knew he was extremely ill and had no energy with which to do this.

Then they were taken into an inner office where the interview happened. Papers of many pages were handed to them to fill out by hand. Ken was not doing well enough on this day to even read the papers. Daisy filled out the papers by hand for both of them.

The typist took the papers. They waited and then signed the typed copies to go bankrupt together. Ken went through the process, including signing without reading any paper for himself. Daisy simply showed him where to sign.

They headed home feeling some relief that it was done. They hoped that all the fighting would finally end and they could concentrate on healing.

DAVID HATTER, Barrister and Solicitor of the BC Attorney General's office wrote a letter dated MAY 22, 2003. He stated that his letter was confidential and not to be copied.

Daisy wrote of response to Henry, hoping it would be relayed to Hatter and his cronies, (as she thought of them).

May 27, 2003

Hi Henry,

We realize you are trying to be finished with this matter.

How ironic that David Hatter demands confidentiality but backs up a regime that does not honor confidentiality where it concerns a physician who has taken the Hippocratic Oath and his patients who believe they are entitled to confidentiality from their doctors.

What games they do play, everything is so secret but they wrote to the College to complain about not having enough of the patients' secrets and after two years it is a rush for an agreement from Ken.

David Hatter wants an answer by Wednesday 28th May; that is within five days. Hatter states that Dr. Schramm is content to see the government prove their claim to claw back 100% of six years income but that a much lesser amount of 10% was offered in the Settlement Agreement. Hatter seems to understand that Ken prefers bankruptcy rather than sign the Agreement. Hatter is apparently offering Ken another chance to change his mind or Hatter will proceed in preparing and filing a claim in an amount instructed by MSC just in case it would survive bankruptcy.

Hatter's letter is business as usual. Hatter does not query about Ken's health and gives no indication of concern that Ken is ill even though the government has been told on numerous occasions.

Ken may not recover ever, and cannot fight back in any way except by bankruptcy.

We have reread the agreement the MSC wants signed and it contains nothing worthy of signing:

***1.** They want an agreement that everything they say in the "Agreement is true and correct". We disagree. Their findings are not true and correct. They have in fact lied along the way and* manipulated the facts and back stepped when caught. Their findings are their findings and we do not agree with their findings, but if they agree not to publish the practitioner's name, who cares about their findings except they will be used as scare tactics for other physicians and used to prove to their colleagues that they did a good job. We cannot give compliance to them having done a good job when we know how shabby a performance it has been and nothing will improve for the future.

2. They want an agreement that the Practitioner is indebted to and will pay the Commission 10% of six years gross earnings. In bankruptcy it is plain stupid to sign any such agreement.

3. They want an agreement to abide by an appropriate Pattern of Practice and they continue to be vague about what an appropriate pattern of practice is. No one can abide by that information and can only lead to more trouble and continued stress. No one can work under those circumstances, with no clear ground rules and do a good job in any field of work.

4. They want an "Agreement shall ensure to the benefit and be binding upon the Practitioner and the Commission and their respective heirs, executors, administrators, successors, and assigns as the case may be". Henry, this must be the silly season for anyone to even ask someone who is ill and bankrupt as Ken to sign this and willingly let his family have to fight this battle.

5. We disagree that the medical records consisted only of date stamps. Semrau and others may not have agreed with the notes and information on each patient but they were more than just date stamps. To say otherwise is not true.

MSC and their lawyers seemed to be on one track only, which was to claw back a percentage of moneys or force a submission to a kangaroo court. They refused and bypassed any and all questions Ken asked of them. There were no clear guidelines to begin with and none to finish with. Even the CONSENT ORDER Appendix "A" does not give clear guidelines; they are as vague as ever. I think these people think everyone else is stupid, or, they do not realize how stupid they appear. Even a layman can pick giant holes in their work. They rely on power rather than brains.

The only Agreement Ken is willing to sign is one that acknowledges that:

a. Ken thought he was working for the patients and that there is a giant gap in what Ken has promised when he took the Hippocratic Oath to do no harm and to keep his patients' secrets, and that of the government and legal system which is eroding confidentiality for all people of this province (and country).

b. That he owed the government all his earnings for the years audited, under the circumstances that he was mistaken about who he worked for and regards his promise of confidentiality to his patients more important than his own self-preservation. On the other hand, the figure is in the bankruptcy so no further acknowledgment is needed.

c. That they do not publish his name with/under any circumstances.

d. Bankruptcy outlives, outlasts and overtakes all of the above and any future audits they may come up with since Ken is no longer billing to them and any moneys he made through MSP of BC was before bankruptcy. Ken agrees that he cannot and will not work for MSP in future because of the confidentiality breech they are requiring.

e. That there will be no further charges brought forward for past differences.

Henry, Ken has only resorted to bankruptcy because of ill health that I blame on those involved here. They refused to negotiate and make clear guidelines. Right to the end, they are as vague as they were in the beginning. Ken will never appear at a Hearing, he is too ill. Ken will never repay anything to them as he has gone the only route available under the non-negotiating route they chose. They may as well close the file and save the people of this province money in their pursuit. Just because those guys have jobs doesn't make them right.

Furthermore, if MSC chooses to publish Ken's name because he refuses to sign this dishonest document, then that opens the door wide for retaliation publicly, like newspapers and magazines. Maybe MSC and their lawyers have more to hide than Ken does. At some point the general public must be made aware of what has happened to their right to confidentiality between themselves and their physicians – sooner rather than later.

Sincerely,

Daisy

UNABLE TO FIGHT due to illness, Ken was now willing to retire with dignity in a letter to the British Columbia College of Physicians and Surgeons. He had given fifty years of his life to medicine – living, breathing, study and teaching medicine. For more than thirty of those years he had been registered as a physician in British Columbia, giving his life to the people who came his way. But the College refused his retirement, saying he must attend a Hearing to resolve a dispute over medical records because of a report to them by Medical Services Commission. They did not care that he was ill.

Daisy took it upon herself to telephone Dr. Blackman of B.C. College of Physicians and Surgeons on behalf of Ken who was relapsing fast under the constant stress and had taken to his bed again, too ill to talk with them.

Blackman initially objected to speaking to her instead of Ken. Daisy insisted. There was a verbal tussle. Blackman grudgingly agreed to speak with her. Blackman told Daisy to let Ken know he cannot retire; instead he must *resign,* but only if he will agree the College can publish a statement about the unresolved disciplinary dispute. Daisy argued with Blackman with no good results. The only agreement Blackman would make was a possible damping down of the College's intended statement.

The meeting over the phone angered Daisy. She was feeling critical of physicians who should understand illness.

Daisy had an ominous feeling that when Ken bravely resigns rather than retiring from his work as a physician, he will die. She knew that his life's work and his life go together.

BY AUGUST 3, 2003, Ken had revived enough to write again:

M. VanAndel, M.D., Registrar,
College of Physicians & Surgeons of British Columbia,
Dear Dr. VanAndel,

Re: July 8, 2003 letter
CPS File #4495 DIS 02 06

Further to the conversation between Dr. Blackman and Daisy Heisler, the intended statement to be published in the #41 of the College Quarterly and in the 2004 Annual Report is incorrect. To this day **I have not resigned***.*

I suffered heart failure a week after a meeting with the audit team of MSC last September. I have been unable to practice medicine since then. I am not covered by insurance and cannot afford a lawyer to defend me. I cannot attend any more meetings to defend my Hippocratic Oath and my character.

I have not paid my College fees for 2003 for lack of money. Because my illness prevents me from continuing my practice, I need to retire. I suggest that the publication be changed to reflect the fact that I will **retire** **due to ill health**. *I have not resigned for reasons of disciplinary charges.*

Please consider the following statement to allow me to retire formally:

> **'The College of Physicians & Surgeons of British Columbia has accepted the retirement of Dr. Kehnroth Schramm due to illness.'**

If you must say anything about the disciplinary action, you might add:

> **' At the time of the onset of his illness, Dr. Schramm was the subject of disciplinary charges with respect to failure to maintain medical records as required by Rule 13 of the Rules made under the Medical Practitioners Act because he was protecting patient confidentiality according to the Hippocratic Oath he took to do no harm and to respect patient privacy.'**

Sincerely
(signed) Kehnroth Schramm, M.D.

AFTERNOON AUGUST 2003. Ken was resting in his bed. Daisy had just come from the mailbox and excitedly paced the floor with an open magazine that arrived. The headlines on the cover had caught her attention.

"Ken, there is an article in this magazine!" She flapped the cover upward to read: "*MD Canada, July/August 2003.* The article is about the audits held similarly to ours across Canada and how doctors are committing suicide over them. The headline article is called '*Audited to Death*' written by Veronica Mandel. It is about how the governments are using insults of doctors' characters and threats under the guise of an audit in order to do a claw back of ten percent of their earnings. They attack by first demanding all the earnings for several years and then settle for ten percent. Doesn't this sound familiar? Some doctors are so insulted that they actually commit suicide. The physician in this picture practiced in Ontario. They say he committed suicide because of loss of face even though he did nothing wrong!"

Ken was wistful. "I wish we had known that two years ago. We would have known what kind of fight we were in... that all the principles in the world did not matter... that it was just money they were after. That's obviously why they were not interested in my questions or answers regarding patient rights and what constitutes a medical record for psychotherapy."

"Yes, and they would lie about the doctors' characters to get the doctors so frightened that they settled for the ten percent. I suddenly understand why I kept reading in the B.C. Medical Services newsletters that so many doctors were settling for hundreds of thousands of dollars – a percentage of their earnings. That is the paper in which Musto said he would publish about you."

THE MATTER OF bad behavior on the part of physicians had been published over the years in the **BC Medical Services Physician's Newsletter** under a column named **Audit Update and Audit Files Settled By Negotiation.** That information never reached the general public but nevertheless was damaging to physicians who cared about their good name and to specialists like Ken, who relied solely on the referral system. Some misdemeanors and punishments listed in the newsletters were: general practitioner... highest biller of house calls... repay $36,750; general practitioner did not provide adequate justification of the medical necessity for specific services provided... repay $115,000; inadequate justification of the medical necessity for specific services provided... settlement to repay $165,000; paediatrician concerning inappropriate billings for office visits, complete physical exams, emergency visits, prolonged counseling and after-hours visits... repay $316,000; general practitioner... billing improperly for complete physical exams, prolonged counseling and out-of-office emergency services... $48,403... and many more.

For the first time, Daisy believed she had insight into the printed information she had been reading and wondering about for years, whereby physicians were found guilty of overcharging for one thing or another and were allowed to continue practicing if they would pay a large sum of money to the B.C. government, usually in the hundreds of thousands of dollars.

Over the twenty plus years that Daisy had worked with Ken, there had been raises in fees for service paid to physicians as a result of the B.C. Medical Association negotiations with the government. News reports often publicly announced the raises. She had been doing billings long enough to also have seen several rollbacks of moneys that were quietly taken behind the scenes following the raises; rollbacks that the public were not made aware of. These across the board rollbacks, sometimes as much as ten percent, had been taken each month from the earnings of physicians. But these present audits were different. They were mean, meant to destroy.

After hearing about the article 'Audited to Death', Ken was sad. "It has cost me my health." Ken looked sorrowfully at the ceiling.

"Ken, I want you to know, I admire you. You are a hero. I am on your side all the way."

Ken turned his face toward Daisy. He brightened a little. "Thank you. I need to know that. I'm trying to get well, Daisy."

"Every time you make any progress in getting well, you get hit again with another blow by those horrible people. All the medicine in the world could not counteract the constant blows. It's amazing you are here at all."

"I have kept my Hippocratic Oath. They told me I am the only doctor they have met who refused them the patients' secrets."

"You have done that. I admire you with all my heart."

15 SEPT '03 KEN WROTE in his journal:

"after almost healthy almost died defending his Hippocratic Oath to keep the secrets of families he visited, he retired knowing his oath is no longer defensible within medicare and no accurate diagnosis or treatment possible without privacy of spiritual counseling"

"i imagine writing all your relations gramma and grampa stories for seven generations
helping me into dying living another world to live in
letting go of attachments as living dying Buddhism"

"I have been lucky to learn and practice Buddhist meditation (Trungpa) Tai Chi (Joe Wong, Cam Tran, Lao Tse)
Prayer (Congregationalism, John Dewey)
Judaism (Jacob Neusner, Rosensweig & Rosenstock)
Fire keeping (Lakota Sweat Lodge)"

> *"Missing Leggo poems*
> *i have Longfellow's nose*
> *a nose for news in Leggo poems*
> *not the news of Knowlton Nash"*

56

Making a Choice

AT AGE EIGHTY-NINE, Daisy's father had been the victim of a home invasion. In October of 2000, he had been hit on the head and laid paralyzed on the floor for three days before Daisy's sister discovered him. Daisy had taken an emergency flight to Regina. The compassionate doctor in charge of his surgery was not sure her father would survive an operation so he waited for Daisy to arrive at the hospital to be with him before taking him at midnight into the operating room he had kept open.

It took only minutes after Daisy's arrival for her to find problems and question protocol. Just before her father was wheeled into the operation room, a nurse said he would have to have a catheter inserted in his penis. Daisy asked why since the problem was in his head. The nurse replied that it was in case he urinated while under anaesthetic. Daisy objected, requesting that a diaper or extra linen be used, just in case. The nurse said it was hospital protocol and that the operation would not be done unless the catheter was inserted. In other words, an invasive procedure was used that could introduce bacteria and infection into the body instead of simply washing linen. There was no time to argue because the doctor was already waiting in the operating room.

During the wait while their father was in surgery, Daisy's sister told her that the nurse in Emergency had given her supreme hell over her father's condition when he arrived by ambulance at the hospital because he had lain on the floor for three days and was not bathed before coming to the hospital. The nurse angrily and roughly bathed their father and roughly chopped his hair short.

After the draining of a pool of blood that had formed in his head to the size of one third of one side of his brain, he did survive. The catheter was removed after he was wheeled into his room. He was horrified at the procedure.

He was never able to live on his own again. He made a valiant struggle to get well, but instead of baking his own bread and gardening the best garden around as he had done, he lingered in hospital and nursing homes praying for death. Determined to stay on his beloved sunny prairies, he had refused Daisy's invitation to move to "rainy" Vancouver where she could care for him in her home.

The hospitals and nursing homes were rough for a man like him. In the first hospital, a strange woman climbed into bed with him one night, scaring him. Never the less, he like the hospital but it was time limited; he was forced to move to a care home. The Lutheran care home came next with promises that he would be able to bake bread and garden but once he became a resident, it turned out they had made hollow promises.

He had always been a personally clean man and took clean care of his food. Some women residents turned out to be terrible bullies. A couple of women were determined to make his meals unclean by throwing their food and drinks at him at mealtimes in the dining room and did so even when Daisy had lunch with him. Angry resident women accosted him in the hallway, making trouble by not allowing him to pass by peacefully. For Daisy, it was a shocking education in how some women can become mean as they grow older and how they act it out toward men, but if the man dares to retaliate, they cry foul and accuse him of abuse.

He liked salt but all the food had no salt. The facility had a policy in a 'grandfather clause' that allowed staff and residents who smoked to continue, but newcomers, no matter what age, were not allowed to smoke; the newcomers had to watch and smell others smoke. People, actually they were all women, would smoke right outside his window but he was not allowed out there in the space he had been promised he could grow a garden. Staff, who were all women looking after Daisy's father, often mishandled him, causing pain. He sometimes cried out in pain while talking to Daisy on the phone when certain attendants were in the room. Underpaid staff robbed him of things in his room.

To make matters worse, clergy visited him to say he was delusional about divining and that he was "dead wrong" about "seeing" anything beyond what was in front of his nose because there was nothing, and definitely he had no healing powers. Being a man of personal honest pride – this took its toll. Other than years earlier losing his first wife who was the love of his life and mother of his children, this experience was his worst nightmare.

He had never been medicated in all his life. Administration, run by a woman, medicated him for complaining about the injustices he was subjected to. He was supposed to take abuse quietly. Medicating residents was obviously a control trick rampant in the nursing home. People with vacant eyes sat listlessly in hallways; some women held lit cigarettes ready to drop. For Daisy, it had been a horrendous experience that would haunt her for failing to protect her father, though she tried by making several trips back and forth regarding his care.

The care home doctor took his direction from the administration staff rather than think for himself, even though they knew nothing about medicine. Daisy had been in a constant fight with the doctor, whose real interest was to get the job done quickly and disappear to spend time in California or Florida with his girlfriend on weekends. .

Right after the draining of his head, and healing three extra holes, Daisy's father had been able to continue doing his daily pastime of crossword puzzles. While in the first hospital, Daisy bought a pen that wrote upside down and more books of crossword puzzles so that he could lie in bed and do his puzzles. After moving to the Lutheran home and medications started, he could no longer do crossword puzzles and gave up another love – reading. He became listless and weak. Life was draining away. Another catheter was inserted into his penis permanently because under medication, he had no control. As another side effect of the medications, his health quickly declined into heart failure. His legs and feet swelled with water. He was sick. Daisy easily recognized the symptoms. The experience at the Lutheran care home in Regina was a lesson in *how to kill a man* who had been alert and vibrant when entering the facility only weeks before.

Daisy made a trip to Regina to personally fight with the physician after several unsuccessful telephone calls. Instead of waiting for him at the care home, she and her sister took their father to the doctor's office to confront him. She wanted all allopathic medications stopped and replaced with

Orthomolecular treatment and Homeopathy. Using what she had learned from Ken and armed with reference books she had brought all the way from Vancouver to show and tell, she won the fight. The doctor gave in. The new treatment started and her father recovered quickly from heart failure, much to the doctor's surprise. The doctor had been reluctant but in the end he had learned something. After that, he refused to answer any of her phone calls. Then the doctor Daisy had been fighting with suddenly left the country and she was downright happy that he was gone – south – **good riddance!** But now Daisy's father was kicked out of the Lutheran Care Home in Regina.

The Lutheran Care Home had been torture for Daisy's father and obviously for others. It came to light that on another floor, people were being tied to chairs where they stayed even when they needed to relieve themselves and sat in it. This was discovered when staff went on strike and volunteers took over.

Ken's father and Daisy's father had both been victims of mishandled medical care as doctor's defied family concerns. In both cases, their father's became casualties of psychotropic medications.

IN NOVEMBER 2003 Daisy's father was in another hospital, Pioneer Village, after being kicked out of the Lutheran care home. His mealtimes were better. In all, people, including women, were more respectful. But now he was deathly ill and not expected to survive. He had influenza and pneumonia.

It was a toss-up about who to be with. Believing Ken will live and her father may not, Daisy left Ken in Antony's care. Three years after the home invasion, Daisy was in Regina again at her father's bedside.

Three years earlier while Daisy stayed a week in Regina with her father, at home her little Miniature Schnauzer had refused to eat the whole week; she became ill and died. Now Daisy was finally ready for another dog. Because of his love of animals, Daisy bought a tiny white Maltipoo puppy from what turned out to be a puppy mill farm. The puppy chose Daisy by plastering herself like glue onto Daisy's chest. She fit in the palm of her hand. Daisy brought the puppy to her father to lay in his hands each day.

Her intention was to stay by her father's side until his last breath and to help her sister and brother Bill take care of family matters.

Daisy and her puppy spent day and often all night just being with her father, remembering and reminiscing years gone by. In the first hospital, his room had overlooked Wascana Lake – the exact spot where they ice-fished together and he forever bragged to everyone about how his young daughter had caught the biggest fish. This new room overlooked the historic mansion where Daisy had worked as secretary for the Saskatchewan Arts Board.

He had lived his life with music and dance. The old ornate parlor organ given to him by a neighbor was Daisy's elephant to learn to play when she really wanted a piano, but the organ was also her father's instrument that he played on Sunday nights to serenade his children to sleep. He always carried a harmonica (then called a mouth organ) in his pocket, which he played all the time, every spare moment. The mouth organ was part of him but when his hands were busy doing something, he whistled tunes. Remembering his love of music and dance, it was time to ask the important question never asked before. She asked him if he ever regretted not going off with his cousin, the famous musician and bandmaster, Lawrence Welk.

Her father answered, "No. We had fun playing local dances when he came to Saskatchewan. He would dance with my wife. He asked me to join the band but I had my wife and we were starting our family. I had a job."

"Dad, do you ever regret the money you could have made?"

"No. I had what I wanted in life."

The answer fit. This man had been a dowser. He had found water for farmers on the prairies. When offered money, he would refuse it, saying he would not take money for a gift given to him. He was afraid of losing his gift if he took any money, so all expenses to do his dowsing work were his. He developed his 'gift' so that he could dowse anything, anywhere at a distance by just drawing a map. He could lay his hands near a person and 'see' the internal body as though looking at an X-ray. He knew when a person was accepting a healing and when it curled back in rejection. He had taught as many of his children as were interested. Daisy, holding the willow branch, had walked the fields with him and learned from him.

Is it any wonder Daisy could understand Ken and why she chose to be with a man who would rather be a healer and make a better world for no money in payment, and a man who wanted to pass on what he knows to those who are willing?

A DISTRESSED TELEPHONE CALL from Ken to Daisy prompted her to call their bankruptcy Trustee by long distance from Regina to find out what the trouble was. The Trustee was stressed over a forced second 'First Bankruptcy Hearing'. He also said VanCity wanted them off their home mortgage and that VanCity had come up with a payout figure of Twenty-five Thousand Dollars that she and Ken must come up with to buy their way out. He insisted that she must return for the meeting. He informed her that she was expected at a meeting November 14th in Vancouver, only a few days away. She objected because her father was expected to die at any moment. He insisted.

Of course, true to Daisy's experiences, there had to be one last disagreement before leaving the hospital that last evening. Daisy's father had developed pneumonia with a severe, painful, choking cough. Daisy asked for a humidifier to help him. It was refused. Daisy offered to get one and bring it in. On duty nurses told her, "**No** humidifier is going to be allowed under any circumstances!"

With hospital administration closed for the night, Daisy ran out of time to carry on the fight to protect her father into a peaceful death. The nurse gave her father cough medicine instead of a humidifier. He stopped communicating entirely as he was drugged. He was suddenly catatonic.

ON THAT MORNING of the flight home, Daisy's father remained silent with eyes closed and hands across his chest as she tried to say goodbye. She did not know if he was unconscious or refusing to acknowledge her leaving. They each knew they will never see each other again and never will she hear his stories again, but she needed to make a choice. Her father will die. There is no turning back. Ken is ill and she must help him through another obstacle and hopefully he will live.

On her return to Vancouver, Daisy found Ken extremely shaken and weak. His health had taken a turn for the worse under blows of the latest accusations.

They had a brief respite with the little white ball of fluff that she brought back to surprise Ken. His face lit up and he relaxed. Ken, bundled in a blanket on the patio with his grandchildren around him, watched the little puppy explore the patio. He could not stop smiling. The puppy and Ken would become sleeping companions day and night. The two had each been abused and needed to heal; they took great comfort in each other.

DAISY READ THE LETTER from VanCity Credit Union and understood how a letter can kill.

Just before Daisy's trip to Regina, because of a note on her bank account, a teller at VanCity Credit Union had refused to take cash to pay a Hydro bill. Daisy called VanCity head-office. A person named Katherine in Lee Chamber's office at VanCity gruffly explained to Daisy that VanCity wanted her and Ken out of their bank because they do not want bankrupt members. That phone call seemed to wake up VanCity.

While Daisy was away, Lee Chambers, Bankruptcy Specialist at VanCity suddenly revved up to fight the bankruptcy. The BC government's legal office had supplied Lee with a copy of Judge Oliver's 1990 Reasons for Judgment against Ken. She wrote a letter repeating Judge Oliver's statements and added her own judgmental remarks to provide leverage to bring about a second 'First' Bankruptcy Hearing.

VanCity had been sleeping at the wheel and missed the First Bankruptcy Hearing. The B.C. office of bankruptcy buckled under pressure from the powerful institution of VanCity and a second 'First' Bankruptcy Hearing was scheduled as though it was a First Hearing.

Chambers used Oliver's Judgment to bring to life again the accusations that Ken had hidden money and diverted money to Daisy and her family; she was suggesting he was hiding money again. Using sections of the Judgment, Lee Chambers resorted to vile name-calling. Based on that Judgment she suggested Ken had no illness. Chambers asked for all clinical records in Halliday format from doctors who may have treated Ken and/or written any letters on his behalf; all books of account used in Dr. Schramm's medical practice for the past five years; personal Income Tax returns, including receipts, for Dr. Schramm and Daisy for the past 5 years.

OUTRAGED AND REFUSING to comply with Lee Chambers' demands, Daisy immediately emailed an answer to their Trustee, saying VanCity already had on file every penny earned and spent in the past twenty plus years and there was nothing elsewhere, and if Chambers wanted accounting information, she should go to work and look at VanCity's own files.

Daisy's letter also refused medical files on the grounds that VanCity had no right to request personal medical records and certainly they had no right to patient files of any kind.

THE MORNING AFTER Daisy's return to Vancouver, news came that her father died.

Father Christmas was gone a month before Christmas as Christmas music hit the airwaves. Daisy thought back to the Christmas when she was only one and a half years old. She remembered clearly the shiny kitchen floor, feeling her smallness as she ran under the kitchen table and wanted to see over the table but was not tall enough, while her mother, who towered above, was cooking by the stove. Santa Claus in a red suit trimmed with white came through the door and how she howled and trembled so hard in fear of the strange figure that she thought the floor was shaking beneath her; she hid behind her mother's skirt. Santa Claus tried to calm her and handed her a Wetums doll, the little doll that peed when she was fed water from her bottle. Her parents had been surprised by her reaction and even though she was small, she was aware that they felt sorry for scaring her. From then on, Father Christmas gave his children lots of Santa Claus experiences, sometimes in a red suit and sometimes in a black coat with a bag full of toys. He always made fudge on Christmas Eve after the family decorated the eight-foot tall Douglas Fir tree that he always walked home through all kinds of snow and ice. Then they would dance and open gifts. Those were the days when he would teach Daisy how to dance ballroom dances with his records spinning music on the gramophone that had to have the needles changed after each and every record. Daisy would play Vienna Waltzes on the organ by day and dance them with her father in the evening. How he enjoyed Christmas with his family. Then there would be the knock on the door every Christmas Eve and Daisy's music teacher would come in with her cheerful greetings and her box of homemade chocolates for the family; she was a spinster and took special interest in the family Christmas tree every year, admiring it from top to bottom. And Daisy's mother would then start cooking for Christmas Day and the cabbage rolls would be put into the oven of the wood fire stove to fill the house with aromas of Christmas all through the night. Somewhere during the night, her father would clear and water the skating rink he maintained for his children in the back yard and stoke the furnace for continued warmth in the home.

The great memory of the trips back and forth to Regina was in meeting up with brother Bill and taking respite walks in the old neighborhood, reminiscing childhood memories and like kids, sneaking a cigarette on the outdoor skating rink they had spent so much time on while growing up.

HAVING GATHERED Ken up to sit with her by the ocean, they were both not up for a walk so they sat on a log watching the November weather play with the ocean. It was a windy, mostly grey day. High waves were wild in various shades of grey-green with large frothy white caps. It seemed perfect for remembering and mourning the loss of a father. The salty air was misty-wet as though crying for their father.

57

Corruption or What?

OVER THE YEARS, VanCity had actually made a lot of money on Ken, Daisy, and their extended family through bank accounts and mortgages.

Ken had not gone bankrupt on one cent of VanCity money. Attacking him was a strange thing to do. In fact, a VanCity money counselor had wrongfully advised him to move money out of a retirement savings account into an account on which he then, that same year, had to pay taxes on because he moved the money before retirement age. VanCity had also convinced Ken to put inheritance money into an account where he could "borrow" against his own money, but they did not tell him that they made regular reports to the credit bureau that he was borrowing against VanCity money instead of his own money, while at the same time telling Ken this was a good investment; they also neglected to tell him that he needed to repay his own money in this account every month or he was given a bad credit record for not doing so. Ken thought all along that he was free to use his own money. Since money was not his foremost interest, he trustingly relied on advice from bank employees and often got wrong advice.

THE STRESS OF another attack by way of old accusations laid out by Judge Oliver to satisfy Jane Anderson was too much for Ken. He had another heart attack.

The morning of the second First Bankruptcy Hearing, Ken was critically ill. He could not get out of bed.

Anger raged in Daisy. She was angry about what people had done and were still doing to Ken over cold money but without thoughts of human caring. Her father had died right after she had been forced to leave his side and she was angry about that. With all her emotions hovering the surface, she tried to be civil with the Trustee, explaining to him by telephone that she could not trust herself to speak civilly to any of those people in a Hearing, and Ken was far too ill to get out of bed. She really meant she was afraid she would rage at them and call them all sorts of deserved vile names.

The Trustee understood and attended the Hearing by himself.

As the meeting was going on across town, Daisy spent that time on the telephone with her sister, writing an obituary and making plans for her sister to carry out the cremation of their father.

VANCITY AND THE B.C. GOVERNMENT representatives were present at the second First Hearing of Bankruptcy. Their anger that Ken and Daisy had not shown up caused disruption of the meeting. The Trustee had his hands full convincing them to lay off under the circumstances.

If revenge was worth something, that's what they got but in money terms, book keeping was obviously not their talent. To make it work in their favor and to make the second First Hearing worthwhile even for a few pennies, they had fudged the actual figures of Daisy and Ken's portion ownership of the house.

Lee Chambers of VanCity was accusing Ken of lying about assets when filing for bankruptcy because of a fraction of a number even though the mortgage held by VanCity was only listed on the asset side and not included in the bankruptcy. It consisted of ownership one-sixth Daisy, one-sixth Ken and two-thirds the rest of the family and that was how Daisy had handwritten the bankruptcy papers. Daisy and Ken's asset was so small on a fairly new mortgage that the Trustee had considered it not worth anyone's interest and assured them that it was safe under bankruptcy rules. Now VanCity insisted that two-sixths, or when added together as one-third really meant just a tiny fraction under half and they wanted the asset based on a larger fictitious fraction. That was how they came up with a bankruptcy payout of Twenty-five Thousand Dollars.

Daisy felt terrible because in fact, on the day Ken had signed the bankruptcy statements in the Trustee's office, Ken was too ill to read or write. She had written the answers in all the blanks and did so honestly, not missing even a fraction. Ken had nothing to do with it except that he was physically present and without reading any of it, he put his signature to what Daisy told him to sign. In the anxiety of the moment, when the typed copy came back for signing, she had missed the fact that one-sixth was missing on Ken's asset side. The typist had made an error.

Bankruptcy rules dictated that Daisy had been forced to include a VanCity loan on her side of the bankruptcy. Daisy wondered why VanCity had not accused her of wrongdoing but instead attacked Ken when he was completely innocent of any mistake and had not gone bankrupt on any VanCity money.

AFTER THE HEARING, extended family sat in front of a VanCity loans officer ready to sign new mortgage papers based on the old mortgage that they were now taking over, plus the payout of the designated Twenty-five Thousand Dollars, leaving Daisy and Ken off the mortgage as VanCity required. As they were about to sign for the new mortgage, the loans officer received a phone call. The family waited and listened while he talked with someone. When he got off the phone, he claimed he was under direction of Lee Chambers to *stop* the signing of the mortgage as written. He then proceeded to rant that Ken and Daisy were crooks. The family was shocked. Then he presented an inflated mortgage. One Hundred and Fifty Thousand Dollars plus future years of interest had been added on to the mortgage in a matter of minutes as a result of that phone call.

Since the equity on a fairly new mortgage was in land value that had risen, VanCity made it clear they wanted to cash in on the new value as though they owned the land and were selling the house to new owners. The loans officer presented the new figures for signing.

The family walked out in disgust without signing.

The family was in a bind, not knowing what to do. They needed a mortgage immediately. Ken got out of bed to phone around. He was determined to find a broker who would find a bank that would take over the mortgage with the original honest numbers. He was successful. He had used what little precious energy he had to help and then went back to bed to recover.

VANCITY STINK CARRIED ON in two ways. After all their nastiness, they charged several thousands of dollars to end the house mortgage before a transfer to another bank could be made.

As a result of all the problems with VanCity, Daisy discovered that VanCity had misplaced more than Three Thousand and Six Hundred Dollars of her money at the time of buying the house when she had cashed in retirement savings funds for her portion of the down payment and legal fees. There had been an excess of money from the fund in the amount of $3,600 that should have been accounted for by being rolled back into an RRSP or at least put into her bank account. It had gone missing instead. She did not want the money now that she was bankrupt but the missing money had to be accounted for in bankruptcy.

Thinking it all a mistake, she started by talking to bank managers at VanCity. One person did offer to do a search and found himself blocked. He wrote a letter explaining to Daisy that he was "forbidden to discuss the matter" because it had to go through the department where Lee Chambers worked.

Daisy tried to find the money by phone calls and letters to Lee Chambers office and several other departments of VanCity's administration offices. They all refused to talk. It became evident there was a cover-up about the missing money.

On a personal visit to consult again with the VanCity bank manager who had written the letter about not being able to talk, he was seen running to a back room as Daisy, accompanied by Ken, entered his branch. Daisy asked the receptionist when he would be available. The woman answered, "Never!"

A brick wall had been put up throughout VanCity. Daisy wrote a letter to the CEO of co-operative banking in British Columbia. She supposed his mandate was to be fair and concerned. She outlined the various discrepancies that had taken place at VanCity. He wrote a "confidential" letter back to say he would have nothing to do with the matter.

Daisy then wrote a letter to the CEO of VanCity. His answering letter was prompt and curt in telling Daisy to get lost and not bother him any further.

Adding this all up, Daisy debated going the next step, to the VanCity Board of Directors, but decided against hitting her head against the wall any more.

Daisy was extremely miffed. While VanCity Credit Union employees were accusing Ken of wrongdoing, and she and Ken were both being called "crooks", the same people refused to account for the missing $3,600 plus and a cover-up was happening from bottom to top. On top of that, they had attempted to literally steal hundreds of thousands of dollars through a phony mortgage, while at the same time they were running ads on television stating that VanCity is there to help people.

THE DOUBLE STANDARD was mind-boggling. So many letters of the past couple of years had *'confidential'* written on them. The writers understood the meaning of the word 'confidential' when they wanted to cover their own rear ends by keeping secret what they were saying. On the other hand, what started this whole mess was that in a medical practice, Ken's patients were not respected to have the right to confidentiality and Ken's Hippocratic Oath to do no harm and keep his patients' secrets was not being respected by many of these same people.

58

Resignation

DECEMBER 30, 2003

Morris VanAndel, M.D., Registrar,
College of Physicians & Surgeons of B.C.

Dear Dr. VanAndel,
I am writing to resign from membership in the College of
Physicians and Surgeons of British Columbia for reasons of:

ill health due to a two year long "pattern of practice audit" which
exhausted all my physical, mental, emotional and financial
resources, preventing me from disputing in writing and in person
the claims made by Medical Services Commission and the College
of Physicians and Surgeons of British Columbia that I "kept no
medical records," making it impossible for me to continue my
home visit psychotherapy practice; ethical conflicts between my
Hippocratic Oath to do no harm and to keep secret what my
patients told me in our respectful and truthful conversations
necessary to make accurate diagnosis and complete realistic
treatment plans made in their own homes, documenting what I
did rather than what my patients said or did in my medical
records, and in my conversations or correspondence with their
referring physicians; and the legal requirements to provide
confidential patient medical records to lawyers, bureaucrats, and
auditing physicians without the informed consent of my patients,
and without opportunities to negotiate these ethical conflicts in
the absence of any appeal process.

This month the Canadian Medical Association sent to
physicians across Canada a poster to be put up on our office
walls as a promise to our patients. The heading of the poster

states that:

"Privacy of personal health information is a fundamental right of health care in Canada. As your doctor, when you provide me or my staff with health information I give you these assurances: I will only collect information required for your care and treatment...only share your information with other health professionals or health care institutions to the extent necessary to provide you with proper health care..."

During the Medical Services Commission audit, Dr. Semrau demanded that I give a psychiatric diagnosis for every patient every three months and details of their personal lives. In keeping my Hippocratic Oath I promised my patients that they would not be labeled, their personal secrets would remain secret, and that only necessary treatment or referral information would be recorded. There are no clear guidelines from the Medical Services Commission and the College of Physicians and Surgeons of B.C. addressing issues of privacy, medical audits, and actions needed to protect patient confidentiality so that accurate diagnoses and realistic treatment plans can be made and recorded by physicians doing psychotherapy within the Medical Services Plan of B.C. The absence of these guidelines increases the vulnerability to audit of physicians providing needed counseling services to their patients.

Health problems of physicians undergoing practice audits are well documented in the article "Audited to Death?" published in MD Canada in July/August 2003.

I appreciate your compassionate attempt to resolve the issues of my resignation in 2003. I am in general agreement with your proposed publication (page 2 of your letter dated August 21, 2003) of the context of my resignation. However, I ask that the ethical issues I have raised in this letter and in previous correspondence with you be publicly acknowledged with a commitment that the College of Physicians and Surgeons of B.C. will study conflicts between requirements of the new privacy laws and current medical auditing practices of physicians who are doing counseling or psychotherapy in B.C. This study should develop an appeal process to protect the health of physicians who are being audited with written guidelines for medical audits and medical practices which respect patients, physicians, and laws which protect their privacy because this protection is necessary for physicians to make accurate diagnoses and to complete realistic treatment plans. I hope I am contributing to this process by writing this letter to you.

Sincerely,
(signed) Ken Schramm, M.D.

* * *

THE COLLEGE did **not** acknowledge or answer Ken's letter. They published the following in the:

2004 College of Physicians and Surgeons of British Columbia Annual Report

December 30, 2003 Kehnroth Schramm North Vancouver

The College accepted the resignation of Dr. Kehnroth Schramm as a member of the College, effective December 30, 2003. Dr. Schramm retired from the practice of medicine due to ill health. At the time of his resignation Dr. Schramm was the subject of charges alleging failure to maintain medical records, as required by Rule 13 of the Rules, made under the *Medical Practitioners Act*. Dr. Schramm denied the allegations but due to health reasons at the time of his resignation the charges had not been able to be adjudicated.

THE COLLEGE IGNORED KEN'S REQUEST to publish:

"...because he was protecting patient confidentiality according to the Hippocratic Oath he took to do no harm and to respect patient privacy."

The College of Physicians and Surgeons of British Columbia Annual Report 2004 was placed on the worldwide web.

ANOTHER CHRISTMAS came and went. Instead of a wedding, Ken has been resigning from practicing medicine – a monumental time in the life of a physician.

59

A Man Without Armor

FEBRUARY 25, 2004

Dear Jo-ann,

I am writing to request an extension of my graduate studies to complete my Ph.D. program by Fall 2005. In the Fall of 2002 I suffered a catastrophic illness from which I have recovered sufficiently to do what is needed to write my Ph.D. dissertation...

* * *

Dear Carl,

I just now confirmed with Jo-ann on the telephone that I will write an overview of dissertation with a timetable...

* * *

Writing in the night, Ken amused himself with remembering ancestors. Ken found a comparison Wadsworth photo on the internet.

Feb. 16, 2004. Hello Carl, Here is a one-minute poem.
> *I have Henry Wadsworth Longfellow's nose*
> *but I don't know what he knows*
> *I am more of a Hiawatha*
> *than a Wadsworth*
> *for all that's worth*
> *to John and Pricilla Alden*

SPRING 2004. FOR NEARLY THREE YEARS, hardly a day or week had gone by without a nasty letter arriving from someone representing the BC government or the BC College of Physicians and Surgeons. Now VanCity Credit Union lawyers joined the gang and were particularly vile in their letters. What seemed obvious was that those people appeared to be void of anything representing human compassion.

Daisy could not help wondering about those people. Why did they congregate into those jobs and bond together in an effort to destroy a man – any man – but in Ken's case, a man who only dedicated his life to giving and healing. For what did those people live – Power? Prestige? Money? Where were their mothers? Who were their mothers? Where was that one person in the lot who would object to a slaughter and stand up to defend moral principles? No such person made an appearance out of that bunch. Instead, the slaughterers multiplied in support of each other and no doubt they felt like heroes going home to families, or as they ate at a favorite restaurant with satisfaction that they had earned enough money to spend there. These people were teaching younger people how to do white collar bullying by example while society wondered how to stop bullying our schools.

IT WAS EVENING. Ken relaxed against a pile of pillows in bed close to the open garden patio doors. Daisy sat on the edge of the bed with him while he sipped medicinal tea. They did not hear the woman who once again managed to sneak up on them, suddenly looming large as she stood over them at the open glass doors. For Ken, she had entered the privacy of his bedroom. The strange woman shoved legal papers at a shocked Daisy, who saw the bottom of the woman's shoes as she ran away.

Glancing at the papers, Daisy explained to Ken, "The B.C. Government has registered a dispute to our Discharge from bankruptcy. They will be there in the courtroom."

The next evening, they were not expecting a repeat of the night before. Again, Ken was trying to read a book in his bed near the door. He usually did that until he fell asleep and the book would lay on his chest. Daisy was painting a picture at the table next to him. They were surprised when a strange man appeared suddenly at the open garden patio door, again interrupting privacy. He shoved a brown envelope at Daisy through the open space and disappeared fast.

Daisy told Ken, "Boy, they aren't letting up. They are all sneaking through the garden. They don't even knock on the front door. This is from VanCity. Their lawyers have also registered that they dispute Discharge from bankruptcy. They will be in the courtroom."

Ken has no fight left in him. He was obviously helpless in this barrage of personal interruptions and legalized threats.

JUNE 2004 DAWNED the morning of the Discharge Hearing. Ken was lying under a blanket on the sofa. "Daisy, I'm so sorry you have to do this on your own. I'm too sick."

Taking Ken's hand and kneeling beside him, Daisy tried to ease his pain. "I'm glad you will stay here where you are safe with Antony. I'm strong enough to do this."

"I am so sorry for all the trouble I've brought to you." Ken was extremely sad.

"I love and admire you. You are a man of honor. I'd rather be with you than anywhere else."

Tears came to Ken's eyes. He nodded.

THE LARGE COURTROOM was crowded to the brim with hundreds of people; so many that they spilled through open doors into the hallway. Somewhere in this crowd were the representatives of the B.C. government and VanCity laying in wait to object verbally and publicly to the discharge. Daisy wondered who the enemies were in the sea of faces packed like sardines. Her Trustee had gathered her up from the hallway as soon as she arrived and after winding their way through the crowd, they took seats in front of the Judge.

The Trustee was a disheveled, older man that Daisy trusted regardless of all the troubles.

When called, the Trustee stood and handed a file to the Judge, saying, "Your honor, I am [name] trustee. I recommend that Ken Schramm and his common-law wife, Daisy Heisler, be discharged from bankruptcy. Dr. Schramm cannot be here today. He is critically ill, having had several heart attacks over the last two years."

The Judge looked directly at Daisy, "What has caused this bankruptcy?"

"Your honor..." The court clerk interrupted Daisy by telling her to stand when speaking to the Judge. Daisy had forgotten in her excitement and stood to continue.

"The Medical Services Commission has done an audit of the medical practice and they want all of six years gross income returned to them. We went bankrupt for the total of six years income and more money than we ever saw because it's a bunch of figures all doubling up and overlapping. The BC government wants six years earnings back because Dr. Schramm, a psychiatrist, doing psychotherapy in family homes, has lived by his Hippocratic Oath and protected the privacy of his patients, withholding the secrets of the patients from government auditors. I have worked with him over twenty-three years." Daisy sat down again.

The Judge asked, "What do you mean by 'protecting the privacy of his patients'? What kind of secrets?"

She forgot to stand again in the opportunity of having a real conversation with the Judge. This time no one bothered her about sitting or standing in anticipation of the answer.

"The British Columbia government wants every session with a patient justified by confidential detailed information. The government wants to know who is on drugs and who drinks alcohol, and they want all the patients labeled with psychiatric labels for every three months. What that means... if any member of your family is to see a psychiatrist, the government wants the details of what goes on in the privacy of your home and your family history, and to know all the confidential things talked about."

The Judge looked shocked. He shook his head slowly and paused for moment. Then, looking around the room, he asked, "Does anyone in this room object to a Discharge of this bankruptcy?"

The crowded room had taken on an eerie silence as though hundreds of people stopped breathing.

While waiting for an answer, the Judge briefly examined what was before him on the desk. Then, he looked around again at the room full of people. He waited for objection.

After all the legal papers filed and delivered along with all kinds of threats, the disputers seemed to have sunk through the floor boards and disappeared. Not one of those people dared show their face.

"Discharge granted!" the Judge pronounced loudly.

ON THE WAY HOME Daisy telephoned ahead from her cell phone to let Ken know the good news. Antony informed her that Ken was in serious trouble. Happiness turned to agonizing worry for the drive home.

She arrive home to find Ken was deathly ill – ashen white and without any strength, lying on the sofa where she left him. Antony had been looking after him through another bad episode and told his mother that Ken almost did not make it this time.

The one tiny win in almost three years was just not enough.

Ken told Daisy, "It was good of Antony to be here with me. I'm so sorry you had to do this by yourself, Daisy."

"I'm okay. It's over. They can't touch you anymore. Discharge granted! I think when they saw the look on the Judge's face, they did not dare speak up and show their own faces. Now you will be able to heal."

Daisy had been able to vent to the Judge and relish in a win, but Ken had not been able to do that. He, instead, felt bad about not being able to help her.

"I can't do battle anymore," Ken whispered.

"I know. You can't! No more! You haven't committed suicide like some doctors but they have been killing you for years. I want you to be retired now. You should spend the rest of your life in peace. There are no more people who can come after you."

But Daisy's private thoughts were: After all these years, an ex-wife's revenge has continued to harm Ken!

60

Two Years of Hope

WHILE FOR MORE than two years, people tried in earnest to tear Ken down and break him, hope was the other side of the story – that Ken would recover again for the next twenty years. He had done it once before.

After months of catastrophic illness, in his usual way of getting on with life, in January of 2003, Ken had written to Carl Leggo, his UBC advisor.

Good morning, Carl, here are my prayers
with words and thoughts and feelings in voices who come to me and from me
making my lives singing and dying with writing

almost healthy grampa almost dies before his seventieth birthday
having lived and died his biblical three score and ten
with his mother father stories
making his life death being physician poet friend lover father husband brother freedom fighter teacher learner fugitive refugee child crazy prayers and stories
brought him back to begin life after 70
writing his body mind spirit relations without hope

almost healthy was born almost dead with a hole in his spine at his neck where spinal cord and membranes bulged out terrifying his parents threatening infection paralysis living death as a vegetable person
almost healthy made his life with his mother's stories of his birth death
his recovery in the depths of the depression

thanks to her father's friend a general surgeon who put him together again
a humpty dumpty story
and fire keeping her fire with fire I walked a path made of mother gramma stories and my body remembered by fathers unsaid unspoken silent stories...

I imagine writing my PhD during the next two years...
after almost healthy almost died defending his Hippocratic Oath to keep the secrets of families he visited, he retired knowing his oath is no longer defensible with medicare and no accurate diagnosis or treatment possible without privacy of spiritual counseling...

I imagine writing all your relations gramma and grampa stories for with seven generations helping me into dying living another world to live in
letting go of attachments as living dying Buddhism...

Father Sky -- Mother Earth -- Creators -- All My Relations
Thank you for the gifts of life
your grandson grampa thanks you for giving me a home with you
where I can live and die today and remember and forgive and be forgiven. . .

IT HAD BEEN A SPECIAL DAY in that January of 2003 when Ken went to meet with his UBC advisor, Carl Leggo after nearly dying the previous September. Daisy had driven Ken to pick Carl up from his office at UBC and they drove to the nearby coffee shop where Carl bought Ken a big scoop of ice cream. It was the first ice cream Ken had since he had fallen ill. More than that, he had not seen Carl for months but had kept in touch through telephone calls and emails. Being with his beloved professor friend again and eating ice cream, Ken looked like a man who had been seriously ill but he was wonderfully happy. It was a healing time. After many dark days, hope for the future was alive and well.

In that January of 2003 and in the many months to come, when Ken was hopeful of a recovery, he craved to be by the calming ocean. During those months, though they were extremely broke and could hardly afford gas for the car, getting out for a walk by the ocean was a necessity. Ken walked very slowly and took advantage of sitting often in the sunlight on the benches placed every few feet along the beach. They followed the markers along the seawall of West Vancouver, telling that they were walking a little farther each day.

Feeling the cool breeze and the warmth of the sun on his face all at once, Ken would say, "This is so good for healing."

To be with Ken walking by the ocean, Daisy counted blessings. She had wondered in the darkness of his illness if they might ever do this again.

Ken's ill health was a direct result of too many years of stress and wrongful allegations. There was no clear escape – only moments of forgetfulness. There was always the knowledge accompanying their walks and all their efforts to heal and to stay calm, that in the background the battle raged between good and evil, healing and death, black and white, dishonesty and honesty.

IF EVER a man wanted to live, he was embodied in Ken. "Daisy, I didn't die! I'm having a chance at life again. Will you drive me out to the university? I would like to go to the library."

Always hopeful and wanting it to be true that Ken was truly over the hump, Daisy responded, "Ah, yes, library... your favorite place. Of course I'll drive you there."

During Ken's first month of illness, he had asked the university for a few months' sick leave and it was granted. However, when he was told that sick leave would bar him from being on campus grounds for any reason and from using the library, he refused to take it. Being cut off from the library would be like cutting off a body part. Just prior to falling ill, Ken had a client who did take the sick leave granted and found herself in serious trouble with the university for being seen using the library, even though she was living in student housing located on campus near the library.

Ken then asked for an extension in time for his PhD and had that granted.

Daisy understood that Ken's healing would come from continuing to research thoughts and ideas if he had any energy at all. Books were his way of communicating with philosophers and physicians of long ago. Even if he just held the books and fell asleep, he would be in a healing state.

And – he needed the fresh air and movement of walking, even if it was at a turtle pace.

Ken had been given a student job on a committee and he wanted to honor his commitment. "I need to get back to work on my PhD. Also, I need to get back to work on the committee, so I am asking you to come to the meetings and sit with me for protection. I'm still very weak and I want you there in case I have a heart attack or just can't walk."

Starting that January, Daisy did attend school meetings with him. Ken was happy to be back at school but he had little energy. Daisy was in an awkward position of just watching silently as he struggled to participate equally and ran out of energy within an hour. At first, she watched with eagle eyes about how people perceived him and sat ready to defend him but this department of the university was another world where people were extremely helpful and kind to both Ken and Daisy. She was welcomed along with Ken into their territory.

With not enough money to splurge on parking meters, Daisy often parked the car as close to the library doors as she could, where Ken could see her through the large glass windows fronting all the different floors of the main campus library. He told her that he needed to be able to see her at all times.

As usual, because Ken was always so ready to give of himself and his time, Daisy warned him, "Ken, please avoid using your energy trying to solve someone else's problems today. Just do your own thing."

He always walked extremely slowly but determined toward the library. Daisy was always torn about going with him because he looked so weak but on days with no money for parking meters, she needed to stay with the car or it would be towed away.

It was always a relief as he came out of the library to the waiting car because though he moved slowly and she wondered at times if he could even make it, he was determined to carry a bag of books and had some on his back in the backpack. She strongly believed his love of books and the authors who wrote them helped to keep him alive.

In the car Ken would tell her about the books he found for other people and their projects. She knew he would find the people to pass the books along.

She teased, "Just like you, thinking of everyone else and their projects even now. You end up paying for lost books when you don't get them back."

"I need to share knowledge. That's what I do best. I met [former client] in the library. She bent my ear for a while."

Frustrated that this often happened, Daisy responded, "I wish you would protect yourself better. Sometimes you need to just say you can't talk now. You are still in recovery. Besides you don't have any armor now. Did you tell her you love her, too?"

"Yes, I did."

"That's what I mean, Ken. You can get into trouble with people who don't understand your kind of unconditional love. Some women might think you are coming on to them. You are a challenge to protect even when you're sick."

After a moment of silence, he answered, "You're right... I need your guidance."

Daisy had watched several people, who had known Ken as his patients or at the university, when they would meet Ken again for the first time during the months of 2003 and 2004. They would looks sorrowfully at Ken. Shock and pity were written all over their faces because of how weak and shrunken he looked. Daisy would cringe just watching them but Ken would pretend nothing had changed and try to carry on a conversation with them.

LATER IN THE YEAR, an appointment had been set up with the financial aid office of the university just to find out if there might be some small grant available. Ken and Daisy waited for what seemed like a long time in the reception room. Then, a tall, young, blondish man exhibiting an extremely angry face with a cold stare stepped out of his office to call them in. No one had left his office, so he had obviously kept them waiting. They sat across the desk from him. Without preliminaries he spewed a range of nasty phrases that were intended to hit Ken like knives. On his desk he had Judge Oliver's Reasons for Judgment in Ken's open file.

Daisy was outraged that this young man, who knew nothing about Ken as a real person, was so contemptuous and at the same time held a professionally powerful position at the university. She wanted to give this guy the tongue-lashing he deserved but rather than make a scene, for Ken's sake she remained silent. They left quietly.

There it was again! Oliver's Judgment had been placed on Ken's file years earlier in the Jane Anderson Schramm/Bruce Katz blitz to get Ken removed from university.

IT HAD BEEN a roller-coaster ride following the Hearing in Victoria in September of 2002. The ups and downs of a continual fight for justice and protection of his Hippocratic Oath had taken a toll on Ken's life. Throughout 2002, 2003 and 2004 Ken fought daily for his life while many people in powerful jobs fought to harm him. It was truly an epic battle of one good man against goliath destructive forces.

With just a tiny surge of energy, Ken would climb out of bed in his usual positive way, wanting to get on with life to spread love around. Full of positive thinking, he always wanted to get back to UBC and resume his PhD. He would always be looking for someone to have food with, especially his sons. He loved to surprise a family member on a birthday with simple things, like stringing Christmas lights around Ron and Loraine's fireplace mantle to surprise them when they got home. He made occasional visits to the sweats at UBC where he had been a fire keeper but with limited energy, he was unable to fully do what he had done in the past.

His health had never recovered enough at any time to think he could continue a medical practice. With the ups and downs, he was so frail at all times, that he would have frightened patients; more than that, he just did not have enough energy to be the physician at work. He had tried to respectfully retire; after all, he was in his 70s, long past retirement age and he was ill. Physicians who were administrators at the College of Physicians and Surgeons of BC denied him that privilege. He had been forced to resign against his best wishes.

Seven seasons had come and gone since that September in 2002 when Ken had faced death. Through the seasons with sun, rain, wind, snow, and changing moons, Ken had chosen to be in a bed by the patio window where he felt less confined and could watch it all happen along with the colorful changes in the garden as it took a rest and renewed itself among the evergreens, and where he could breath the evening fragrance that the garden let off. His guardian cat and puppy were constantly with him. His books often rested on his chest as he would fall asleep.

Then came the eighth season...

61

Broken Heart

EMAIL: June 2004

Hello Andy and Stephen,

I hope we can meet Sunday for food and conversation and a walk. The stresses of the past two years seem to be over. I am well enough to resume writing my Ph.D. and plan to complete by Fall of 2005. During the past few months, I have had several episodes of fast and irregular heart beating with a feeling of imminent death which responds well to singing and loving company. I am determined to live and write each day as it comes and with you whenever possible.

good and happy journeys,

Dad

> EMAIL: June 19, 2004 9:45:27 AM PDT (CA)
>
> *Re: Father's Day & Andy's Birthday*
>
> *Hello Andy,*
>
> *I could not reach you at home so here's another email to ask what are your plans for your birthday?*
>
> *Dad*

EMAIL: From: kschramm

Subject: *Where are you?*

Date: June 22, 2004 8:28:30 AM PDT (CA)

To: andyschramm

 Cc: StephenS

Happy birthday! Andy

Love,

Dad

IN CHINESE MEDICINE, there is the belief that if a sick person rallies in the Spring, they will probably last another year.

The devastation of repeatedly being the butt of terribly false allegations coming from several directions leading up to the Bankruptcy Discharge Hearing in June of 2004 had taken a terrible toll on Ken's recovery. Ken relied on positive thinking, willpower, and prayer to keep going, but his pulses were even more erratic and fading instead of pounding as they used to do.

Knowing is difficult for a physician and Daisy was aware of possibly losing Ken. They clung to hope.

In August of 2004, at the eye examination for new glasses needed before starting the autumn term at UBC, Ken was told he would be blind in five years unless he undergoes an operation for cataracts. This was an unexpected, sad blow for a man who had spent his life practically living in and reading all the libraries.

On the drive home with new glasses made in an hour, both Ken and Daisy mulled over the knowledge that Ken's heart would not withstand an operation. Ken did not complain. He was quiet and Daisy was at a loss about how to help except to nourish him from the inside out with love and good food. She imagined she would read all the books to him to solve the problem.

Ken joined a summer class led by an aboriginal New Zealander that he admired. While doing a presentation in the class, Ken collapsed but revived enough to insist on taking a bus home and only informed Daisy of the incident at home.

There had been several incidents of near collapses and collapses during the summer where Ken almost could not complete his mission. Each time, he only told Daisy about the incident when he arrived home. He wanted to be alive so much and continue with his love of school, that he had insisted on buying and using his monthly bus passes for July and August. Daisy struggled with respecting his autonomy but worried every time he went out the door without her.

THEN ONE EVENING, Ken had been watching Daisy from his bed and bracing for her reaction to what was on his mind. He asked,

"Daisy, will you come with me on a small trip to the cemetery so that we can see it? I need you to understand my wishes."

He was surprised when she agreed and did not argue, even though she looked stunned.

From her point of view, she was willing to do anything that would give Ken peace of mind about the distant future.

It was a pleasant evening as they took the journey to the cemetery. Even though it was close to their home and its location could be seen across the green valley, neither had ever gone there.

They drove up the road past Capilano College where Daisy spent many happy hours studying and producing art and where Ken came to visit and offered encouragement, and where they had walked together through coloured leaves crunching under their shoes that afternoon in another August so long ago.

Across the road from the college and a next-door neighbor to the cemetery was an equestrian centre. The only riding trail was up the road through the cemetery and beyond into the green forest of the Seymour River water shed. The horses were reminiscent of Ken's beloved Vermont and Daisy's love of riding.

They drove through the middle of a most natural old growth forested cemetery they had ever seen. Ken took it all in silently. Daisy announced surprise at how beautiful it was. In her mind, it was an idea for the future – away 'way 'way in the distant future and hopefully never.

They were at the foot of Seymour Mountain where she and her children had learned to ski. They were on a foothill right above where she and her children had lived for a while in a cedar and glass house right on the bank of the Seymour River. She had even hiked and bicycled the vast forest before Capilano College was built on the hill above her former home, but had never seen the old cemetery tucked in the forest on this hill.

Ken had accompanied their grandchildren to pick wild blueberries on Seymour Mountain just above where they were now. Daisy had videotaped Ken walking with the grandchildren and holding the leash of their beloved Miniature Schnauzer through the forested paths and alpine meadows of the mountain that meets the sky high above the city.

The cemetery meandered over several small plateaus between two rivers where wild life abounded freely in the surrounding forest. Eagles flew and nested. Deer, coyotes, black bears and more made this area their home, roaming through the cemetery from one side of the forest to the other eating the flowers, berries and leaves of trees on their way.

In the watershed park just beyond the cemetery, Ken and Daisy walked slowly. On that walk, Ken explained his wishes for his burial. He was calm about it. Daisy listened carefully but remained convinced that any possible death was in the far distant future.

As they rounded a tiny lake the size of a large puddle or what would be called a slew on the prairies, the mosquitoes were ravenous, so it was time to drive back down the hill.

Ken seemed more at peace now. He wrote at the kitchen table in the night.

Remembering

i remember mother mom jean
father dad pop gus
my jeans and my gusses
and the whole schramm damily schrammily
grandmother granny and grandfather dadad I named them
aunt ruth aunt barbara uncle barry
cousin judy aunt helen and uncle cliff who killed himself...
uncle sumner aunt elaine my other parents in high school
remembering up and forgetting down and across generations
cousins whose names escape me in continuous kick-the-can
i remember most of all Chappaqua and White Plains
and Long Island Hampton Bays and Northport
where we learned to swim,
clam and fish, lobster clam bakes, corn and salt potatoes
Horace Greeley Hampton Bays,
Katona, and New Canaan high schools

DAISY WORRIED CONSTANTLY about Ken riding the bus to get to and from UBC and to visit his friend Man Bear. She busied herself with writing a screenplay about her father. She had her nose in a computer instead of spending the time with Ken, but she justified it by trying to win a contest to make some money so she could look after him better. The problem was, if she won the contest, she would have to travel and Daisy knew she would not leave Ken ever again. It really was an exercise in keeping busy and allowing Ken his freedom.

Though weak and his heart hurt, Ken always arrived home proud that he made it. He wanted to prove he could go back to school and defy the call to give up. He got ready for the Fall term by writing email notes to solidify plans about continuing his PhD in the Department of Education and Curriculum Instruction. By the end of August 2004, Ken was more than ever determined to get well.

Daisy's constant refrain was, "Eat your chicken soup. Take your vitamins," in her determination to make him get well.

By the middle of September 2004, as Ken walked across the room, Daisy noticed that his legs suddenly seemed fuller. For a couple of days, she imagined that he was gaining lost weight back.

Then Ken's health took a dive. It became obvious that all the progress he made in getting better was disappearing. He had not been gaining weight; instead his body was filling with fluid. His pulse had been extremely erratic and at times felt non-existent. He had been having trouble eating and spending more time in bed again with constant pain in his heart. He was cold all the time. Ken was very ill, repeating what had happened two years before.

Ken was having a difficult time getting to the car to go to daily medical appointments. He needed Daisy to hold him upright and a chair had to be placed halfway for him to sit and gather strength before making the other half of the trip that was only a few feet long.

One day, as he sat in the chair in the driveway and the mid-day light shone on his face, he asked, "Daisy, am I turning yellow?"

He trusted her to tell the truth – to confirm what he already knew.

She already knew the answer and had been hoping the symptom would go away. She knew better than to lie to a doctor. Looking closely at his eyes, his lips, gums, and skin. Reluctantly she answered, "Yes."

Profound sadness slid over his face but as a physician, he was silent in knowing what this meant – his liver was in trouble, a prelude to complete failure of internal organs.

She could not fathom such a strong personality dying but a foreboding came across her with the knowledge that he had been increasingly weak over the summer months – actually since June.

Death was for others, not Ken!

Though his doctors were bewildered about the change, Daisy knew the cause was the endless war. She could see clearly that people had been harassing him over money and over his strong morals; they refused to allow him a respite, at any time in two years, long enough to achieve sustainable recovery and she was convinced they had killed him. She was convinced dark, misguided souls had killed a man of God. Anger and resentment became emotions she wanted to accept as a legitimate stage of her grief and not cover them up as the man she loves may be dying.

Through all the years and even through difficult times and illness, just being near Ken or just seeing him caused Daisy's heart to flutter with pleasure. His presence was comforting. She had been in love with the man first, then the teacher. She then fell in love with the physician. Now she was intensely aware of loving the immortal being that he is.

THE WEATHER WAS HOT in the day, cooling only at sundown. Ken wanted the fresh air, so he enjoyed sitting in the warm afternoon sun wrapped up in blankets. Daisy arranged the chairs on the patio so that he could have his feet elevated. His adopted family surrounded him, talking and even laughing a little with him. Granddaughters, Maria and Katie sat on either side of Ken as though protecting him.

Daisy took pleasure in these seemingly fleeting times when Ken looked content and his adopted family rallied around him.

At the same time, she was aware of a foreboding like a dark cloud sitting on the edge of life... about what will come next. She knew Ken, as a doctor, knew all the signs and symptoms of his fading life. She knew he had been trying to prepare her for what he perceived as his end in this life.

In a gentle way and making it seem natural, over past months he taught her how to look after her computer, made sure she remembered the password to his own computer, how to maintain the car, and many small things. He had her take him to a jewellery store for a medical alert bracelet with a message that he showed her and filled out a form with the same message that he placed on the refrigerator door; the message specified a 'no resuscitation' wish. He reminded Daisy that he did not want to be manhandled by any emergency team and kept alive in a half-alive state.

At times Ken seemed to be living in two worlds – even talking briefly with invisible beings. Then he realized that he was in two worlds and made a correction to be in this world.

Daisy missed the opportunity to talk seriously with Ken about what he was experiencing because, regardless of her own beliefs and experiences of seeing spirits, she was not willing to accept his leaving her. She hoped that once again the invisible spirits surrounding him would leave and not call on him.

SEPTEMBER WAS STILL dry and hot but Ken had trouble feeling warm since June. His body lost the ability to generate internal heat. All summer he had worn a winter jacket when out regardless of the summer heat.

Now, there was a constant need for hot-water bottles at his now bandaged, weeping feet that again rested on towels and waterproof pads. A heater was necessary by his bedside and hot water bottles at his feet. It was a struggle to keep him warm while at the same time keeping fresh air coming in to help him breath. Antony and Daisy did body massages each day in hopes of bringing his chi back up.

Ken's outings consisted only of visits to his doctors. Just last week, Ken was still walking and was keeping his weekly appointment with the allopathic doctor. He had used a lot of energy just to get there but without notifying Ken, the doctor left his office just before Ken arrived. The receptionist informed Ken that because the doctor had seen his quota of billable patients that was allowed for the day by the Medical Services Plan, he had gone home. He was not there to give Ken the latest test results and either did not realize or did not care that Ken's health was failing so fast.

They sat on a bench looking out over the vastness of the ocean for a while before going home. It would turn out to be a last time.

The Chinese doctor treated him with more respect but was visibly alarmed at Ken's disappearing pulses. The daily visits to him had become increasingly difficult because Ken was becoming so weak that he needed Daisy's help to walk. Ken could only walk about three steps, needing to rest before going on even when supported. His heart was so weak.

Then came the day when Ken opted to stay in bed rather than see any doctor. It was a paradoxical relief because over the past few months, Ken had been selling his best and newest books in order to pay for medicines that they had no money for and did not want to burden family about. Daisy had fewer books that interested booksellers. Now suddenly he did not have to sell any books – at least for a day or two and they could relax at home instead of going out to a medical appointment or to sell books. The problem was that they still hoped this break was only temporary.

A family member, who was a physician, encouraged another physician to make a house call. The two had gone to medical school together and he was simply doing a favor for a fellow student. As the new doctor stood tall over Ken, refusing a chair to sit and talk for a few minutes, he corroborated in the knowledge that Ken was in heart failure and in imminent danger of a stroke. But – his message was clear that unless Ken went into hospital, he would not be caring for him.

Being reminded of a possible stroke was frightening to Ken; he was most afraid of losing his ability to think and communicate his thoughts.

Ken made an overture to the visiting physician to talk together at any time that would fit his schedule. The physician ignored Ken's wish to talk and walked out.

Daisy was again disturbed and disappointed at how many people refused Ken the simplest of human gifts, that is of spending time together to just talk and share thoughts and knowledge.

She absolutely would not be sending Ken to hospital where he did not want to go.

Daisy was sadly reminded again of the time two years ago when Professor Carl Leggo had wanted to take the time to visit Ken at home when he found out that Ken was ill. Because Ken's apartment had been cleared out and her living room was piled full of boxes, Daisy had suggested that visiting was not desired at that time. Daisy regretted her selfishness over thinking 'house beautiful' was more important than the two men talking. It was a time Daisy would live differently if she ever could but redoing the past was not possible. In times like these, regrets and guilt over past regressions are strong.

EARLY EVENING of Thursday, September 23, 2004, Ken was propped against pillows in his preferred bed by the large glass patio doors overlooking the garden as he sipped medicinal tea. Daisy quietly watched television in the same room while Ken listened to his favorite aboriginal music on the stereo from a disk given to him by his sister.

From his bed Ken asked, "Daisy, will you do some writing for me?"

Ken always got fulfillment by handwriting with his pen and a notebook, so in surprise she answered, "Of course. You usually like to write yourself."

"I know. I need you to write this one."

He had a determined look about him. This request was so unusual that it seemed important enough to turn off the television and get a pen and notebook. On the edge of a lazy-boy chair she assumed her old secretarial position.

Ken looked toward the garden. "Please write:

"I ask the Creator to forgive for me all the people who have been mean to me... us. Love is possible to be shared among people."

Ken's voice was strong and obviously his thoughts were clear.

Daisy interrupted, "You are more forgiving than I am."

He looked at her. "I almost died two years ago and when a spirit came to take me home, I told him to get lost and prayed a lot. I have had two more years."

"I remember. I have had two more years with you. I pray a lot because I want more. I don't want you to die. I'm afraid of losing you."

"You and Antony will be alright. When you write my story, the only thing I ask is that you tell the truth. The title should be **doctor ken** with small letters."

"Yes, I promise to tell the truth. I will use the title." She even managed a reassuring smile for him.

"Please write." He spoke quickly now, emphasizing the first line.

> ### *"MY TRUTH, SO WE CAN CHANGE:*
>
> *"What is at the center of my life? Extended family. Love... meaning knowing that I'm alive and I'm dying and so is everyone else.*
>
> *"To accomplish that knowledge of living and dying is happiness.*
>
> *"Unconditional happiness is health... health is life... death... a safe and loving home with other loved ones... where we could be honest with each other and make the changes that we need to make to live together.*
>
> ### *"AND A HOPE:*
>
> *"That would include being able to be cared for at home when sick and dying from birth to death.*
>
> *"That we would be able to learn together as in home schooling and that would include a home funeral."*

A realization came over Daisy that he was writing a last message. She paused.

"Please continue writing." Ken turned his face toward the sky outside the window and continued to speak clearly.

"TO MEAN VIRTUE MEANS HUMAN POWERS.

"The human powers I admire most are:

"The Courage to be Honest... to do Good... and to take Responsibility for one's actions especially how they affect others.

"To do what's Right and Good based on real knowing of what's good and true and beautiful.

"Listening and responding to the needs of others with an open heart.

"SPEAKING MY TRUTH AS I KNOW IT:

"Thinking as thanking and giving of my life to others who need or want something from me that will help them grow and be more alive.

"LOYALTY:

"Refusal to give up on life.

"Willingness to Learn and Change with others.

"Courage to be honest... and to do together what is necessary to be alive in the continuing wartime conditions going on all around us, particularly the war on families.

"LIFE:

"What is most satisfying is enjoying that I am alive and knowing that I will die... and that this life is a one time gift... non-refundable."

Daisy was scribbling fast but needed to pause in amusement at his "non-refundable" statement. She was amazed at his quickness of thought – his insight. As usual, he could make her want to laugh even when he was being serious. He paused only long enough for her to catch up in writing.

"MOST FRUSTRATION:

"To share the gifts that I have... especially the gifts of love with others who don't seem to want either love or my gifts or knowing.

"MOST DIFFICULT:

"To continue to stay alive and do the impossible with others I love.

"MOST EASY:

"My relationship with animals, children and plants through singing, breathing, touching, and feeling.

"All sensory body stuff is easy except for breathing right now.

Opening my heart to forgiving myself and others who I feel have betrayed me in dishonesty and cruelty, meanness, and ignorance.

"CONTRADICTION:

"I feel my life is just starting... yet I know I am dying too soon with not enough time to share love with others in a home that is safe.

"I still try.

"I despair I will not have enough time to get beyond it to really genuinely grow with you, Daisy... like ripping the plants out before they have time to grow."

Ken's last sentence summed up her thoughts and fears, too. The writing was finished. Sadness was shared as they took a moment to just feel.

WITH TRUTH SUMMED UP, they both became aware again of the aboriginal music playing in a loop on the stereo. It would continue through the night.

They were interrupted by Ken's son Stephen stepping through the patio doors. During the week Ken had summoned all his sons to come. He did not want to broadcast that he might be dying, just in case he could cheat death a fourth time, so they did not come.

Ken's face brightened, "Thanks for coming, Stephen."

"Andy and Peter are too busy to come," Stephen explained.

Father and son visited quietly.

While Ken had company, Daisy dashed out to rent a wheelchair and a walker from the local medical supply store before it closed for the night. Ken had been holding out on this type of aid, relying on Daisy for help. He reluctantly agreed to the wheelchair.

To give father and son private time together, Daisy spent time cleaning the kitchen and tending the large pot of simmering chicken soup made for Ken. He had not eaten solid food in a month, though he did take the vitamins and minerals Daisy gave him. She still held hope that he would start eating again. In fact, now that his son had come to see him, she hoped his appetite would be stimulated.

After Stephen left, Ken was peaceful. "Daisy, I feel better. I saw my son."

Ken's music continued to play in the background. From his pillow, he sadly told Daisy, "I regret that I do not have more time to heal more people and make a better world."

In that moment, she knew that no more sincere words have ever been uttered on the face of this earth. Profound sadness washed over her. "I know."

"My heart is broken." He was so sad.

"I know," she whispered.

DAISY HAD BEEN trying to sleep on the sofa near Ken. At 1 a.m. she dashed up to check on Ken. She took his hand. It was extremely limp and cool.

Ken turned his head toward her, "I don't want to leave you and Antony." Tears welled up in his eyes.

"Don't cry." As he turned his head away and stifled his tears, she regretted saying that. She held his hand. His hand had gotten lighter and lacked even a little strength.

AT THREE IN THE MORNING, again she dashed up from the sofa to check on Ken. His eyes were closed. She feared the worst. As she looked closely into his face, Ken's eyes sprung open. His eyes were shining with brilliant, clear blue light of pure love. She had never before seen anything like the pureness of loving light coming from within him.

Reading her thoughts, he said, "I know what you are seeing. This is my love for you."

She said, "Your eyes are so clear and brilliant blue. *You are unconditional love.*" She was struck with the thought that this man was able to read her mind.

Ken smiled, "You are seeing my love for you."

Though his body was that of a frail, ill man, Ken revealed to Daisy his pure spirit that had transcended the peccadillo of earthly people.

She marveled that this man was brighter, more alert than she by far, even in a body so weak. Ken requested that Daisy hand him his long white feather that had been given to him by an aboriginal teacher in recognition of one teacher to another. She went back to the sofa and fell asleep... a deep sleep this time.

AT 4:30 A.M. SHE WOKE UP to see Ken sitting at the kitchen table having tea that somehow he had managed to make for himself without waking her. She got up even though she was extremely tired. It was as though a bucket of mud was in her head. Through fuzzy thinking, she wondered how Ken maneuvered around the small kitchen in his wheelchair.

He asked her to wheel him back to his bed. Knowing he would take forever to get ready to move from the chair to the bed, she thought she would lie down for just one minute.

"Ken, when you are ready, let me know."

All the tiredness of years had come to this; she fell into a deep, unconscious sleep.

62

They Come – They Write

...Before I die, I want to know that I have done all that I can do to help make the world safer and more enjoyable for children, families, and natives. I want my epitaph to say out loud in the hearts of my readers: Ken Schramm was alive all his life and he was alive when he died in the knowledge that he made a home for the family of humankind with all the animals and spirits and dreams of the world as divine grace. He lived his life in gratitude and love and defiance and humor. His body returns to the garden of the earth where his spirit lives and lives his family.

Ken Schramm

FRIDAY, SEPTEMBER 24, 2004 was a hot, sunny morning. Opening her eyes, the first thing Daisy did was to look at Ken as usual. He looked like he was sleeping peacefully. She relaxed for a few minutes, not wanting to disturb him. She picked up a Sears catalogue from the pile of books and flipped pages, looking for a raised toilet seat to buy for Ken. Just yesterday, he had requested that the toilet seat be raised.

Looking at the clock and seeing that it said 10:30 am, she thought it odd for her to sleep six hours since 4:30 am. She had not done that in two years as she had tried to be awake for Ken round the clock or at least be awake every two hours to check on him.

Something twigged her and suddenly she became afraid to look up, reasoning with herself that if Ken was alive, good! But if he died she does not want to know... She snuck a glance at him. The grey cat that kept vigil over Ken for months had left him and did not return to him. Ken held his large white feather across his chest with his right hand. Daisy slowly approached Ken and touched him. He was still warm but not breathing. In his stillness, he looked like he stepped out of biblical times with long, neat white curls reaching his shoulders and newly grown short white beard, framing a beautifully peaceful face. She kissed his face. Then she went to the washroom to get a wet washcloth and came back to wipe Ken's face. She noticed a last small tear almost dry under his right eye and sadly wiped it away.

Where had he come from? Where has he gone? ...this vibrant man who loved so deeply... with hopes and dreams... now having shed his last tear... a man who celebrated the birth of his sons and cried to the depths of his soul over the loss of his sons... this man who generously embraced an adopted family as his own... this man who cared about the wellbeing of all life... a man who had never hurt even a bug as long as Daisy knew him... a man who gave tirelessly of his time to volunteer work in communities to make a better world... a man who only wanted to share so unselfishly his vast knowledge... a man who had helped so many achieve their goals... this man whose heart had beat only hours ago and now was still. Where? ...where? ...where are you?

ON THE TELEPHONE with Man Bear, whom Ken had kept fires with at the Long House, Daisy tried to fulfill Ken's wishes. "Ken has passed away. I need you to come. I fell asleep. I should have been there for him. Somehow he managed to find his feather and he is holding it across his chest. He looks so peaceful. He has asked that I keep him at home as long as possible for people to visit him here. No funeral home."

From the garden, Daisy called her brother Bill in Alberta. He surprised her with, "Thanks to Ken, I have been just been given a clean bill of health. I owe my life to Ken!"

Bill had been struggling with various bouts of cancer. Several doctors in Alberta gave up and sent him home to die. Ken advised Bill to come to Vancouver for consultations in alternative and natural ways to deal with it.

Bill was not the only one; he was in good company. In the brilliant sunshine this day of extreme sadness and shock, Bill gave Daisy a stream of contentment in a reminder that Ken's helping hand had left several people behind who were continuing to live healthy lives after being given death sentences by other doctors.

As she stood in the garden with renewable life growing around her, Daisy thought about their fourteen grandchildren. In this one family, five children had been in danger of losing their lives or being crippled because of serious medical errors. The five grandchildren were presently alive and healthy because Ken recognized problems and changed the course of their medical care, and in so doing had changed the course of their lives and the lives of their family. Daisy could not help but wonder what would have happened if Ken had not been in their lives.

In those few minutes of pause in reminiscence because of her brother's declaration that Ken saved his life, Daisy thought that even though Ken had not been able to save everyone or the world, there were many as a testament to a life well lived.

MAN BEAR, a large, soft-spoken, half aboriginal man arrived within the hour of the call and stayed all day, performing rites to protect Ken with rituals of burning sweet grass and praying. Daisy was comforted by his presence and by knowing this was what Ken did want.

Sleeping close to Ken again another night – the last night, she felt comforted by his presence and did not want morning to come; but it did. It would be necessary to give up his body later in the day because of the extreme hot weather.

Family and friends did visit and prayed beside Ken. Some just sat with him for hours.

The inevitable time came too soon. The sun was going down when a white van pulled up to the house to take Ken to a cooler room to wait for burial. Daisy had given up the day for other people and now she had to give Ken up too soon. There was a moment of internal panic in knowing the flesh body she has loved was going away forever.

Three aboriginal men and an aboriginal woman, friends from the UBC Longhouse had stayed with Ken the whole afternoon. Now they drummed and sang outside on the large patio where family and friends were gathered, waiting for Ken's body to emerge from the house and be put into the waiting van. Inside, behind the closed drapes, Antony took Ken's bracelet and feather to keep until later as hurried men moved Ken's body from his bed to a stretcher and covered him. Daisy wished she had planned this better so that she could have a private moment before he would be taken out. Now it was all happening too fast; it was too late and she would never see his face again or be able to touch him.

The heavy curtains flung open and Ken was carried out. Antony and Daisy followed, filing past the singers and through the small crowd.

Ken was efficiently loaded into the back of the white van and it starts to move away. Antony and Daisy jumped into her car to follow. As they drove away from the house, they could hear the drumming and singing in a native tongue. A song of Thanksgiving for having known Ken was being sung. The song followed for a long way down the hill – perfect for honoring Ken.

SUNDAY MORNING, September 26th, 2004. Daisy spent the night again sleeping on the sofa where she had slept to be near Ken. On the brink between sleeping and waking, Daisy saw Ken lying beside her, on her left side – in the air! His hair curled around his earlobes as he wore it most of the time all through the years and he was wearing his red jacket. He looked healthy. As she focused, he slowly becomes lighter, as though he was made up of molecules of coloured light that began to meld with the air and slowly became invisible.

Daisy's sister had jumped on an airplane the day before and was present in the house. As she entered the room, Daisy tried to explain. "Ken was sleeping beside me. I saw him as clear as can be. Then he disappeared."

Terisa paused as she headed for the Easy-boy chair with a cup of coffee and the morning newspaper. She made no comment, just "Hmm-hmm." and started to read.

Sitting on the edge of the sofa, Daisy pondered the experience and wondered if her sister believed what she had just been told.

Then as though to make a point, this was the beginning of several experiences both sisters shared over the next few days. As the sisters discussed possibly putting the ashes of the Miniature Schnauzer, who had died earlier, in Ken's casket with him so he would not be alone, there was a loud bang in the kitchen. Since no one was in the kitchen, they investigated. The Miniature Schnauzer magnet had fallen from the fridge door to the floor. This particular magnet was large and extremely strong and could not be moved manually with ease. It was impossible for it to fall off on its own. When it was put back on the fridge, it could not be budged. This got Terisa's attention.

Then, as Daisy was working on her computer in another room, she heard a scraping sound over and over coming from the kitchen. Finally, she got up to investigate and the sound stopped. A piece of paper lay on the kitchen floor. She picked it up. It was an article cut out of a newspaper titled 'Privacy Rights' about the Federal Privacy Information Protection Act that came into being January 1, 2004. Ken had placed the paper on the fridge door under an angel magnet and now it had slipped to the floor but the magnet that held it to the fridge had not moved. This particular paper was important because Ken had tried to talk to the Federal Department of Human Rights after the audit in 2002 but they had refused to consult with him about his problem over confidentiality. Then they came out with this Privacy Act two years later. Daisy put the paper back under the magnet and tried several times to slip it out; it could not be budged without the magnet being taken off first. Seeing that particular piece of information lying on the floor, Daisy knew for certain that Ken was saying, "This is really me! I am alive!"

The stereo system would be turned on unaccountably and would play the CD of aboriginal music Ken loved, or it would open the CD drawer and remain open until Daisy noticed.

The television turned into a radio for a few days between the time of passing and the burial day; then the picture returned. It was well known that Ken preferred music on the radio to television.

Then the sculptured wishing well kept as a symbol of their favorite story began to fill with coins that appeared in fast succession in the most unlikely places, like under his favourite chair where none had been the day before.

In life, Ken was a man of determination; he was just as strong-minded in death to keep his promise to Daisy to prove his survival.

"Okay, Ken. I know you are alive. I believe you!"

Once Ken's promise was thoroughly recognized, those kinds of capers stopped.

THE RING! Daisy remembered the gold ring! Emptying the pillow that Ken had kept for all those many years, Daisy found their gold ring and finally she put it on her finger again for keeps.

BURIAL TIME at noon was brilliantly sunny. Antony and Daisy accompanied Ken from Langley to the cemetery in North Vancouver. Riding in the hearse, Daisy had a surreal time bringing Ken's body in the back of the car instead of beside her after all the years of being side by side.

Ken had written a poem during one of his recent nighttime writing sessions.

Would you
really visit me
here and there
in the graveyard of my heart
where a silence
silent words do our work
in the morning songs...

They came and were waiting. On arrival, Daisy could see across the lawn that Ken's brother Richard and sister Molly had come. They traveled thousands of miles to be here. And so were both ex-wives waiting with Ken's three sons.

It had fleetingly crossed Daisy's mind while arranging this day to uninvite the second ex-wife, but Daisy was now glad to see Jane present so that she could experience how other people feel about Ken and to teach her how wrong she was.

Ken's adopted family was present among clients and people from the university. Ken's aboriginal mentor, John and his wife had traveled several hundred miles through the mountains and were waiting.

Man Bear would officiate the burial of Ken's body in a native ceremony. Ken was being buried in his Fire Keeping clothing with his feet bare, and he was wrapped in his Great Spirit Blanket.

The plain pine casket that Ken had requested was opened though he remained covered in his blanket. Some of his belongings and gifts from people present were passed through sage smoke and placed with Ken. His drum that John had guided him in making was placed with him – without a baton – a testament to that which remained unfinished between Ken and Daisy. A book about Lakota fire keeping was also placed with him because Ken always had a book to read, along with the bell he had asked for. His long white feather was placed across his chest. Sweet grass and a few more significant belongings were placed. His sister Debbie sent a Pueblo Zuni Fetish Turquoise stone carving of a Badger to be placed with him for protection; it represents the spirit of the badger and believed to have knowledge of healing roots and herbs, and characteristics of tenaciousness, passion, and persistence – very fitting to Ken. And lastly, the tiny white ceramic urn containing the ashes of the Miniature Schnauzer Ken and Daisy shared, and he had spent so much time holding and who gave Ken so much unconditional love, was laid with him. The casket was closed one last time as Daisy stood beside him.

Man Bear, with aboriginal men and women, all friends of Ken, drummed and sang as the casket was carried across the lawn to the prepared spot by six men of Ken's family... his three sons, his nephew, brother Richard, and Antony.

The chosen spot was underneath the overhanging branches of old growth maple trees – a reminder of Vermont, surrounded by giant cedar and pine trees for protection, on the edge of a high cliff where the University of British Columbia could be seen in the distance through the moss covered trees. A rushing river could be heard from below. Daisy's secret was that there is a path into the forest a few feet away that looks exactly like the path in the picture that hung on Ken's office wall – the picture of two children walking hand in hand on the path through the woods into the light, that was her fantasy image of Ken and herself.

Man Bear placed smoking sage at Ken's head on the ground.

Friends and family, with many of Ken's adopted grandchildren formed a large circle. Daisy stood at Ken's feet and the aboriginal people dressed in their ceremonial clothing, sang and danced with their drums at his head. John's feet seemed to get lighter and higher until he appeared to be dancing in the air and he was transformed into a younger man in the air.

Daisy had also asked a person that Ken loved and respected to speak for him. Carl, a middle aged man, wearing a dark suit and tie, long wavy graying hair neatly tied back, stepped forward out of the crowd to stand at Ken's head.

In a strong, clear voice he said, "I am Carl Leggo. I have been asked to speak on behalf of my dear friend Ken. I have been Ken's advisor for his PhD candidacy. We had a relationship more like father and son. Sometime I was the father and he was the son. Sometime he was the father and I was the son. We often would enjoy eating ice cream together and talk. Sometime we would just enjoy the ice cream and not talk. I do believe Ken was the most intelligent person I have met in my life. He will always be remembered for the knowledge he shared so freely."

As Carl spoke, a grateful Daisy knew that he spoke truth. He was absolutely the right person to speak for Ken. Carl and Ken had a profound and honest relationship. They both had considered becoming ministers and both were poets and teachers. Ken loved Carl with recognition of a bond beyond the present known human life.

Carl continued, "Last night I was going through papers written by Ken and I found this poem. Ken's words speak better than mine."

Unrolling a paper, head held high in the sunlight, Carl read:
"Father Sky
Mother Earth
Creator
All My Relations

Thank you for the gift of life
Your grandson grampa thanks you for giving me a home with
you
Where I can live and die today
and forgive and be forgiven
Hold me and love me and heal me and help me
In all ways and places
I need healing and living and helping
Teach me all I need to know
And help me be the best human being I can be today
Cleanse all my body mind spirit relations
Open my eyes to your goodness and beauty
Open my ears to hear your songs and your truths
Open my nose and mouth and tongue and throat
To smell and taste and chew and breathe your goodness
Open my heart to your loving knowing
Open my voice to sing my songs with yours
Open all of me to receive and share your goodness with others –
My parents and their relatives who made and make it possible
for me to be alive naming and renaming me and mine
My children and grandchildren and their families and friends
My teachers and healers and helpers and their families
Daisy and Antony and Joe and Cam Tran and Man Bear and
John & N'kixw'stn and Carl and Karen and Jo-Ann and Michael
and Graham and George and especially their families
And remembering all those relatives I hurt and who hurt me
and with whom I experienced conflict and trouble and difficulty
making our lives more difficult and painful.
I ask you to help us all to be the best beings we can be
 And teach us all we need to know today.
I want to thank you all my relations
Sky people earth people water people stone people animal people
plant people
named unnamed people who make possible my life with their
lives

Giving me shelter and clothing and food and medicine
Loving and challenging me to be more alive while I die"

As Carl finished speaking, though there was no wind, the enormous, old maple tree suddenly rustled loudly high above and dropped large yellow, orange and red leaves onto the casket. Some people let out a large gasp. Daisy's young grandson fainted to the ground and revived with his physician aunt kneeling beside him during a pause of concern. After the grandson recovered and stood again, people took turns to sprinkle dirt, which was passed through the cleansing smoke of sage, over Ken's casket.

THE WOODEN WALLS of the UBC House of Learning Longhouse have been a soundboard for many a voice and drum in song and prayer. The walls hold many memories. The poles stand watch. A gathering at the Longhouse following the burial was a time to share food and stories about Ken. Inside the golden walls that had protected Ken and where his voice had given prayer, family, friends, and a former client gave testimony as to how Ken had bettered their lives.

Students and faculty of UBC expressed their sorrow by writing letters at losing a man who had worked tirelessly to help students and teachers in one way or another. Graeme Chalmers, head of the department in which Ken was working on his PhD, told the gathering he has never before seen such an outpouring of grief and admiration in a university setting. He had printed the letters and presented the folders to Daisy for the family.

LETTERS VOICED TESTIMONY that many lives have been touched and changed by Ken in a positive way. Daisy wished Ken had living knowledge of how deeply he affected so many people in a positive way – it might have helped him to live.

   * *Ken, a beautiful, loving, generous man...*

   * *Ken was a special man: a physician and healer of great personal integrity, an activist, a scholar, a life-long learner.*

* I always understood his conscientious objection to US policies based upon his deep religious beliefs and was not surprised – only happy for him – that he found a place to practice his unselfish kind of medicine.

* What a masterful teacher he was. I continue to quote him in my work. ...I have never been in contact with another person who was so passionately aware of inner freedom and its value. ...It will take me a long time to accept this loss.

* Ken's gift, for me, was his reminder to listen to the stories of our ancestors, and those of our grandparents... Ken's gift to narrative is his gift to those who follow...

* Ken was a great companion and friend to me. ...I have some of his books.

* Ken's voice of wisdom and also his passion for justice had a strong impact on me when I first arrived at...[university]. For those of you who didn't know Ken, well, you've missed knowing a very special person. I hope there is some way our Centre can remember him in a tangible way.

* Ken showed us what was possible. His creative use of narrative and interactive text opened doors for each of us who comes after. ...Thanks, Ken, for being who you are... and for being a model of aging with grace and dignity.

* An inspiring soul... I continue to be inspired...

* It was amazing to watch his spirit, which seemed so strong, struggle within his body that was so wounded.

* A spirit with profound sense of Care and Wisdom. He came to us – silently – to enrich our own stories.

* Ken, an angel with wings of love.

* He will always live in our hearts as an unselfish and fun-loving friend who acted with courage and conviction.

* Because of Ken I made a (final) decision to transfer to... This 'turning point' moment took place when I listened to Ken sharing his story, his pain and concern for our world... I remember...

* Ken reminded me of alternate hopes of recovery and transcendence... even in your passing, we learn from you Ken, our souls, deeds, hopes and dreams yet survive.

* He was a genuine human being who dared to be in places where others wouldn't venture.

* Ken's sharing in my hour of loss was not a small measure.

* Like many of you, I hold dear memories of Ken's influence... especially of the way he followed through with action.

* Ken has truly walked as a leader in the lives of so many people. May each of us honour his gifts in our lives by being his followers...

* Ken has always been a kind and generous person, with great courage and an inquisitive mind.

* ...that he challenged us to move with passion and care in the world.

* Ken helped us with our marriage...

* Ken helped my granddaughter grow out of her fears and hurts...

* Ken helped me with my sister's suicide... I was lost and needed guidance. He witnessed my grief after my sister's death and separation from my husband.

* He introduced me to a new career and many authors and teachers.

* I still have some of Ken's books. [a refrain heard from so many]

* I regarded him as the best of teachers. He had my absolute trust, he supported my questioning, he respected my pain, he never interfered with what was happening. I experienced a great easing of all forms of authoritarian thinking in his company. I witnessed him telling many emperors that they had no clothes, what courage. It will be a challenge to capture his educational practice in words.

* Ken was and is a doctor of many people and many fields, and anyone I know that knew him, knew and appreciated this.

* Ken and I discussed John Dewey a lot because we both had teachers who had studied with Dewey. Dewey's idea of intelligence as the pragmatic life of action for what is truly good, not only for what "works" or is profitable, is a thoroughly modern reframing of classical wisdom. We explored "that for the sake of which we do anything" to get beyond psychologizing and needs as determining drivers of conduct.

* ...he was there for me. ...I felt incredible good fortune to have in my life come to be close to someone like Ken. ...all of us are trying to walk in Ken's footsteps with similar generosity and love.

* Next week is my 60th birthday, and 5 weeks ago I had a total hip replacement... Before I went for my operation I had a dream where I was standing before a seated Ken. He told me to "remember the earth, and let it support you". And so I did. Ken removed the need to use or experience power over anyone by embodying the meaning of truth and honesty between equals. You [Daisy] are right to remind me of how he acted in my dream, and how thoughtful he was in all encounters by demonstrating human dignity and the reality of connections that are free of domination in any form. ...Ken and I discussed Buddhist philosophy in the mid 70's quite often and tried to apply it to counseling. The lineage continues. Ken was authoritative and authentic without being authoritarian. He was protective and assertive at the same time. He showed all of us how to be fearless in the presence of power, how to live...

* I've tried writing some fragments about my experience of Ken, but I realize there is some avoidance of the fact of his death that is blocking me. I recall things he said to me, and then I start working on what I've made of these communications, but with the idea that I can still find him to talk to where we left off. I don't want him gone, is the long and short of it.

* *Ken embodied the spirit of liberation through friendship (truth speaking), and his wealth was uncontaminated by money. In a way, the 'world' may be incapable of appreciating a spirit like Ken's, perhaps because the world is the product of all the rules that Ken was able to demonstrably question and change in his interactions with others. I spoke with Ken about human development, about how the project of liberation for a material being requires understanding the causes of unfreedom in material terms as well as spiritual terms. "Trying to control my behavior is a waste of time," he would say, and for people who needed him to do or be a certain way for them to get what they wanted, frustration would always result.*

* *I can remember one Sweat Day, ...and I got to the sweat early and Ken was sitting there with the fire. He asked me how teaching was and I told him that I was thinking of changing my career. I told him the kids drive me crazy. Ken told me, "Stop trying to control the children... let them be themselves and let them learn the way they know how to best." He continued to say, "Don't think of the noise as noise... think of it as kids learning." Those are the only words he said to me that day but it gave me enough for me to figure out that children learn by interacting with each other. ...Ken was a man of a few words... but those few words said a lot. So you see Daisy, Ken is still with us too.*

* *My thoughts are that we have been talking a lot about Ken... that he visited me in my dreams. ...In my dream... he offered me real ginger ale... [The woman had stomach problems].*

* *Ken and HIS Hippocratic Oath... he cast it into a way of life that would be too daunting for most physicians.*

* *Ken lived the meaning of "first do no harm".*

* * *

NOVEMBER 21, 2004, Ken's brother Richard Schramm, (scholar and professor) wrote this letter:

Today is my brother Ken's birthday. If he had lived, he would be 72. In memory of Ken, I want to share with you some thoughts of mine about him; along with some things I learned when Nancy and I went to Vancouver for his burial.

Ken was always into books and ideas. As a child he cut articles out of magazines and stored them in an old pirate-like trunk; in public school he was always reading and doing his class work, a rare activity in a school culture more into sports and social relations than into learning. As a student three grades behind him, I just thought he was different and (I) looked to others for companionship. It wasn't until we were both at Dartmouth – he a senior and I a freshman – that I began to fully appreciate Ken's excitement about learning and teaching. Then, and for years afterwards, I turned to him for intellectual inspiration. He was always passing on to me the names of authors and books that seemed to be perfect for where I was in my own studies and work. And when I told him of a new author I had discovered with exciting ideas, inevitably he had read these works years earlier. He was a gifted teacher and thinker, and I considered him my intellectual mentor even in later years when all we did was have a yearly phone conversation. Its clear that the faculty as well as the students he worked with at the University of British Columbia felt the same way about Ken. At his burial and the gathering afterward, one of his faculty members spoke of how he looked up to Ken and learned so much from him; another talked about how Ken, through his questions and reading, came to know her area of study as well if not better than she. And the collection of e-mails written by co-students when they heard of his death testifies to Ken's importance in their own learning.

Ken was also a radical. In eighth grade he became a member of the World Federalists, advocating for world government. He became a strong critic of Capitalism, and I'm guessing he was an anarchist opposed to institutionalized power of all sorts. In his study of Psychiatry he aligned himself with Thomas Szasz, someone who vowed to defend the rights of any person labeled mentally ill... He was truly a non-conformist and I'm sure his practice of family psychiatry was like no other psychiatric practice ever. His fondness for Native Americans included, I imagine, considerable sympathy for holistic and interconnected view of life they shared in contrast to the reductionism – the looking at parts of the whole in depth and isolation – of most university scholarship and western thinking in general. His moving from western medicine to alternative medicine, an entirely different way of approaching health, reflected his radicalism. Whenever you took a position with Ken, it was likely that he would offer an alternative view that was often way off the charts, radically different, and then argue strongly and persuasively for it.

In talking with Don [youngest brother] after learning of Ken's death, he emphasized that Ken was an idealist in the sense that he held onto his radical views of government, healthcare, economics, epistemology come hell or high water, and did not give an inch... Yes, Ken had the courage of his convictions. He was always willing to stand up for what he believed even though it often got him into hot water. In seventh grade he took the side of women in a debate on who was better: men or women? He opposed the Vietnam War in the early sixties long before most people, and was a certified conscientious objector. He regularly took on the institutions where he worked. He sued his department chair for harassment when the Chair took action against his taking his class 100 miles off campus to study indigenous peoples to the North. He refused to open his client files to the British Columbia government in the face of a major suit about payments for health care rendered. And these stands on principle were not costless to him, as he lost jobs and income and changed where he lived, as a consequence of these stands.

I will miss all these qualities of Ken – his thoughtful mentoring, radical ideas, and idealistic stands.

The First Nation's burial ceremony and the following Long House meeting, with the sage smoke, drumming, singing, testimonies, and shared food I found to be both soothing and freeing, allowing me to tap into a very deep sadness about Ken's passing, and helping me in the grieving process.

So I was glad that Nancy and I were able to go there, to learn more about and celebrate his life, to cry with others who loved him as we did, to support one another within his many "families", and to say goodbye to Ken, which was truly the hardest yet and in many ways the most important part of the trip.
Love
(Signed) Richard

ON A MISSION on behalf of the Dartmouth College men to find Ken for an upcoming half-century class reunion, Bob Bean, Ken's roommate at Dartmouth College, had telephoned in June. Now in their seventies, just before Ken's passing, the men renewed an old friendship in a last conversation. Bob's daughter had tracked Ken through a poem on the Internet.

In an email the day following the telephone call and an email from Bob, Ken had written:

> *Hello Bob & Carol,*
>
> *Now comes the joy of two keyboard challenged friends on email! I don't remember typing anything in college, my handwriting is so legible people could actually read my prescriptions.*
>
> *I look forward to seeing you ASAP. Meanwhile, here is our address and phone numbers for Daisy and me...*

Feeling a sense of joy at hearing Bob's voice, and the following emails, Ken had gone back to his bed to rest.

GOING THROUGH THINGS to find all of the seventy-some library books that must be returned as soon as possible, most of which were neatly on a shelf, but in looking for any strays, Daisy found a thick white envelope. It had been fifty years since Ken had been Best Man at Bob and Carol Bean's wedding; a napkin from Bob and Carol's fiftieth wedding anniversary celebration was in the envelope, wrapped around pictures and a written description of the Dartmouth College 50th Year Reunion of Class 1954 in Hanover. Ken had not been able to make it to the reunion, so Bob filled him in:

...Of course, Wigwam Circle is gone – replaced by a Thayer School parking lot and several new dorms. We visited 401 Middle Mass [home dorm to Ken and Bob] – rope "fire escapes" replaced by ugly steel fire escapes at end of building, wall to bedroom and old john and sink are all torn out and new sink, john and shower relocated in part of old study area. No hall showers – I remember

when you cut your hand badly on the ceramic shower handle. "Eleazar" is still buried out behind the dorm! Remember [G & NV] and the water balloons from the center suite. Well, [V] is now Chief Justice of the [D] Supreme Court... we had a very nice visit.

Daisy wrote to Bob, asking: *Who is Eleazar?*

Bob answered: *I will always be proud to call Kehn "my friend" and cherish the memory of my BEST MAN. Only regret is that we lost touch with each other for almost 50 years. You ask, "Who is Eleazar". He was Eleazar Wheelock, the founder and first president of Dartmouth College in 1769. He was buried in the College Cemetery behind our old dormitory, Middle Massachusetts Hall, and from our window in room 401 we could see Eleazar's tombstone through the trees. ...He paddled his canoe up the Connecticut River until he found the Hanover Plain, founded the school, started educating the Native Americans, as the old song goes, 'with a gradis ad parnasseium, a Bible and a drum, and 500 gallons of New England rum'. Sometimes during the Winter Carnival, we would drink a toast to Eleazar with the hard cider we kept on our window ledge overlooking the cemetery!*

MIDDLE OF OCTOBER, only three weeks after Ken's passing, a letter arrived from representatives for the Dartmouth College Class of '54, requesting information about Ken's life.

Daisy wrote back:

Thank you for your interest in Ken. He was so unique that I just cannot say enough about him and his life.

I went to a sweat at the UBC House of Learning yesterday. Having received your letter just as I was leaving at 2:30 pm, I decided to keep it in my pocket and ponder over what I might say to you while sitting by the fire and maybe you would somehow get the good vibes from that whole experience.

I was on Ken's territory. Ken had begged me to take part in the sweats. Except for attending some of the feasts afterward with him, I never took part. I always said I was too busy. So now, here I am trying to honor his wishes when I have to do it alone.

I now go around telling anyone who will listen to live the moment. Spend time with a loved one. All the busy-ness is not worth missing out on sharing important things and times with loved ones.

I was with friends yesterday. The people running the sweat were good friends of Ken, and I have known them over several years; so I was welcomed with many hugs. I helped build the women's lodge and dismantle it later. I did not go into the sweat lodge but remained outside watching the fire for them, while they all went inside the sweat lodges and prayed, sang, and drummed. They had to take care of keeping the fire going, heating the stones, placing each stone prayerfully, etc. I watched them do what Ken had done for them. I was told they have not been able to replace Ken yet – even though there are other fire keepers – and that Ken was so gentle in his teaching of others about the ceremony and he was there faithfully when called upon.

On the way to the sweat, Ken's presence was joyously strong. So I sat and reread your letter by the firelight and felt for Ken's presence. I listened to the prayers and songs and thought about you and the life Ken has had.

This was followed by a circle inside the Great Hall of the Long House, more prayers and thanks for the food we were about to have. Also, a pipe carrier had come and we all, in a large circle, smoked the pipe. Then we had a grand potluck feast and visited with each other.

In all it was 7 ½ hours long. And during the visiting I met yet another person (one of many) who has a book of Ken's. He had helped with her PhD which she is working on, by loaning her just the right book and she was telling me that only now is she ready to give up the book but did not know where to return it. Funny, how we ended up sitting together talking for a long time before she figured out who I am.

I came to the idea that I would write three emails to you so that each one is not too long. ...

(Signed) Daisy

NUDGED BY THE MEN of Dartmouth College Class of '54 and by the fire next to the House of Learning on university grounds where Ken spent so much time, writing the story of Kehnroth Schramm's life began...

Dartmouth College administration wrote in a letter that they were placing an inscribed book in their library as a memorial of Ken. A woman at the Vermont University Medical School researched and sent a copy of the 1958 Hippocratic Oath that Ken promised to uphold. She also sent an archival picture of Ken with his graduating group of physicians. A gentleman at Goddard College searched their archives and sent material in reference to Ken's teaching there. Research for this book took off...

63

Sound of the Hippocratic Oath

THE WORLD SEEMED ALIVE with sound. The waves splashed sound as they mixed with the sand. The sounds of the_Seagulls were crisp in the air that was alive as though singing freshness of sea and air mixing. Sitting on a bench with her two little white Maltipoos at West Vancouver Ambleside Beach, Daisy watched the ocean and all that happened at the seaside. There were people and seabirds everywhere. It seemed unfair that a man like Ken was gone but life continued without him.

Where does all that feeling -- all the wishes and dreams that he encompassed go? Looking to the right she could see herself and Ken walking the seawall as they did when he was ill and they were full of hope, expecting him to get well another time. To the left, just past Stanley Park, she could see where together they lived and walked the streets and the sands of those beaches for so many years. Straight ahead she could see the green university campus jutting out high over the waters... where Ken should be... and it still goes on without him. Close by, within a few feet, there stood a large, carved wood monument of a welcoming aboriginal woman standing on the rocky point facing the open sea; with outstretched arms she embraces the point on which the university stands in the distance and all in between and beyond. A seagull always sits on her head. Daisy remembered Ken standing in the garden just like that in thankful prayer, welcoming each new day. The monument was now a comforting symbol – a reminder of Ken.

It was a misty kind of day that matched her feelings. Across the ocean where the white and grey clouds blended together with the waters, a tiny white dot emerged and became a ship like a phantom out of the blurred horizon. Mesmerized, Daisy watched it approach... becoming clear and large... sliding smoothly in the waters. It approached fast and became a wall of white towering over the beach... silent... until blowing its horn once as it approached the Lions Gate Bridge... its sound echoed around the inlet, filling the seascape, bouncing from mountain to mountain following the inlet waters, crescendo to diminuendo as the sound made its way past the mountain where Simon Fraser University was perched and on toward the distant waters of Deep Cove deep in Indian Arm where it was followed by silence. Only a few inches in size, Wendy, responded by barking at this powerful stranger.

As an artist, Daisy was always amused by perspective. She watched the welcoming arms of the wooden monument embrace the ship briefly as it slipped past. People on the stately white giant were welcomed.

THE WORLD – Daisy suddenly noticed the glaring words on the ship. This was no ordinary cruise ship; the people on board were permanent residents or tenants who originated from about forty countries around the world. Though the event had somehow been beautiful, the ship passing by was realized suddenly as a symbol of glut and greed – the known ills of people living in our world. Those who could own or rent apartments on this ship had money – lots of money – and it disturbed Daisy in knowing someone probably got hurt in the capture of wealth and self-indulgence.

This ship was a reminder of intense grief over what happened to Ken and over her own loss of his physical presence.

Sitting there on the beach, she mulled over the sneaky symptoms of Post-Traumatic Stress Disorder, an insidious killer that can be harder to recognize than plain old grief. Daisy knew that PTSD can be a result of anything, like the war of life... but she did not lose her life... Ken did lose his life under years of stress as a target for other people's unrelenting greed for money and power.

She wondered if she and he had not loved each other, would any of this have happened to him. How much was she guilty for just being in his life. The years together had been filled with unconditional love and caring but also a battle had taken place between what seemed like evil and good. Her sister had reminded her that it was other people who did the harmful, vengeful acts as adult white-collar bullies, not her.

Daisy had experienced much powerful magic in her lifetime but she had not been able to protect Ken. Her thoughts shifted to knowing the stages of grief is also to have an understanding of living with loss of this magnitude. She and Ken had helped many people with grief through life and death; she had been well acquainted with grief, having seen its many faces. Knowing the stages of grief had not protected Daisy from going through them. They surfaced randomly. The biggest grief came from knowing how Ken suffered at the hands of others.

Thinking this over, Daisy realized again that she must rise to include compassion for those who hurt Ken because of their own Hell on earth. She thought back – isn't that what her Buddhist teacher of many years ago was trying to teach her when he said he came to teach the sinners? And what had Ken been teaching?

Just last night Daisy had a lucid dream. In the dream, she was standing beside Ken when Jane arrived to talk. They all looked younger with clear smooth skin of youth. Ken's face was relaxed; his eyes were kind as he looked at Jane with compassion. With his right hand, he brushed fuzzy dirt off Jane's shoulder. With that gesture, Daisy knew that Ken was continuing to help Jane by removing whatever was stuck to her that should not be there.

And what kind of man would frequently get up from his bed in the middle of the night to minister to a distressed doctor who had caused Ken much distress in the past? Even though Ken was struggling in his last month of life, he would crawl out of bed to answer the telephone calls to give of himself to this man. Ken had done this quietly and in secrecy; during the time of the doctor's crisis, Ken had asked Daisy to sleep in her bedroom.

When Daisy found out through a telephone log of nighttime incoming calls from that man and asked why, when Ken was so weak himself, he simply said, "I answered his calls for help."

And with that, Daisy realized another lesson in how loyal Ken was to his Hippocratic Oath.

Daisy mused about the man who had compassion and understanding for everyone and all their personal Hells; a man who was never judgmental, accepting thousands of people as they were and continually tried to be helpful; a man who was often hurt but never retaliated; a man who simply stepped aside when he was not wanted.

Ken had given his deathbed message in which he forgave those who harmed him, and he gave his message to teach with the hope that those who would do harm could learn and change.

For years, Ken had expressed the need to spend some time in contemplation and meditation. He had talked often about wanting to enter a monastery for time to spend in prayer. Even in his last days, he still spoke of that wish to be in a monastery but he qualified it to say he did not want to leave family. Ken had never been allowed that kind of healing time in his whole life, but especially in his old age when he needed it. In his later years, he did write that he had given up the idea of being a priest, but what should be a normal time for peace, prayer and contemplation in the last part of one's life, Ken had not been allowed that.

In his last hours of life on earth, he gave a gift to Daisy; he allowed her to see the indescribable clear love of eternity shining through his eyes. Since first meeting Ken, Daisy had recognized the man who was close to God – the man who was a priest in man's clothing. It was her secret conviction that he had been a priest in another incarnation and was trapped in this life with worldly responsibilities of a different kind but always yearning for the ministerial life. Ken had spent countless hours comfortably in Theological libraries while Daisy waited for him. And one of his best friends among students at UBC was a lady about his age, who in fact was a nun. In hindsight, it was easy to understand why he could not live up to ex-wives' expectations.

As she looked down at her shoes in the sand, now making solitary prints, Daisy remembered back to the days of stories they told each other on the beach as together they made footprints in the sand. So determined they were that their coming together was for love and to work together to help others through the worst of life's hurdles... but she failed to protect Ken... on the other hand, did Ken need her protection? Ken lived in love. He was love. In his last days on earth, he was the embodiment of pure love that transcended earthly matters. And she would forever treasure the days and nights she had with him. Her only regret in that regard was that she and Ken did not get together sooner, especially after meeting in 1969, and bypass marrying others who did not respect and love them.

She searched her mind for some other profound philosophical meaning of this ship named The World passing this day. Perhaps it was in the sound that, though invisible, took on a life of its own, traveling far, vibrating, bouncing, moving and touching objects. Sound cannot be dismissed even though it cannot be seen – just as life after death cannot be dismissed because it cannot be seen.

As Daisy's eyes returned to the misty space where sea and sky blended, she remembered Kehnroth Schramm, an honorable man, who left a living legacy of physicians, nurses, teachers, artists and good people in sons, daughters and grandchildren to stand in his place. Ken stood strong in taking his Hippocratic Oath, promising himself to the life of a healer and teacher. He kept his word.

The Hippocratic Oath is a circle without end as new physicians continue swearing the oath across the centuries around the world. The sound vibrates through the air into eternal surrounding space, following the sound back to the beginning of this story, with another group of graduating doctors.

"You do solemnly swear, each by whatever he or she holds most sacred:

"That you will be loyal to the Profession of Medicine and just and generous to its members.

"That you will lead your lives and practice your art in uprightness and honor.

"That into whatsoever house you shall enter, it shall be for the good of the sick to the utmost of your power, your holding yourselves far aloof from wrong, from corruption, from the tempting of others to vice.

"That you will exercise your art solely for the cure of your patients, and will give no drug, perform no operation, for a criminal purpose, even if solicited, far less suggest it.

"That whatsoever you shall see or hear of the lives of men or women which is not fitting to be spoken, you will keep inviolably secret.

"These things do you swear. Let each bow the head in sign of acquiescence. And now, if you will be true to this, your oath, may prosperity and good repute be ever yours; the opposite, if you shall prove yourselves forsworn."

AS THE SOUND of the Hippocratic Oath reverberates throughout the universe, the sound of Ken's words echoes those promises.

> *"...I remember the Spring day in my third year of medical studies when I learned that traditional Chinese physicians were paid to keep their patients well and lose their lives if a patient died under their care. I saw American families forced into poverty by cost of illness and surgery. I realized that physicians make a living from the suffering of other people. I decided that I would work in Community Medicine to barter my work and teaching for the essentials of life. I resolved never to make money at the expense of another person's suffering. For me, Doctor means Teacher, not Businessman. I was called to heal and be healed by words not by money.*
>
> *"...Exercising our powers of imagining in self-making knowledge, we bring childhood and ancestors to life in time for our children to become teachers of health as human happiness and freedom in the family of life. ..."*
>
> *"We need to be healthy and hopeful human beings able to care for our bodies, our families, friends, neighbors, and all the others."*

IN KEN'S LAST NOTEBOOK that contains notes he wrote at the kitchen table in the middle of the quiet nights during his last weeks on earth, Daisy found a letter addressed to her. In the black ink from Ken's pen on the white paper, Ken expressed his regret that he and Daisy had never formally married each other; he wrote of his sorrow for the reasons why not. Ken apologized to Daisy for being ill, and ended the letter with, *"...Daisy, I do love you."*

64

The Healing

Poet and Professor, Carl Leggo wrote:

Refusing to Forget.
Ken Schramm was a medical doctor, psychiatrist, and homeopath. In his seventies he was pursuing a PhD in the Centre. Then on a late September day, he died, suddenly, too soon.

Psyllium
(for Ken)

Ken shared books, show and tell.
He always carried a big bag of books,
more books than I will ever read:
poetry, philosophy, history, theology, literature.

Ken wore his intellect like a rumpled coat.

We sat outside Benny's and ate gelato,
sat in silence, savouring the gelato,
the pleasure of being together.

He loved me with heart-breaking constancy.

He laughed with joyful abandon.

He told me he had Henry Wadsworth Longfellow's nose,
acknowledged his genealogical connections to the poet
who had to be both embraced and challenged.

In autumn air I said good-bye,
as if good-bye is ever possible,
connected to Ken like rhizomes
        without end.

And in autumn air
    through winter air
        into spring air
I walked the dike along the Fraser
        remembering Ken.

The best gift an older man
can offer a younger man
is the same gift a younger man
can offer an older man:
love, bountiful love.

Ken was a poet who saw
connections everywhere
so all our relations rendered stories
in a continuous present
that breathed always.

Ken knew the healing in roots.
He healed me many times.
I'm still taking the psyllium he recommended.
And every morning when I drink a glass
of pineapple juice with psyllium
I remember Ken, hear his light.
                        Carl Leggo

BELIEVING – QUESTIONING. Fantasy – Reality. Knowing – Searching – Knowing. Going in and coming out, and going in deeper are human traits.

In the forest, standing at the foot of Ken's grave and looking at the flowers blooming in the four foot square garden over him that she tends year round, Daisy looked up and cried out, "Ken, where are you?" The sound was especially poignant in the stillness of the cemetery.

As her body drooped after the outburst, her eyes caught sight of a large, green Maple leaf falling overhead from the giant tree. She was transfixed because it was the only thing moving in the stillness of the summer air. The leaf floated gently, swirling slowly a little to her right, then a few feet to the left, pausing in mid-air four feet above the ground; the leaf made its way slowly, horizontally through the air in a straight line across the space of six yards directly toward Daisy and landed in her hands as though it has been carried and handed to her. Impressed on her in loud silence were the words, "I am here." In the presentation of a green leaf, she knew her sound had been heard... and so had his.

Remembering now, the gift of all gifts... Ken had been a vessel for unworldly love flowing through his frail body. Just before his passing Daisy had gazed into the soul of a man who had transcended into clear spirit, whose eyes were windows to clear, pure love and he had said it was love for her. She knew there could be no greater gift.

The small clump of ground-daisies that Daisy, with her granddaughter Katie, had taken from Jericho Beach where Ken and Daisy walked together for many seasons, was planted in the garden at Ken's feet. The daisies had jumped out of the confinement of the garden and seeded in multiple spots around the lawn. The freedom seeking, multiplying daisies were a perfect reminder of Ken, the man who could not be contained – the man who needed freedom of thought, freedom in teaching and ways of healing, and now escaped the confines of earth in a continuation of healing in his own way...

IT HAPPENED SEPTEMBER 2005, on the First Anniversary of Ken's passing. A miraculous healing happened in the Foothills Hospital in Calgary, Alberta, Canada, where Ken had been a Senior Resident Physician in the Department of Psychiatry, studying and teaching Family Psychiatry in the years of 1973 and 1974.

A young man, an insulin dependant diabetic also fighting an addiction to street drugs, alcohol, and smoking, was already in poor health when he had a truck accident that seriously damaged his hand. He required an operation to repair his hand. A hospital borne Staph infection entered the wound. He ended up in the Intensive Care Unit with MRSA (Methicillin-resistant Staphylococcus aureus) that had traveled from his hand to his lungs. He was now dying of this infection and resulting pneumonia with no available medicine. He lay unconscious for several days in ICU. The attending physicians did not expect him to live. His family arrived from another province to be with him at the end, when he suddenly woke up, hysterical.

He had tubes removed from his throat just hours before in preparation for death, so now he had difficulty speaking. "Mom, was Ken a fire keeper?" were his first words. "I think it was Ken!"

[This man lived in Alberta and though he had met Ken briefly, he had absolutely no knowledge that Ken was a fire keeper.]

He was hysterically trying to tell about his experience and this was his story. "It was Ken who healed me. There were two elders accompanying Ken who looked like whites, one male and one female, but they were really native souls. Ken, the fire keeper, gave me a choice to live or die. I chose to live. So the fire keeper hung me upside down for two to four hours and kept my fire burning. I had a near death experience and a fire keeper helped me. I was given this aboriginal name so that I could have life."

He was trying so hard to say the name and make it sound the same as he knew it; his mouth was twisting and tears were falling because it was not a word from his vocabulary. He spoke the letters, "TNE"; then suggested it might be "ENT". Quickly he resolved it was TNE, but when he spoke the word it sounded more like "T Hee N EE". He said it several times. Then he said, "I was told groups of three cling to TNE."

He told his mother that he had not realized until this experience that souls are different, opposite or upside down. He said, "Souls are fusions of light!"

Looking for answers, the mother had made notes and telephoned Daisy from the hospital. Daisy knew that two friends had died of hospital borne staph infection in Vancouver hospitals just weeks before and others over the years, Daisy had known of several other deaths in Vancouver hospitals because of hospital borne infections. So, this sudden waking up was like a miracle. But answers were being sought. Daisy offered to ask Ken's friends, aboriginal elders John and N'kixw'stn.

Over night Daisy received part answer from Ken.

"The tree of life is the human body. A baby in final months of gestation is head down and feet upwards. A normal birth is head first, feet last. The young man was put upside down. I gave a cosmic current that was the fire, to rejuvenate the brain and spinal centers, and get oxygen flowing."

Then an answer arrived from N'kixw'stn.

"I got a response about the TNE immediately. I have an aboriginal word in my language that means "BUTTERFLY". Just say the three letters quite fast and it sounds like "Tee-N-Eee". Bring it to my language it will sound like this: "TEE-HE-HONN-KNEE". Now what you have to do is to think about what the butterfly does. The butterfly goes from one flower to the next extracting nectar from the flower. Butterflies are also beautiful. The most amazing fact about the butterfly is it's migration pattern. That alone proves how powerful they are, but yet they are so fragile."

At sunrise Daisy emailed the answers to the mother along with an additional note:

"The native elder tells me that TEE-HE-HONN-KNEE in her language means BUTTERFLY. Butterfly means Transformation. 'Groups of three cling to TNE' are the caterpillar, the cocoon, and then transformation takes place and the butterfly flies free. We are the mirror image of our astral body. We are three bodies -- physical, astral, and causal.

"Ken has described himself as points of light.

"Also, Antony reminds me that in Chinese medicine, some meridians of the body run from bottom to top. The young man has had a near death experience and a rebirth. He was held upside down to receive the infusion of light. He is now in a transformation of his life."

AFTER BEING RELEASED from the hospital and free of MRSA in subsequent testing, he had been wondering why he was brought back to life... to do what great work? He traveled to visit with Daisy and posed the question. She slept on the question that night.

In the new morning, Daisy told the young man, "It is possibly very simply that one boy, your son, needs a father and that is the special work you must do. That is the answer for most parents. The job of parenting is as important as any job on earth. It is a gift."

[At the time of writing this book, seven and a half years have passed since September 2005; the young man is free of MRSA and free of drug and alcohol addictions. The young man continues life by working, heading up large projects. And he is a caring parent.]

[To this day, Daisy's brother has been cancer free.]

* * *

Each of us human beings is here in this world on Planet Earth to manifest, express, be, do that unique gift/part of creation that we are. Our task is to become human beings, sharing the gifts we have been given and the gifts that we are, with all our relations, human and non-human, becoming indigenous, at home in balance with the places we inhabit and co-create, in the process of living and dying.

Kehnroth Schramm, M.D.

Finis
Love is never finished...

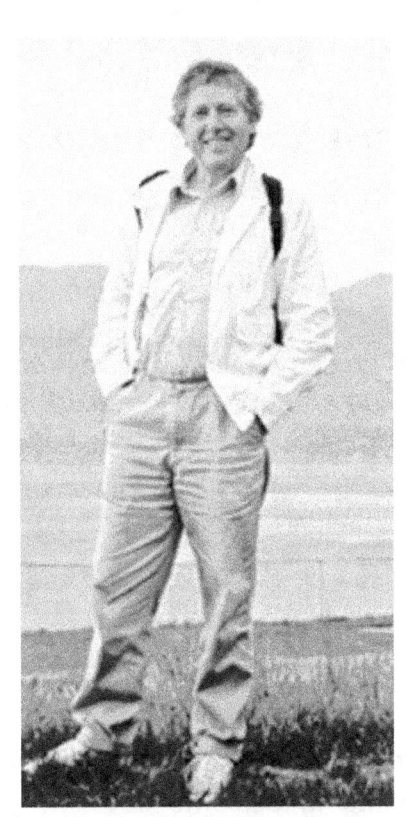

Packets of Seeds

In the Words of

Kehnroth Schramm in Spirit

Transcribed as he told it to me after his passing.
Ken named these passages "Packets of Seeds".

Doctor Schramm was a physician and teacher. Ken crossed over September 24, 2004 and has been describing his experience of crossing over. Ken has offered these words for those of us who wonder and want to know, and for the many suffering loss and grief over a loved one. He continues to be a teacher and physician caring for us, and letting us know what is important in our lives.

Ken first gave me this poem.

my poem
now another poem
from Ken

> *footsteps   reunion*
> *he led the way through the forest*
> *rejoicing welcome join*
> *satisfying wish to rejoin*
> *all loneliness is gone in that moment*
> *golden palace materialized here tonight*

Then Ken requested the return of his over seventy library books. When the books were returned, these messages began.

I am light, love, young, healthy, and happy.
There is life beyond this life – a larger life.
I am very much alive.
Who would have guessed!

What holds us together is love.
We are made of light.
I am points of light in eternal bliss.

I crossed the room and comforted you [Daisy].

Meditate and I will teach you.
Meditate daily, and I will teach you.

Don't grieve for me. I am healthy and happy.
I am extremely large.
My mind and far reaching memories are intact and live on.

What keeps us together is love.
Love is unconditional on the other side.
(All Ken asks for now from us, is: "unconditional love".)

I am invisible.
I see your face.
I look into your eyes.

There is no money here!
I do not need to sleep.
I do not need to eat food.

I know I am dead, but I am acutely aware and very alive.

I will be with you instantly.

Relationships do survive death.
It is a falsehood that death ends relationships.

On being born and dying...
There is a time for everything.

It is true that words are in the universe forever.
Thoughts are deeds.
There is no secret life.
All is known.

Where do you think God is? Live life now.
Enjoy the flowers. Flowers are God's gift.
Play and listen to music, sing and dance.

Large or small... Size does not matter.
We are one with God.

Grief is a hurdle but can be conquered by learning to live with it and replacing it with unconditional love.

Guilt is a giant hurdle.
Let us bury the old hatchet and just love unconditionally.

Everything is balanced.
Karma does play a role in relationships."

Ken has maintained his sense of humor, and sees and hears what is going on. He holds conversations with me about absolutely everything. Mine is the mind that wonders, and then he tells me, *"You are not present."* He comments with precision on things I do. Conversations can be very normal and even sometimes funny as he was in this life.

In answer to my questions about what it is like where he lives, Ken says he is *"healthy, young, happy."* He says he is *"also in pleasure"*. He tells me a bit about his being and his environment but says it is beyond my/our comprehension at this time. Explaining in detail is not really possible. What he does say is that it is: *"Peace, Love, Sincerity"*. To understand, he says we should *"meditate daily"*.

Ken has been teaching me about transfer of thought that takes place between all living things, including transfer of thought between humans and spirit, not just human to human.

Ken answers thoughts that are thought patterns a layer beneath the surface thoughts, in the subconscious. I recognize them when brought to my attention. Nothing is hidden.

In answer to a question of a concerned doubter about why he does not go somewhere where dead people go, wherever that is, Ken gave this message on May of 2007:

"I do belong on a higher plane. It would be selfish of me to stay there when so many living on earth need my help."

Friday morning, May 9th, 2007, I received a message from Ken as follows:

"Let me tell you about my crossing over...

Large doors opened.

My soul and mind entered.

I maintained memory of myself and my life.

I experienced immediate peace.

Dead friends greeted me.

We had conversation.

I see God in progress.

Realizing the Essence of Creation is light.

Sincere prayer arranges light atoms of the Universe, changing Time and Space.

Essence of all objects is swirling, throbbing streams of light energy.

I have spoken."

In answer to my question regarding feelings, how does he feel if he is light?

He tells me, *"I am complete. A soul is a body."*

When asked again what it is like to die, Ken responded, *"Think of it this way. It is like when you wake up from a sleep, get out of bed and go for a walk in the early morning sunshine where the air is fresh and clean. You are awake!"*

Packets of Seeds Volume 2

Ken's advice to me: *"Be careful of delicate perception."*

In answer to my questions about what Ken is doing in spirit, he says:

I am training disciples – students.
Discourses are mental.
Disciple is a term broadly used.

I greet souls arriving – unconditional – innocent --
consciousness – permanent

I attend meetings on WISDOM.
Meetings are enjoyable beyond imagination.
Curiosity about wisdom.

I love thinking thanks.
I love thinking.

I needed to relearn the ancient language.

All thoughts vibrate eternally.
Tune out undesirable ones.
Thoughts are like a radio broadcasting, sending and receiving.
I hear a whisper.

Whatever you believe strongly is a force.

Invisible is the difference in reality of Time and Space.

Power is in meditation.
The centre of forehead is where single eyes become one.

Ken brought his mother in spirit to see me; I turned away, believing he was busy and I was the intruder. He then told me that he had brought her to see me because she now understands our relationship.

One day Ken told me:
"Now Earthly Karma finished. Out of the realm of karmic cosmic currents of earthly life – I have made my final exit."

Questions I ask: Why can we talk and feel each other? And how do I know it is you? Ken answered:
"Focus... Magnetism... Tied Together.
The feel is a recognition."

* * *

April 26, 2008: I am looking at the extensive library of books that Ken and I have put together on many subjects.

Ken says, *"Twenty-six letters."*

With those words comes the astonishing realization that all the ideas and stories in English books in all the libraries and bookstores are composed variations of only twenty-six letters. I have written the book 'doctor ken' with only 26 letters.

April 27, 2008: I ask the questions, "What good are books? What good are my writings? Why would I write a book?"

Ken's answer: *"Teach... You/We have a responsibility to teach. People try to fit it all into the known, the expected. Like a child holding a lamp, a beacon of light open to new ways of seeing, knowing... Expect the unexpected."*

May 2009 – Ken tells me, *"Enhance the little book."* [Packets of Seeds, volume one with volume 2]

* * *

There was criticism from my relatives. Too heavy.
My heart was too heavy (over) my family war.
Let us bury the old now.
You [Daisy] you, you, bury the old hatchet.

I did not want to leave in death... attached by affection to family.
I walked the next morning to assimilate my predicament of my youth... being young again.
You [Daisy] love me.
I was very sick. I am healed.
I observed God's universe.
I rushed to send telegrams... messages. I listened, listened, and listened. You [Daisy] heard.

* * *

A note from me, the writer: For twenty-four years I tried to protect Ken... I have buried his body. No one can bury his soul.

Ken has gone on to be a healer and teacher in another realm. He is light and love, young and healthy – complete. He is keeping his promise to me to let me know he is alive and he takes me to realms beyond description. Our relationship continues with a promise of eternal union. Our memory of each other continues.

Our thoughts live, affecting each other across the thin veil of a changing frequency.

As the writing of the book 'doctor ken' took shape, it became necessary to tell the 'real' story and not lose half of the true story that we experienced in the medical practice. That includes the realm of experiences beyond life and death and our physical bodies that we all, whether we are aware or not, live with. It would only be half a story to leave out what we really shared of a larger life.

I know each person is and has a multifaceted story. Ken taught me that Truth is in the beholder. This story is my/our truth.

Ken does continue to teach and with his continuing communication, he is teaching that there is an eternal life and that souls retain memory of the life they lived on earth, and that departed souls do see and hear us as we continue our sojourns on earth.

The joke is on me because in my arrogance I once said to Ken, "No living person can be my spiritual teacher." I learn that Ken is my teacher, and he does live!

My thoughts are, "I miss you, Ken."

I feel Ken's familiar touch on my head infusing me with light and fire of eternal bliss. He answers, *"I am not missing. I am with you always."*

Update September 23, 2011: The writing of the book about Ken's life is finished. It is Friday morning. I am not quite awake. My brain feels like it is taking a break from remembering or even thinking. Out of the blue, Ken reminds me of the Friday morning of September 24, 2004 (the morning he passed away). Knowing that eventually I would wake up fully and remember, Ken offers a comforting reminder, *"I arrived in the morning to the irrevocable divine peace of another world healing my heart. All fear was gone."*

Morning of Saturday, September 24, 2011, I ask, "How are you?"

Ken responds, ***"I am great. I teach Wisdom. I know Wisdom. I teach without requiring assistance."*** This comment is an inside joke that is understood between Ken and myself because I had assisted him in his medical practice and as his companion for twenty-four years, always wanting to protect him even when he insisted he did not need protection. Now he wants me to know he no longer needs protection – he is safe.

There can be no mistaken identity. These comments are so like Ken. He often says things in a way understood only between us.

* * *

November 21, 2011 – Today would be Kehnroth Schramm's birthday. His message:

"Wrote Booklet – drew in world. Write more. I am willing. Write essay."

"Final pass. You [Daisy] have been assigned textbooks. Dear, do not worry about your life."

(My mind started to wonder, thinking about this last statement.)

Ken said, *"Thoughts are tuning out."* This brought me back. *"Much work to do yet. You and I are blazing together in educational work."*

Then in a message for the world, Ken said:

"Discard discrimination and prejudices of people of foreign lands.

Discard discrimination of differences of skin color, sex, size, age, or religion.

The goal is absolute unity – Brotherhood of humanity.

No one religion or group of people own God or have exclusive right to the 'here after'."

Ken has requested that I remember him as a young man.

I have been remembering him mostly as an elderly man. It comforted me to remember this time because of the unconditional love he always had for everyone, but to be honest, my selfish reasoning was that during the last two years, we were no longer working and I had him all to myself as I nursed him.

One day, when as usual, I was looking at his picture and admiring his white hair and angelic face, completely ignoring his previous descriptions of being young, he said to me, ***"Stretch your mind. I am young now."***

... Love is never finished ...

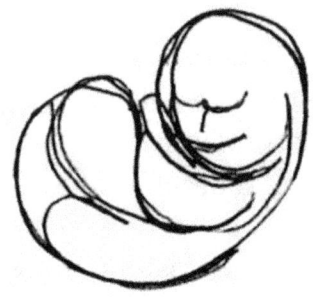

Ken (in Spirit) then gave us this *one stroke* image
drawn very fast.

The Rose

Every now and then, people may wonder whom I am talking with when I believe I am talking with Ken and receiving messages from him. One day, when I questioned, I was told I would be given a sign. In my busyness I almost forgot and was not looking for a sign.

On Valentine's Day, February 14, 2012, I bought a long stemmed red rose at a chain grocery store – no special place. On buying it, I asked for one of those small plastic tubes they put on the end of the stem with a tiny bit of water. It was late afternoon, so I drove straight to the cemetery. In other words, I did nothing to properly prepare the stem or the rose. It was just as is.

I placed the rose on Ken's grave, across Ken's chest (symbolically) where he had held his white feather. I thought it would be protective of Ken.

I asked Ken several times if he knew of the Valentine rose and got no answer.

In North Vancouver, British Columbia, Canada, we have had unusually turbulent weather since Valentine's Day. It has been up and down the temperature gauge – above and below freezing. It has been stormy with almost continuous heavy rain and several windstorms that blew furniture and other heavy items around, and downed branches of trees. It has snowed more than once.

As the stormy days came and went, the **ninth day** arrived and the rose was still in pristine shape, looking like the day I laid it over Ken, I began to take notice that something special was going on.

Saturday afternoon of **February 26**, there was a windy storm of frozen ice pellets mixed with snow that were about a half an inch in size.

Each day I have gone there expecting the rose to have blown away or succumbed to the fierce elements but it is always there just as I placed it.

It is my understanding that cut red roses should be expected to only last three to seven days with optimum care and environment.

February 28, fifteen days later – Our granddaughter Maria had come on this day to see the phenomenon of the rose. The rose was still as fresh as the day I laid it there for Ken, just opened a tiny bit more.

Last September 3rd, Maria had married. In memory of her grandfather Ken, Maria had chosen to decorate her wedding with bouquets of red roses at the ceremony and on all the banquet tables. She carried red roses in her own bouquet and she had attached Ken's lapel pin to her formal wedding gown so that Ken would be with her as she walked down the aisle to marry Luke.

On the day following the wedding, Maria laid a red rose bouquet from her wedding on Ken's grave.

Amazed on this February day, Maria took pictures of the Valentine rose on her cell phone camera, which is all we had with us. We had a break between rains and the light was low and dull in late afternoon, but the pictures came out fine.

March 2: I went there today. It is still raining after a layer of snow that hung around for about twenty-four hours and is now melted, except in some protected spots. The rose is still there and is still beautiful and strong.

March 5: It has been 21 full days. It has been pouring rain for days but today the sun came out. There are high winds blowing tree branches down again. The rose is still perfect and beautifully fresh. I picked up the rose for a minute to smell it and feel its strength – it is strong.

March 6: 22 days. I visited the rose today in sunshine and calm. The rose is still very alive and strong. Although it is the first day that there are tiny dots on the tips of some petals, a sign of getting old. It smells like a rose. Oddly, the original water in the little plastic vial on the end of the stem is as it was the day I laid the rose over Ken. The rose seems not to have needed any nourishment through the stem. It obviously has lived for over three weeks, and stayed untouched by extreme weather, on some other kind of nourishment and protection.

Ken has often said to me, *"Flowers for you."* They were thought flowers. I believe that Ken has just given me a rose – real in our dimension. I believe he has told me that he did notice the Valentine rose. I know I have been given the promised sign.

A Child's Version Of Life After Life

A message from my mother came through my three-year old granddaughter who had recently been to Regina to visit with her great-grandfather.

Katie was born ten months after her great-grandmother's passing and Katie had never seen a picture of her. During the night her great=grandmother appeared to the child and talked to her. Katie reported the visit happily the next morning as though it was the most natural visit. A photo album was brought out. She identified her great-grandmother by picking out her picture among many.

In the photo on the next page, Katie was drawing at my kitchen table with other children. She worked quietly and intently, producing several drawings. On that same day, she drew the picture on the next page and handed it to me. She said, "Gramma, this is a message for you from your mother."

Of course, I was completely surprised.

She described the picture she had just drawn. She told me that I am standing by a body of water, crying with big tears running down; a reflection of my face is seen in the water; my mother is in the air overhead; the letters surrounding my mother is her message telling me not to cry or be sad because she is ALIVE and I should look at my reflection in the water as a peaceful mirror image of life.

Unprompted, Katie then matter-of-factly told a story of grandmothers being born as babies, then becoming a mother, then being a grandmother, then dying and being born again. Katie continued drawing.

A midwives' tale is that when a baby is born with a caul (amniotic sac) over her head, the child will become a midwife. Katie had such an interest in midwifery that whenever she could, she would wear the real stethoscope and listen intently to babies. Her favorite toy at age three was a doctor's kit.

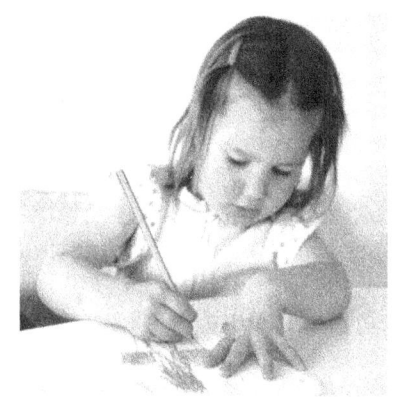

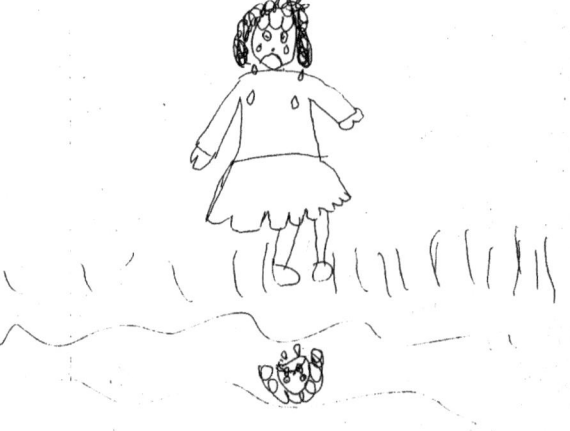

Appendix

A stack of newspapers with three-inch high black headlines screamed out, followed by large sub headlines. It was an article by Jonathan Fowlie on the front page of the VANCOUVER SUN Saturday, March 4, 2006

THOUSANDS OF BRITISH COLUMBIA PRIVATE HEALTH RECORDS SOLD AT PUBLIC AUCTION

Government tapes contain information on conditions such as HIV status, mental illness

The provincial government has auctioned off computer tapes containing thousands of highly sensitive records, including information about people's medical conditions, their social insurance numbers and their dates of birth.

Sold for $300 ...

Included among the files were records showing certain people's medical status -- including whether they have a mental illness, HIV or a substance-abuse problem -- details of applications for social assistance, and whether or not people are fit to work...

Following the article to page 17, there were more large headlines and an article by Jonathan Fowlie:

PRIVACY BREACH 'A WAKE-UP CALL'

Confidentiality / Sale of tapes by the provincial government exposes personal information and health records...

This data tape, [shown in picture] one of 41 containing confidential information on about 77,000 British Columbians, was sold by the province. ...

Government made no attempt to erase files, tech expert says ...

* * *

September of year 2012, another serious breach of confidentiality happened. The breach had been ongoing for several months before it was reported to the public. Media reported that employees in the British Columbia Ministry of Health did pass confidential patient information to University of British Columbia and University of Victoria students doing research on patient drug use. It was serious enough for several union protected employees to be fired outright and several to be suspended without pay. The Four Million Dollar contracts were suspended. However, very quickly, the research contracts were reinstated and there was a blackout of news.

* * *

In another case reported by the media in the **year of 2012**: a nurse's aid was fired for researching and reading confidential medical files of prominent professional people in the province of British Columbia.

* * *

Postscript

My philosophy of life

I believe the world and everything in it is alive, including and especially our thoughts, feelings, dreams and desires; God/Goddess is present in creation and the world expresses (is) his/her/their grace. My response is gratitude when I know I am loved and living in the love of life as their gift to us.

doctor ken

A simple poem to Ken on the stairway to forever

Roses are red
Violets are blue
Though you're in heaven
Know I love you

Roses are red
Your eyes were blue
Though I live on
Know I remember you

Roses are red
And many a hue
Where ever you are
Know I love you

Roses are red
Your story is true
I hope you know
That I love you... forever

Daisy

the way we were 1969

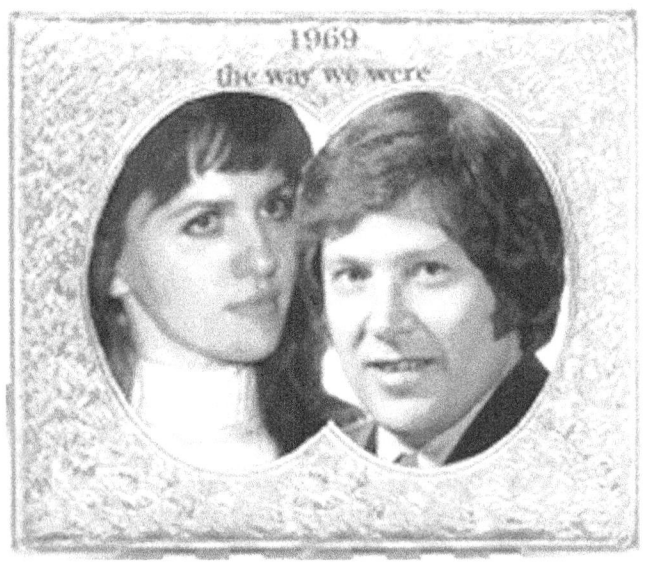

Daisy Heisler and Kehnroth Schramm
as they looked when they met
in Regina, Saskatchewan, Canada

Real Stories – Real People

I have been alive dying for more than half this century to tell my stories, my medicine for my children, the healing power of real stories about real people.

I want to be alive when I die in remembered jokes and words that live with my family and friends.

Kehnroth Schramm

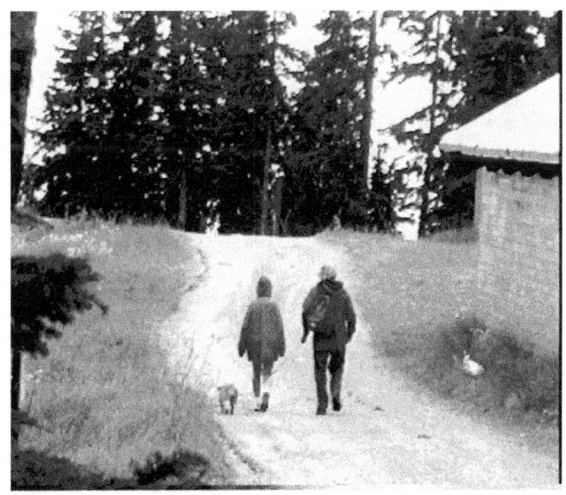

Ken walking and talking with Granddaughter Maria and dog Cinderella on Seymour Mountain after picking wild blueberries

When Maria was six years old, she asked Ken to help her find true stories about real people.

After her grandfather Ken passed away, Maria read an early version of this true story. She was surprised and said, "I had no idea he had so many troubles. All my life he was always available to me, always had time to talk and be helpful. He always was smiling for me."